Whitewash

…Joseph Keon has done us all a great service in writing this book.
His research is meticulous, his writing is lucid, and his conclusions are
reliable. *Whitewash* is a doorway through which you can enter into
a world of far greater health for yourself and your family. If you heed
its messages, your body will thank you for the rest of your life.

— John Robbins, from the Foreword

Most of us grew up with the idea that milk is healthful, if not essential.
And yet research has shown a surprisingly different side to dairy
products, linking it to a broad range of serious health problems.
Whitewash takes a comprehensive look at the problems associated
with drinking milk and the industry that promotes it. This book
has the potential to dramatically change your health.

— Neal Barnard, M.D.
President, Physicians Committee for Responsible Medicine

Human beings need to learn what all other animals instinctively
know: milk is for infants. Despite the fact that allergies, disease, and
obesity can all be linked to our obsession with cow's milk, we have
bought the milk lobby's fable hook, line and sinker. Dr. Keon's
scrupulous research and meticulous documentation will wipe
those sinister milk mustaches off all the smirking dairy execs.
Whitewash is nothing less than a lifesaver.

— Rory Freedman, author, *Skinny Bitch*

Joseph Keon's *Whitewash* is another authoritative and well-referenced
nail in the cow milk coffin. Having discovered firsthand the adverse
effects of milk in much the same way as Dr. Keon, I can say that
without relentless taxpayer-funded USDA support, shameless
advertising (with IRS tax deductions for same), milk products would
finally stand exposed only as an expensive way to make yourself sick.

— William Harris, M.D. Author of *The Scientific Basis of Vegetarianism*

In my medical practice, I have watched children with eczema, allergies, ear infections and chronic upper respiratory congestion lose most or all of their symptoms when they stopped drinking cow's milk. And whole cow's milk is also the food most to blame for the huge increase in obesity in America's children. *Whitewash* is an excellent, well-researched book. Read it and don't drink your milk!

— Jay N. Gordon, MD, FAAP
Assistant Professor of Pediatrics, UCLA Medical School
Former Senior Fellow in Pediatric Nutrition,
Memorial Sloan-Kettering Institute

If cows bought books, *Whitewash* would become an instant and perennial bestseller. The truth about dairy has never been so clearly told. Every parent and pediatrician needs to read this book. We should be raising our children to cherish truth telling and to be on the lookout for effective whitewashing. Joseph Keon has done a remarkable job in revealing the most effective (and expensive) propaganda campaign in US history.

— Patti Breitman, co-author of *How to Say No Without Feeling Guilty* and Director, Marin Vegetarian Education Group

Anyone, health professional or lay person, who pushes either dairy or calcium pills really needs to read this book. Unfortunately, this includes most of the health professionals I've come into contact with. Whether you're a novice to strategies to get healthier OR you'd like to stay on top of the latest research, you need this book, not to just read, but to re-read, and keep for the constant references you'll need as you try to educate others as to how they've been "whitewashed"!

—Ruth Heidrich, Ph.D., Ironman Triathlete
Author of *A Race For Life* and *Senior Fitness*

WHITEWASH

The Disturbing Truth About
Cow's Milk and Your Health

JOSEPH KEON

NEW SOCIETY PUBLISHERS

Printed in Canada. First printing September 2010.

Paperback ISBN: 978-0-86571-676-6
eISBN: 978-1-55092-456-5

Disclaimer:

This book is intended to be educational and informative. It is not meant to serve as a prescription for your personal health problems. It contains the viewpoint of its author. By purchasing this book you understand that neither the author nor the publisher are dispensing medical advice. Please do not adjust your diet or medications, or begin any type of exercise program, or adopt any of the strategies presented herein, without first consulting your personal physician. The author and publisher disclaim all responsibility for any liability, loss or risk that may be associated with the application of any of the contents of this book.

Inquiries regarding requests to reprint all or part of *Whitewash* should be addressed to New Society Publishers at the address below.

To order directly from the publishers, please call toll-free (North America) 1-800-567-6772, or order online at www.newsociety.com

Any other inquiries can be directed by mail to:
New Society Publishers
P.O. Box 189, Gabriola Island, BC V0R 1X0, Canada
(250) 247-9737

New Society Publishers' mission is to publish books that contribute in fundamental ways to building an ecologically sustainable and just society, and to do so with the least possible impact on the environment, in a manner that models this vision. We are committed to doing this not just through education, but through action. Our printed, bound books are printed on Forest Stewardship Council-certified acid-free paper that is **100% post-consumer recycled** (100% old growth forest-free), processed chlorine free, and printed with vegetable-based, low-VOC inks, with covers produced using FSC-certified stock. New Society also works to reduce its carbon footprint, and purchases carbon offsets based on an annual audit to ensure a carbon neutral footprint. For further information, or to browse our full list of books and purchase securely, visit our website at: www.newsociety.com

Library and Archives Canada Cataloguing in Publication

Keon, Joseph

   Whitewash : the disturbing truth about cow's milk and your health / Joseph Keon.

Includes bibliographical references and index.

ISBN 978-0-86571-676-6

   1. Milk--Health aspects. 2. Milk contamination. 3. Calcium in human nutrition.
4. Nutritionally induced diseases. I. Title.

RA602.M54K46 2010   613.2'6   C2010-904810-5

NEW SOCIETY PUBLISHERS

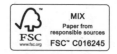

For you, SS

Also by Joseph Keon

Whole Health: The Guide to Wellness of Body and Mind
The Truth About Breast Cancer: A Seven-Step Prevention Plan

Join the Conversation
Visit our online book club at www.newsociety.com to share your
thoughts about *Whitewash*. Exchange ideas with other readers,
post questions for the author, respond to one of the sample questions
or start your own discussion topics. See you there!

Contents

Acknowledgments

I am grateful for the love, support, guidance, and friendship from family and friends, particularly over the last two years, as I worked to complete this book. Thanks to my mother, Peggy, my siblings, Pam, Liese, Susan, Margaret, and Katherine, and to Neal Arnove, Dean Arnove, Mark Arnove, Marilyn Arnove, Christine Berger, Ladd Bogdonoff, Lynnea Brinkerhoff, Joseph Brooke, Stacey Caen, Helen Caldicott, Jerome and Grace Contreau, Margi English, Evan Frank, Koroush Ghadishah, Yosh Hann, Lexa Herron, Abigail Huller, Shane Liem, Trina Lindsey, Thomas Liu, Heather Lugassi, Heather MacDowell, Christi Nees, Guillaume Pruniaux, Albert Retodo, Deborah and Forrest Rhoads, Bob and Grace Salk, Gary and Kezia Smith, Garth Twa, Patti Waughtal, and Marianne Woo.

I am grateful to Joshua Moore for reviewing the manuscript, Patti Breitman for championing this project and being such an ardent supporter, and Katherine Boyle, my agent, who recognized early on the importance of this book and worked steadfastly to find it an appropriate home.

Thank you to John Robbins for his inspiration and leadership and for the enormous contribution he has made to empower us all to live healthier and more compassionate lives.

It will be embarrassing enough if the current calcium hype is simply useless; it will be immeasurably worse if the recommendations are actually detrimental to health.

— D. Mark Hegsted, former professor of nutrition,
Harvard School of Public Health

Foreword

by John Robbins

I might be one of the last people you would expect to find questioning the value of dairy products for human health. Not that this is an easy question for most people. The assumption that dairy products are wonderful foods prevails throughout our culture with amazing tenacity. But in my family of origin, this assumption was held with a steadfastness that was virtually religious.

There was a reason. My father founded, owned and ran what became the world's largest ice cream company — Baskin-Robbins. Our house included a commercial-sized freezer with each of the 31 flavors, one for each day of the month. By the time I was 21, my father had manufactured and sold more ice cream than any human being who had ever lived on the planet. And he groomed me, his only son, to succeed him. It was his plan that I would follow in his footsteps.

So what am I doing writing a foreword for a book titled *Whitewash: The Disturbing Truth About Cow's Milk And Your Health?* It turned out that I didn't follow my father's plan, but instead walked away from the company and the money it represented to become an advocate for a healthy and compassionate way of life. And that brings me to this marvelous book by Joseph Keon. Because if you are looking for the truth about dairy products and your health, if you are wanting to understand what scientific research has actually shown, this book is an immensely helpful resource. I consider it, in fact, the best book yet written on the subject.

One of the intriguing topics Joseph Keon covers thoroughly and clearly is the calcium paradox. Why is it that the countries with the highest consumption of milk and other dairy products, including the United States, also have the highest rates of osteoporosis and bone fractures? Why do so many studies find that increasing calcium intake from dairy products has no positive impact on the body's overall calcium balance? And why do the countries with the lowest consumption of dairy products have the lowest rates of osteoporosis and bone fractures?

Bone health, the scientific literature attests, isn't merely a matter of adequate calcium intake. It is more a matter of how much calcium is retained. Can you imagine trying to fill a bathtub in which the drain isn't plugged? As long as the water is emptying down the drain, turning up the spigot to increase the amount of water entering the tub isn't going to fill it, or at least not for long. Similarly, consuming ever more calcium without addressing the reasons our bodies fail to retain it doesn't lead to bone health.

And there's another problem with our assumptions about dairy products that we need to address if we are going to free ourselves from beliefs that aren't true. In my days at Baskin-Robbins, the walls of every store were adorned with large and beautiful sepia-toned photographs of Guernsey and Jersey dairy cows grazing contentedly in pastures luxuriant with grass. Such is the image many of us still have when we think about where our milk, cheese, yogurt and ice cream come from.

But the reality is very different. With the industrialization of the dairy industry, everything has changed. Many of today's dairy cows never see a blade of grass. They live crowded in dirt feedlots or worse. They are bred, fed, inseminated, and manipulated to a single purpose — maximum milk production at minimum cost.

Of course, the industry doesn't want you to know this. Profit-seeking creatures, they have no qualms about bamboozling the public with talk of "happy cows."

Peter R. Cheeke is Professor Emeritus of Animal Nutrition at Oregon State University, and has served on the editorial boards of The Journal of Animal Science and Animal Feed Science and Technology. "One of the best things modern animal agriculture has going for it," he says, "is that most people… haven't a clue how animals are raised and processed… For modern animal agriculture, the less the consumer knows about what's happening, the better."

You don't have to be a vegetarian or an animal rights activist to be appalled by what actually takes place in modern dairies, if you look behind the veil of advertising and other forms of industry propaganda. Modern milk has become, in the words of a contributing editor at Gourmet magazine, Anne Mendelson, "the milk of human unkindness."

The natural lifespan of a cow is about 20 years, up to 25 if conditions are favorable. But in today's dairies, the animals are so exhausted and stressed by the conditions in which they are raised that few live to see their sixth birthday.

Everything about the modern milk cow, from her breeding to the food she is given, is determined by what is profitable for the industry. No concern is given to the animal's welfare other than how it affects the bottom line. The industry is proud that the average yield per cow today is two-and-a-half times what it was only 50 years ago. But this extraordinary gain in productivity has come at a great cost to the cows. Modern dairy herds are perennially riddled with many kinds of disease, including painful udder infections called mastitis.

Meanwhile, the small family dairy farm is fast becoming history. As recently as 1970 there were about 650,000 dairy farmers in the US. Now there are only a tenth that many. Some dairy farms, housing up to 20,000 cows, are so large they should more accurately be called factories rather than farms.

Modern industrialized cows are fed rations they would never eat in nature, and are confined in conditions that frustrate virtually all of their natural urges. Their calves are taken away at birth, or at most allowed to be with them for 24 hours. Some cows are tied up all day in stalls. Milked on the spot, they spend their whole lives virtually immobilized. Others are allowed a bit of movement, but only between the barn or dirt feedlot and milking parlor. None ever graze on real pasture while lactating.

Does some of the misery modern cows are forced to endure end up in the cheese, yogurt, ice cream or milk that people consume? Are we unknowingly incorporating the biochemical stress and reactions to pain of these tortured animals?

Whether or not this is so, Joseph Keon has done us all a great service in writing this book. His research is meticulous, his writing is lucid, and his conclusions are reliable. Whitewash is a doorway through which you can enter into a world of far greater health for yourself and your family. If you heed its messages, your body will thank you for the rest of your life.

And this splendid book is also a key to liberation from the unexamined assumptions about the dairy industry and its products that prevail in our culture. It will free you from beliefs that have attained the status of conventional wisdom but which hold no scientific credibility. Mark Twain died 100 years ago, but he would be as proud of Joseph Keon as I am. "Loyalty to a petrified opinion," he wrote, "never yet broke a chain or freed a human soul."

John Robbins is the author of *Diet for a New America, The New Food Revolution*, and *The New Good Life: Living Better Than Ever in an Age of Less.*

All truth goes through three stages.
First it is ridiculed.
Then it is violently opposed.
Finally, it is accepted as self-evident

— Arthur Schopenhauer, German philosopher

Introduction

For every human problem there is an answer
that is simple, neat, and wrong.

— H.L. Mencken

I sat in the studio of a radio station in northern California, facing the host of a politically progressive health talk show. Roughly two minutes remained before we went live on air. I had been invited on the show to talk about my first book, *Whole Health: The Guide to Wellness of Body and Mind*. While putting on her headphones, with the red hand of the studio clock approaching thirty seconds till show time, the host paused and looked at me.

"Oh, let's not talk dairy issues today," she said. "There's a lot more we can talk about."

Puzzled, I nodded weakly, trying to understand her last-minute directive. In our previous telephone conversation, she had expressed enthusiasm for my recently published article on health problems associated with cow's milk. We had spoken in depth about the topic. Now she had derailed a trainload of important information I had planned to share with listeners. As she raised her hand to visually count down the last five seconds, I decided I had better abide by her request.

When the show was over, I asked her why she had changed her mind about discussing cow's milk. The radio station, she explained, was located in the heart of a dairy-producing community, and she hadn't wished to offend her listeners. On my way to the parking lot, while reading a promotional pamphlet I had taken from the station on my way out, I discovered another possible motivation. The health program's primary sponsor was none other than a local dairy producer.

Unfortunately, such information-squelching occurs with great frequency, and not only to guests on radio talk shows. Despite our First Amendment right to freedom of speech, our corporate-owned media increasingly discourages people from speaking candidly on issues that might antagonize a variety of special interests. Some states even have "food disparagement" laws — also known as "veggie libel" laws — to prevent people from criticizing particular food commodities. Such laws were inspired in part by former president George Bush Sr.'s public confession that he hated broccoli, which sent broccoli sales plummeting.[1]

Uninformed, Misinformed, and Generally Confused

Commodities and corporations don't need civil rights. But people do, especially where their health and well-being are concerned. Essential information about the products we purchase and the foods we eat should be openly available to all. Yet too often we are misinformed, or crucial health and product information is withheld from us, for purely economic reasons. A key problem is a complicit media that allows advertisers and corporate sponsors to virtually legislate content for financial reasons that override public health considerations. What magazine, radio or TV network wants to offend a company that pays them thousands or even millions of dollars a month to advertise its products? My radio experience is a small example of a pervasive problem.

More than ever before, reliable information about the food we eat is essential to our health. Many foods today contain industrial contaminants, pesticide and herbicide residues, preservatives, and other unhealthy ingredients. Our health increasingly depends upon knowing exactly what we are putting into our bodies. Without such information, how can we make informed decisions and healthy purchases? This simple concept of full disclosure and informed consumer consent is the inspiration for this book.

Most people want to live healthy and vital lives, and many adopt strategies and lifestyles they believe will protect and fortify their health. Yet most

Americans are deeply confused as to what constitutes truly healthy nutrition. Sadly, much of the official information we are given is harmful to our health, the health of our children, and even the health of our planet. Where health matters are concerned, surveys continually point to the reality of an under- or mis-informed public. Most Americans today largely base their health choices on nutritional myths, the food industry's advertising propaganda, and the compromised nutritional guidelines of bureaucratic government agencies enmeshed with and corrupted by special-interest lobbies. This book shows the devastating impact of such misinformation on our health, and how comprehensively the federal government agencies appointed to protect us have failed to do so.

Even oversight agencies sworn to protect us protect the industries that put our health at risk instead. The Food and Drug Administration (FDA), the Environmental Protection Agency (EPA), and the Department of Health and Human Services (HHS), refuse to level with Americans about the contaminants we are exposed to every day through the foods we eat, and also refuse to prosecute criminally negligent corporations that contaminate our ecosystem and food supply. Such bias can reach ludicrous extremes. After the accident at the Three Mile Island nuclear reactor, government officials assured the local public that the exposure level was no greater than what one would receive from wearing a radium dial watch. One nuclear industry official publicly announced that plutonium was safe for human consumption and could be sprinkled on breakfast cereal and eaten without hazard. But when an anti-nuclear organization invited him to prove his claim by attending a plutonium breakfast, he declined to attend.

Unfortunately, when it comes to information, the popular health industry is almost as unreliable as the federal government. Month after month, year after year, countless magazines, books and articles — and now websites and infomercials — serve up new dietary rules, plans and theories guaranteed to dissolve fat and miraculously improve our health. Even major newsmagazines, TV and radio networks offer daily advice on exercise, weight control, cholesterol levels, heart care, and more. But much of this information is contradictory or unsupported by scientific studies. Most of it is market-driven — geared to promote related programs, products, or services. Some of it is downright dangerous. And each approach is generally touted as "the last," "the best," "the ultimate," or even "the only diet you will ever need."

The contradictory health directives of countless nutritionists, physicians, health experts and gurus, credentialed and otherwise, only increase our confusion. It's no surprise that, just a few years ago, the authors of three bestselling diet books admitted to being overweight, with one approaching obesity, while a fourth, a cardiologist presenting the secrets of good nutrition, admitted to having heart disease for which he took prescription medications. No wonder so many of us feel bewildered and led astray on the road to wellness.

As the health of the average American is sacrificed to the profit motive, we are all put at increased risk of serious medical conditions like osteoporosis, high blood pressure, heart disease, obesity, cancer, and a host of others. Today more than ever, what we don't know can make us sick, and eventually kill us, even while we believe we are doing all the right things.

The Calcium Paradox

I wrote this book to try and explain why Americans, among the top consumers of calcium (largely by way of dairy products) in the world,[2] also have one of the world's highest rates of bone fracture.[3] For over eighty years the milk industry, through relentless advertising and the cooperation of our public school systems and the medical professions, has hammered a myth into the collective American psyche: that cow's milk is a healthy, calcium-rich food essential to building and maintaining strong bones and teeth. Surprisingly, our obsessive consumption of calcium derived from dairy products seems to be a detriment to our bones and our general health.

Consider these facts: societies with low-calcium diets and only a fraction of our dairy consumption have less risk and prevalence of bone fracture.[4] Dairy products are not dietary staples in China, Japan, Vietnam, or Thailand, yet the residents of these countries suffer some of the lowest rates of bone fracture. The same can be said for populations that consume just one third of the US recommended calcium intake. The world's biggest consumers of cow's milk, dairy products, and calcium — Australia, New

Zealand, North America, and Western Europe — also have the highest risk of suffering a bone fracture.[5]

For years, numerous studies have shown a link between dairy consumption and a variety of common ailments including allergies, acne, constipation, colitis, eczema, colic, and ear infections, to name just a few. More recently, leading researchers have uncovered an aberrant protein in milk whose presence may explain why it is so strongly correlated to risk for heart disease, Type I diabetes, and symptoms of autism. A host of insidious diseases, including bovine tuberculosis, Johne's disease (implicated as a cause of Crohn's disease in humans), leukemia and an AIDS-like condition, now infect many dairy herds. An extensive list of contaminants routinely found in dairy foods includes poisons like dioxin, pesticides, flame-retardants, dry-cleaning solvent, and even rocket fuel and radioactive substances. And yet official US recommendations for calcium intake, with a focus on dairy products, have increased, as has the incidence of bone fracture and many other illnesses and ailments, some associated with cow's milk.[6]

Ignorance in Health Care

Another key problem is the field of conventional medicine and medical education, with their primary focus on disease intervention rather than prevention and their heavy reliance on, and aggressive promotion of, prescription drugs, surgery, and other modalities that treat existing conditions that might easily be prevented by proactive health choices and lifestyles. This is true even of many of conventional medicine's most esteemed practitioners.

The ignorance of, and lack of focus on, proactive, "preventative" health strategies and habits is most apparent in the area of nutrition and its relationship to disease. Seventy percent of all chronic degenerative diseases in America are rooted in the dietary choices we make.[7] Yet in an intensive education lasting a minimum of five years, most physicians receive only two-and-a-half hours (at best) of nutritional education.[8] This means that most doctors lack essential, in-depth knowledge of the impact of diet on the health of their patients, and so are unqualified to properly diagnose and treat the numerous ailments that stem from poor dietary habits.[9] Too many doctors recommend prescription drugs and surgery for ailments that could be remedied through simple lifestyle and dietary changes.

Many otherwise legitimate health professionals, including well-credentialed nutritionists and dieticians, were brainwashed, as we were, regarding dietary matters, and perpetuate unhealthy dietary myths in good faith. In short, those professionals to whom we confide our most intimate and serious health concerns, and to whom we at times entrust our very lives, are often ill-equipped to give us wise counsel regarding diet-related issues, diseases and cures.

America's Health Paradox

America is the wealthiest and most health-conscious, health-obsessed nation on Earth. Yet it also has one of the least healthy and most overweight populations.[10] Two of every three American adults, and more than one in three children and teens, are now overweight* or obese.[11] Americans will spend a staggering $40 billion this year alone on a vast array of diet books, pills, herbal formulas, and branded weight-loss clubs, in an effort to finally resolve their ongoing weight problems. Yet every indication is that this costly effort will continue to prove futile.[12] Ninety-five percent of dieters regain the weight they lose within three years.[13] In a sad irony, Americans spend on weight-loss efforts fifty times the amount the United Nations spends on hunger and famine relief.[13] Meanwhile, eight hundred million people in the developing world go hungry and undernourished.[14]

But our weight is not our only problem. Twenty-three million Americans have diabetes, and another forty million have a condition known as pre-diabetes and don't know it. The Center for Disease Control and Prevention now predicts that one in three Americans born in 2000 will develop diabetes.[15] One in three Americans has hypertension (high blood pressure), and one in three of these hypertension sufferers hasn't been diagnosed.

---

* The terms overweight and obese reflect a range of body weights that, based upon a given height, are considered to be unhealthful and have been shown to increase risk of serious disease. When one-third or more of a person's body weight is composed of fat, they are said to be obese.

The number of Americans diagnosed with osteoporosis leaped fifty-five percent between 1995 and 2006.[16] Some form of cancer will now affect one in three women and one in two men in their lifetime,[17] unless they adopt those lifestyle changes shown to lower risk. Seven million Americans will suffer heart attacks this year, and many of these will be fatal. Sadly, most of these health problems are self-inflicted through dietary habits and other lifestyle choices we make each day.

Our diet, level of physical activity, and exposure to certain drugs and consumer products are the most significant health determinants. Ironically, many people in less-developed nations who are not obsessed with diet, weight and fitness, eat a simpler, healthier diet, live a more active lifestyle, and enjoy far superior health to average Americans.

Yet this is not a book of doom, gloom and terrible truths presented without hope or remedy. Our decisions and choices are only as sound and reliable as the information to which we have access. In this book, you will discover explosive facts that will permanently change the way you think about the foods you eat and the sources you reply upon for dietary advice.

We'll take a comprehensive look at probably the most destructive nutritional myth of all — the one that says that humans need the milk of a cow to be healthy. We'll also look at the real factors that are contributing to the epidemic of osteoporosis occurring today in America — and I assure you, a lack of cow's milk in the diet is not one of them. We'll see how, in the process of attempting to fortify our bones, we are not only failing to achieve this goal, we are actually accomplishing just the opposite. Because osteoporosis-related fractures cost $17 billion in medical and related costs annually in the United States[18] (£6.4 billion in the United Kingdom, $650 million in Canada)[19] and lead to significant disability and ultimately death, health-care professionals and policymakers are understandably deeply concerned about getting a handle on this disease.[20] Unfortunately, until now, most of our efforts have been self-defeating. One of the key reasons for this failure has been our misguided preoccupation with one micronutrient: *calcium*. Americans have been told that if they can just manage to pack enough calcium into their diet — whether through food or supplements, antacids or aspirin — they'll have healthy bones. Yet surprisingly, the quantity of calcium that one consumes ranks very low on the list of essential strategies for maintaining bone health.

We'll look at the myriad ways in which undiagnosed allergies to cow's milk can compromise health, and can produce symptoms that are often attributed to unrelated factors and therefore left unresolved for years — even for a lifetime. We'll also learn about the extensive list of dangerous contaminants routinely found in dairy foods.

We'll see that after children are weaned and introduced to cow's milk, a plethora of common health problems — such as repetitive ear infections, colitis, eczema, and constipation — become more likely. We'll also examine the role cow's milk may play in the onset of autism in certain children, and we'll hear the uplifting stories of parents who have successfully reversed their children's condition through dietary modifications.

In these pages, I reveal important health information of which many medical doctors, registered dieticians, nutritionists, athletic coaches, personal trainers, policymakers, food industry workers, and other "health experts" are unaware. You will learn why cow's milk and products made from it are not only unnecessary in your diet, their inclusion places you and your children at risk of a host of health problems. You will come to understand why and how the milk myth has been so successfully perpetuated upon us all, and how truly easy it is to leave dairy products behind. I'll also show you how unjustified the American obsession with calcium is and introduce you to a plethora of healthful foods from which you can easily obtain all the calcium and other nutrients your body needs. Finally, I hope that you will take advantage of the Resources section at the back of the book. There you will find a multitude of supportive sources to explore, from cookbooks to websites, from products to organizations, even restaurant and shopping guides. All of these resources will nurture your efforts to achieve and maintain optimal health.

One

Our Love of Milk

*It seems ridiculous that a man, especially in the midst of
his pleasures, should have to go beneath a cow like a calf
three times a day — never weaned.*

— Henry David Thoreau

Mother's milk, our first food, creates a strong emotional tie with mother, and with milk as a life-giving substance. Most of us were weaned from mother's milk to cow's milk, which plays a significant lifetime role in the average American diet. Americans love milk. In America, milk has mystique. More than a liquid, it is a symbol of goodness, nurturing, nourishment, and health. Milk and cookies, the ultimate comfort snack, and vanilla ice cream and apple pie, the homespun dessert of our forefathers, are American traditions.

According to the US Department of Agriculture (USDA), the average American consumes approximately thirty ounces of milk, cheese, and butter a day — or six hundred pounds of dairy products a year. One of every seven grocery dollars purchases some form of cow's milk. Seventy-two percent of our dietary calcium is derived from dairy foods.[1] Milk-vending machines stand in high-school corridors across the nation. These statistics are a testimony to the pervasive messages promoting cow's milk and dairy foods that we receive from our earliest years.

An active weight lifter in my teens, I considered milk an essential ingredient to my muscular development. Milk advertisements equated milk consumption with athletic prowess. Coaches at school and self-proclaimed authorities at the gym all urged heavy consumption of milk, yogurt, and cheese. My consuming a couple of quarts of milk a day was not uncommon for a serious high-school athlete. Even consuming pints of "gourmet" ice cream was justified, because it was rich in calcium and protein.

What did I get for my fanatical allegiance to dairy? Fat. During the twelve-month training period in which I consumed the most dairy products, I gained almost twenty-five pounds of body weight. It wasn't just muscle. I also developed horrible acne and my cholesterol soared to levels more suited to a man three times my age suffering from heart disease. Yet none of these symptoms raised a red flag around, or made me question, my dairy consumption.

Due to a lack of objective information and a non-stop barrage of advertisements, including "educational" health pamphlets distributed in most schools by the dairy industry, my love affair with dairy products flourished, as did my milk-induced ailments. Every source of available information, from health magazines, wellness newsletters, doctors, school coaches, personal trainers and commercials on television, confirmed the same message: Drink more milk! Milk, I was told, was "wholesome," "nature's perfect food," even "patriotism in a glass." Milk was sacrosanct, beyond reproach. To question milk was almost like questioning the American flag. Even today, some people find the suggestion that milk might pose health risks, or not live up to the promise of assured bone integrity, hard to swallow.

Tainted Advice

Every five years since 1980, the USDA and the Department of Health and Human Services (HHS) have published *Dietary Guidelines for Americans* to help American consumers, dieticians, doctors, and the National School Lunch Program, determine how to plan healthful meals.[2] The current incarnation, "The Food Pyramid," is about as vague and unhelpful as it's ever been (the 2010 edition was not released at the time of writing).

You might assume that a government advisory board tasked with setting dietary guidelines would be composed of unbiased doctors, scientists, and nutritionists who understand the critical relationship between diet, health, and disease. But you would be wrong. During the last revisions, six of the eleven advisory board members selected by the USDA and HHS had intimate ties to dairy industry institutions, including the Dairy Council, the National Dairy Promotion and Research Board, and Dairy Management, Inc.[3] According to a *Wall Street Journal* report, at least three members had received financing from the National Dairy Council.[4] Another reason to regard dietary guidelines with suspicion is that the USDA's primary job is not to encourage healthful eating, as you might assume, but rather to promote American agricultural products.

Ideally, public health organizations determining public health guidelines would be non-profit, objective, and not affiliated with industries with a biased view of our nutritional needs. But as the example above shows, that's not how it works. Much of the literature handed out by the American Dietetic Association and the American Heart Association is mired in food myths rather than reliable scientific data. The National Osteoporosis Foundation aggressively promotes the milk myth, strongly advocating the consumption of dairy products in its literature, even when the body of scientific evidence fails to support this as a truly effective way to protect bone.[5] Such examples raise legitimate concerns about the influence of major food lobbies, including by financial contributions.

The US government's significant role in supporting and virtually sponsoring the dairy industry also compromises its objectivity in this regard. Consider the fact that the government subsidizes the milk industry with up to $2.5 billion in tax breaks every year, while promoting our dependence upon milk through discounted surpluses given to public schools nationwide.[6] When government agencies and business conglomerates become enmeshed in this way, and their mutual financial interests are at stake, objectivity is fatally compromised. Such conflicts of interest can't help playing an intrinsic role in the fashioning of public policy, and can't help influencing much of the advisory literature produced by these public/ corporate "health organizations". "We are absolutely drowned in information coming out of the dairy industry," writes T. Colin Campbell, Ph.D., Jacob Gould Schurman Professor Emeritus of Nutritional Biochemistry at Cornell University[7], "Our national nutrition policies are corrupted by the influences of the dairy industry."[8] Contrary to what nature intended, from childhood on we're told by a series of authority figures and institutions that cow's milk is essential to human health. This organized, systematic campaign of indoctrination has been going on for nearly a century. As early as 1922, the dairy industry was already in schools providing "nutrition education materials." This effective marketing strategy is still used today. A 1979 study by the American Dietetic Association found that teaching materials provided by the Dairy Council were the primary source from which teachers derived nutritional information for their classes. Today, an estimated twenty million schoolchildren each year receive the dairy industry's promotional literature in the classroom.[9]

So-called "teaching aids" promoting dairy consumption, with titles like "Delicious Decisions," "Nutrition Nibbles," and "Food Choices to Grow On," are mainstays in classrooms across America. In one such pamphlet, children are encouraged to check off how many glasses of milk they have consumed each day, with space provided in the chart for six glasses. Six glasses of whole milk (consisting of 3.7 percent fat) delivers a whopping 942 calories, 53 grams of fat, 210 mg of cholesterol (the recommended maximum is 300 mg/day), 714 mg of sodium, and 48 grams of protein. And that doesn't include the average three meals a day, plus snacks. As we will see, such "Delicious Decisions" may, according to a growing body of research, be a perfect prescription for future osteoporosis, heart disease, hypertension, obesity, and elevated risk of cancer.

In the industry trade magazine Dairy Foods, Peggy Blitz, Chief Executive Officer of the California Dairy Council, clearly states the goal of this literature. "The Dairy Council of California's nutrition-education programs in schools help children learn to value milk and dairy foods early in their lives, thus laying a foundation for industry promotion efforts ... it's information that, combined with ongoing marketing efforts, can motivate Americans to take the action we want them to take even more frequently — consuming milk and other dairy foods."[10] At one time, the National Dairy Council was offering $30,000 a year in "nutrition education grants" for programs that "help increase calcium intake (presumably in the form of dairy products) among youth."[11]

Just a decade ago, the Washington, D.C–based organization Physicians Committee for Responsible Medicine filed the first of several petitions with the Federal Trade Commission (FTC) asserting that advertisements for dairy products violated federal advertising guidelines. Ultimately, the FTC rejected these petitions. But this was not the first time the dairy industry has been confronted about the health claims made in its advertisements.

The American Dairy Council was challenged over its advertising claims in the 1970s when the popular slogan "Every Body Needs Milk" was found to be "false, misleading, and deceptive." An April 1974 *New York Times* article reported that the FTC filed a formal complaint of false, misleading, and deceptive advertising that implicated the California Milk Producers Advisory Board and their advertising agency. The Dairy Council agreed to modify the slogan to "Milk Has Something for Everybody."

The California Milk Processors Board's nationally franchised "Got Milk?" ads, with the familiar milk mustache, have generated a good deal of scrutiny from some members of the health-care community, who assert that they mislead consumers about the nutritional value of cow's milk. In October 2005, the British Advertising Standards Authority forced Nestlé Health and Nutrition to withdraw its advertisements in the United Kingdom stating that milk was "Essential for healthy bones."[12]

Why all the fuss over slogans? After all, isn't milk simply wholesome food? Even a little too much of a "good thing" couldn't be that bad ... could it?

The Weaning of America

Although still high, sales of dairy-related products have been declining since the mid-1960s. In 1966, the average American consumed 35.5 gallons of milk. By 1976, consumption had fallen to 31.6 gallons a year; by 1986, to 28.6 gallons; and by 1997, to 26.2 gallons.[13] In 1999, the introduction of flavored milks boosted sales 0.7 percent.[14] But between 1999 and 2004, fluid milk sales dropped another 3 percent.[15] Still, in 2006 California's dairy industry alone generated $47.4 billion in economic activity.[16]

It is impossible to know the exact causes of this downward trend. Factors may include the rise in dairy costs, the proliferation of soft drinks and other popular "sports beverages," and increasing awareness and related concerns over dairy-related health problems such as lactose intolerance and dairy allergies and issues like mad cow disease and the use of rBGH, the synthetic hormone administered to some dairy cattle.

The significant decline in sales noted above would send shock waves through any big business. And industry efforts to boost sales and counter "bad press" regarding legitimate health concerns typically involve aggressive advertising campaigns and image makeovers. In this light, the "Got Milk?" ads, many starring notable celebrity athletes, icons of fitness and health, seem to have provided the financial shot in the arm the dairy industry needed. The "Got Milk?" campaign reportedly achieved a 91 percent awareness rating, leading to spin-off licensed products including watches, toys, dolls, apparel, cookies, books, kids' accessories, and even a "Got Milk?" Barbie doll.

From a business and marketing standpoint, the success of dairy advertising campaigns is simply phenomenal. What is not so laudable, however, is the failure to acknowledge the scientific literature with regard to our current strategy for bone health. As noted, these ads leave out important health facts that refute the industry's claims that milk products are an important ingredient in human fitness and health. The ads also reinforce milk-promoting myths, such the age-old myth that osteoporosis is caused by a calcium deficiency, *rather than by excessive calcium loss*. Milk ads are racially biased in their universal recommendation of dairy consumption, since they fail to acknowledge the high rate of lactose intolerance — the inability to digest lactose, a sugar found in cow's milk — among African Americans (75 percent), Native Americans, and Asian Americans (nearly 100 percent).[17] Almost invariably, advertisements for milk and calcium supplements present them as a panacea for weak bones, yet fail to address any of the numerous other factors that play a critical role in maintaining bone health. These factors include our intake of protein, sodium, magnesium, fluoride, vitamins D and K, and other micronutrients, as well as our consumption of coffee and sugar and whether we smoke or lead sedentary lifestyles; even the medications we may take can be a factor.

In the words of Jeff Manning, executive director of the California Milk Processor Board, "This is our objective statement today: Sell More Milk. Everything that we do, every moment that I spend, gets filtered through this objective. If it doesn't sell more milk or have the potential to sell more milk, we won't do it — it's that simple."[18]

Speaking about the success of the "Got Milk?" campaign, Mr. Manning recalls the effect of the ads in which people indulge in some snack — such as cookies or a sandwich — and discover they have no milk left in the fridge. "We gave people the food, took the milk away, and they started to think milk was crucially important."[19]

As we will see, such advertisements for cow's milk present a biased and inaccurate perspective on human nutritional needs, and how best to fulfill these needs.

The Truth Isn't in the Advertising; It's in the Bottom Line

The dairy industry has made clear that its primary objective is to sell as much dairy to as many people as possible. This bottom-line commitment to selling a product isn't unethical in itself. The ethical problem occurs when an industry infiltrates and corrupts public institutions responsible for advising American consumers about their health and skews the information given to the public purely for the sake of profits. The milk industry has also donned the guise of "nutritional expert" to dispense "health advice" that is unsupported by scientific data in our public schools, again, purely as a marketing strategy.

In 2001, under pressure from consumer activists, the US government appointed a scientific panel to examine health claims commonly made in advertisements for dairy products. This panel of physicians concluded that milk "cannot be considered a 'sports drink,' does not specifically prevent osteoporosis, and, in its high-fat, whole milk form, might play a role in heart disease and prostate cancer."[20] Critics in the United States are not alone in the effort to confront milk-promoting propaganda. The Swiss Federal Health Ministry has filed suit against the Swiss dairy industry, complaining that it "failed to provide medical proof for the health claim that milk has a preventive effect against osteoporosis."[21]

You may recall the controversy that erupted in the 1970s over Nestlé's infant formula sales strategy in third-world countries. The multinational company's sales people, often wearing nurses' uniforms and offering free samples in hospitals, urged women to feed their babies Nestlé's infant formula instead of breastfeeding them. The infant formula has less nutritional value than mother's milk and contributes to numerous health problems and even deaths among infants, especially in economically underdeveloped countries.

As the Nestlé example shows, the marketing strategies of major industries selling products that promise health benefits can easily, perhaps inevitably, cross an ethical line. Such strategies have compromised and even corrupted the public institutions responsible for dispensing objective, unbiased, scientifically based health information to the public. They have imperiled the health of the public, and not just the American public.

In the next chapter we will take a look at another industry marketing strategy — the manufactured calcium crisis.

Two

The Calcium Crisis

It will be embarrassing enough if the current calcium hype is simply useless; it will be immeasurably worse if the recommendations are actually detrimental to health.

— D. Mark Hegsted, former professor of nutrition,
Harvard School of Public Health

The various approaches used to promote dairy foods culminated in what has been called a "calcium crisis." There is a serious shortage of calcium in the American diet, we are told, and this portends the serious condition of osteoporosis. Funded by the dairy industry, full-page advertisements in the *New York Times* warned of this "major health emergency."[1] To address the situation, the dairy industry called for a "calcium summit" to be held in New York City, in the way presidents and prime ministers of foreign nations hold a summit to address some pressing political issue. Respectable figures from the National Institutes of Health have also touted this message. When talking about children who consume less than the recommended daily intake of calcium, Doctor Duane Alexander, director of the National Institute of Child Health and Human Development (NICHD), said, "Osteoporosis is a pediatric disease with geriatric consequences," and "As these children get older, this calcium crisis will become more serious as the population starts to show its highest rate of osteoporosis and other bone health problems in our nation's history."[2] Cabot Creamery of Vermont repeated the mantra, declaring in a press release, "America is in a Calcium Crisis: Dairy Supplements Are No Substitute for Milk, Cheese and Yogurt."[3]

There's actually a relative abundance of calcium in the average American diet. The National Health and Nutrition Examination Survey for 1999–2000 showed that boys and girls aged 12–19 were consuming 1,081 and 793 mg per day, respectively. Men and women aged 20–39 were consuming 1,025 and 797 mg, respectively, and men and women 40–60 years were consuming 797 and 660 mg, respectively.[4] By the estimation of the World Health Organization, this is beyond an adequate amount of calcium to protect bones from fracture. Moreover, studies show that cow's milk does not protect humans against bone fractures in the way we have been told. In fact, consuming cow's milk may even elevate the risk of bone fracture. For example, a Harvard University study of seventy-eight thousand women revealed that those who drink the most milk were actually at *greater* risk of bone fracture than those who drank little or no milk.[5]

The obsession with calcium suggests that all bones need to be healthy is calcium, and if we can simply cram enough calcium into our body — through cow's milk, supplements, juice, antacids, aspirin, and everything else to which calcium has lately been added — we will have a healthy skeleton. It's simply not that easy. As we will see, this culture of calciumism is sorely misguided.

One of the most important messages in this book is that calcium is but one of numerous nutrients essential for bone health; and, as we will see later, an abundance of dietary or supplemental calcium in itself has not been shown to assure greater bone density or protection from bone fracture.[6]

The Crisis of Common Sense

The reality is that our present approach to preventing bone fracture is an unqualified failure. It's time we rethought it. We can begin by applying a little critical thinking, if not simple common sense. We need to ask ourselves questions such as: "Why is one industry seemingly so deeply concerned about the health of Americans, while untold numbers of others don't seem to care at all?" For example, why is there no "Broccoli Growers Association" or "National Kale Council" busy holding "calcium summits" and filling magazines and billboards with clever ads coaxing consumers to rely on their products? As you will see, these products are far superior sources of calcium, the primary selling point used to promote dairy products.

If cow's milk is essential for human health, how did so many humans survive prior to large-scale dairy farming, packaging, trucking, and refrigeration? And how do hundreds of millions of people around the world continue to maintain excellent bone health while eschewing cow's milk? Why are humans the only species that drinks the milk of another species?

Loren Cordain, an evolutionary biologist at Colorado State University, points out that the milk-drinking phenomenon is a relatively recent one in human history. So if cow's milk is so important to bone health, we might assume that our ancestors in the pre-milk era must have had terrible bone health. However, after examining the bones of those who lived in the pre-milk-mustache era, Dr. Cordain paints a different picture. "We don't find that at all," Cordain writes. "What we do find are robust, fracture-resistant bones."[7] Other research has shown that though bone disease did exist, the bones of postmenopausal women from the 18th and 19th centuries were generally stronger than those of today's women of similar ages. These earlier women, of course, did not have a stash of yogurt in their refrigerator, nor were they devouring calcium supplements or undergoing estrogen replacement therapy.[8] Later, we'll learn some of the reasons why their bones stayed so healthy.

Although many of the best-credentialed health authorities in America still cling to the peculiar notion that humans require milk produced for another species' offspring, some health professionals are beginning to question or even oppose this notion. There is ample reason for them to do so.

Retired surgeon Robert Kradjian conducted a review of articles about cow's milk in the medical literature, examining an astounding five hundred studies. "First of all," he wrote in his summary, "none of the authors spoke of cow's milk as an excellent food, free of side effects. The main focus of the published reports seem to be on intestinal colic, intestinal irritation, intestinal bleeding and anemia, allergic reactions in infants and children, as well as infections such as salmonella." "In adults," Dr. Kradjian continued, "the problems seemed centered more around heart disease and arthritis, allergy, sinusitis, and the more serious questions of leukemia, lymphoma, and cancer."[9] Can you recall your doctors speaking to you about such concerns?

Mixed-Up Media

It is a downright shame when a weekly magazine such as *Business Week* decides to do a column on nutrition and includes an inset heading in bold type that says: "The best sources of calcium are dairy products such as skim milk and yogurt."[10] To make such a statement to its readers suggests *Business Week* does not understand human nutrition, and should therefore avoid giving advice on the subject.

These oversights are forgivable; but what about when similar food myths are promulgated in a reputable health column? A prime example is Jane Brody's well-respected health column in the *New York Times,* which advised readers: "The best, and best absorbed, sources of these nutrients [calcium and vitamin D] are low-fat and nonfat dairy products."[11] In another column, this one on dental health, Ms. Brody assured readers that "Milk builds strong bones."[12] As we will see, the first assertion is simply untrue; the second would be correct if it only referred to cow's bones. There is no conclusive evidence that cow's milk builds strong bones in humans; in fact, the data that do exist suggest it plays a far less significant role than we have been led to believe.[13]

Then there is *Men's Health* magazine, which tells its readers that cow's milk not only prevents osteoporosis but also helps keep us lean.[14] I have yet to locate the body of scientific literature that supports such claims, yet as you will see, there's ample evidence to the contrary. Another source to which millions of Americans subscribe, the *Berkeley Wellness Letter,* chimed in with: "Milk and other dairy products are the best source of calcium, which not only keeps bones strong, but also may help prevent hypertension, heart disease, colon cancer, and possibly diabetes."[15] If you don't read this quote carefully, you might come away thinking that the editors of the *Wellness Letter* want you to think that *dairy products* provide these potential health benefits. In fact, it is *calcium* to which they are referring, not dairy products. None of the other factors influencing bone health are mentioned, which leaves an inaccurate impression.

I recently read an article in a popular health magazine in which a professor of nutrition told readers they were fat because they didn't eat enough dairy products![16] So should we believe that nursing from another species is the missing piece in our puzzling struggle with body weight? Another health journal claimed that one of the causes of osteoporosis is lactose intolerance.[17]

If you log on to the Internet, you can find a legion of questionable advice on personal health, even from a source as respected as WebMD. This organization has published the claim that "An additional glass of milk or serving of yogurt each day could help many women ward off osteoporosis." They also mislead readers into believing a person absorbs over three hundred milligrams (mg) of calcium from one cup of milk.[18] Again, the scientific literature indicates that this is simply not true.[19]

I wrote and asked WebMD's editors if they could provide me with studies to support their claim that a woman drinking an "extra glass of milk" each day would enjoy a lower risk for osteoporosis. They said they would "look into" the request, but by the time this book went to press, they had not come up with anything to support such a claim. Several months later, they reported that "Dairy products are the best source of calcium."[20] And WebMD is hardly the only source promoting such misinformation.

"Perfect People" Sell a Not-So-Perfect-Food

Well-intentioned health practitioners don't face an easy task in educating their patients and the public. A single voice, no matter how strident, is dwarfed by clever images and slogans that bombard consumers from magazines, billboards, radio and television. Anyone attempting to offer a contrary view is easily blown over by the hot wind of a multimillion-dollar advertising campaign.

What's more, the dairy industry has recruited a host of television and film actors, supermodels, celebrated athletes, and even federal officials to endorse cow's milk as a healthy food. There is a great fixation on celebrities in America. We want to know about their latest haircuts, who they are dating, what kind of cars they drive, and what kinds of foods they eat to remain so glamorous and sexy. For participating in milk advertisements, celebrities are rewarded handsomely, with paychecks in the range of $25,000.[21] You might hope that those being paid so well (even if they donate the money to charity, as some have been reported to do) would be sure they understood the ramifications of the message they are helping the dairy industry deliver to America.

To give but one example, filmmaker Spike Lee's participation in such ads leaves me wondering. Consider that people of African descent have the second-highest incidence of lactose intolerance as a population, about 75 percent.[22] Lactose intolerance means a person is unable to digest the sugar (lactose) in milk. People with this intolerance — in this case, three out of four African Americans — who drink milk may suffer from abdominal bloating, cramping, intestinal gas, nausea, diarrhea, and other symptoms. As an influential role model, Spike Lee's appearance in milk ads sends a direct message to fellow African Americans that it's okay, perhaps even admirable, to drink milk.

Despite the fact that African Americans, Latinos, Asian Americans, and Native Americans have some of the highest rates of lactose intolerance in the world,[23] the US government continues to recommend that these populations drink at least two glasses of milk a day, with no apparent concern for the suffering this advice may cause for millions of Americans. The dairy industry was reported to have lobbied for an increased recommendation of three to four servings a day, and in 2005, the HHS did raise that recommendation by 50 percent, to three servings a day.[24] Walter Willett, M.D., chairman of the Harvard School of Public Health's Department of Nutrition and someone we'll hear more from later in this book, calls that recommendation "egregious."[25]

Where Do Cows Get Their Calcium?

The current fixation on the calcium we can derive from cow's milk suggests that there are no other sources of dietary calcium. As you will see, this is far from the truth. After all, where do cows get their calcium? They get it from the grass they eat, not from suckling from another species.

Peruse any of the multitude of health magazines published in America, particularly those aimed at women, and you are bound to find an article on the importance of calcium and the virtues of drinking milk. Almost invariably, such articles include a stock photo of a glass of milk or a cup of yogurt. I have written to a number of magazine editors asking them why they perpetuate the myths that a large calcium intake guarantees bone health and that calcium comes only from cow's milk. I point out that they could just as easily have inserted a photo of a tempting pile of sautéed broccoli, or one of at least seventy other calcium-containing foods. However, when it comes to nutrition, magazine editors are frequently just as misinformed as their readers, and thus the myths and misinformation are perpetuated.

Pressure on Parents and Children

The journal *Pediatrics* published a study that raised questions about the conventional wisdom that says large quantities of milk build strong bones in children. The study, a meta-analysis which evaluated findings from previous studies, concluded that exercise may be more important to bone strength than increased calcium intake.

"Under scientific scrutiny, the support for the milk myth crumbles" wrote Dr. Amy Lanou, a Cornell University-trained nutritionist and lead author of the study. "This analysis of 58 published studies shows that the evidence on which US dairy intake recommendations are based is scant .... A clear majority of the studies we examined for this review found no relationship between dairy or dietary calcium intake and measures of bone health."[26]

Yet parents who declare that they no longer feed their children cow's milk are often perceived as imprudent by other parents, and downright reckless by their doctors. When I question people about their milk-drinking habits, one of the most common retorts I hear is: "My doctor tells me I have to drink cow's milk," or "My pediatrician says my children *need* cow's milk." What a silly concept — a human child *needing* the milk of another species! If nature had intended children to drink cow's milk, she would have made them into calves, not children.

The process of coercion begins even earlier than grade school. If you read the newsletter *Nutrition Edition*, published by the Contra Costa Child Care Council Food Program, you might think that the editors worked for the dairy industry. One issue, published for the benefit of childcare givers within that California county, advised: "If a child requests a different beverage (usually juice), *you* need to set limits. Simply inform the child that milk is the drink being served, and offer no other choices .... Do not respond further if the child complains."[27]

Further advice to the caregiver stated: "Let children know that milk is a required item at main meals and part of a healthy diet. When you continue to set limits and repeat these procedures, children will understand what is expected of them and will soon drink milk because they know there is no other choice." The letter goes on to describe children who reject milk as "causing great alarm." What should be alarming is that many children instinctively know cow's milk is not for them, and yet they are forced to get in the habit of drinking it! Cows don't need to force their calves to drink their mother's milk, nor do human mothers need to force their babies to drink breast milk.

Three

Udderly Ridiculous

Perhaps when the public is educated as to the hazards of milk,
only calves will be left to drink the real thing.

— Frank Oski, M.D., Former Professor of Pediatrics,
Johns Hopkins University School of Medicine;
Past President, United States Society for Pediatric Research

There are some 5,400 different species of mammals, including cows, and every one produces milk for their young. In each case, including humans, the milk is nutritionally unique to meet the exact needs of the species. In other words, its nutrient composition — fat, protein, carbohydrate, sodium, phosphorus, and so forth — varies in proportion to factors such as the growth rates of the various species' offspring, which differ dramatically. For example, a mother whale produces exceptionally fatty milk the consistency of mayonnaise, so that her calf can quickly develop the blubber it needs to survive in its ocean environment. Rat's milk, on the other hand, is about 49 percent protein, to support an exceptionally rapid rate of maturation. A baby rat will double its birthweight in a mere four days!

Consider the composition of cow's milk compared to human milk. As you will see in the following table, the two are nutritionally quite dissimilar. This is just one of the reasons why cow's milk is not well suited for humans.

Note the calcium content of mother's milk relative to cow's milk. At a developmentally critical time, nature decided that a fraction of the calcium found in cow's milk was perfectly suited for a newborn or infant child.

Grams of Various Nutrients per 100 Grams of Milk

	Protein	Carbohydrate	Sodium	Phosphorus	Calcuim
Human	1.1	9	16	18	33
Cow	4	4.9	50	97	118

Pennington, Jean A. T., *Bowes & Church's Food Values of Portions Commonly Used*, 17th ed. (Philadelphia: Lippincot, Williams & Wilkins, 1998).

Why Not Elephant's Milk?

Where did we get the idea that humans should drink cow's milk? Why is it that so many people find it acceptable to drink cow's milk but not cat's milk, giraffe's milk, dog's milk, or rat's milk for that matter? If I asked you why you don't drink elephant's milk, you would probably reply, "Because elephant's milk is for baby elephants!" Precisely my point.

From a historical perspective, it makes some sense that humans decided to try cow's milk after noticing the nutrition it provided for calves. After all, cow's milk is formulated to enable a calf to double its birth weight in a mere 47 days (as opposed to 180 days for a human), grow to 300 pounds after 12 months, and ultimately reach a body weight of 1,200 pounds! This aspect of cow's milk does not play out well in human beings, especially those who struggle with their weight. Today, this means an estimated 60 percent of the American population, including one in three children are overweight — perhaps the most overweight population on Planet Earth.[1]

Comparison of Calories as Protein in the Milk of Various Species[2]

Milk Source	Percent of Calories as Protein	Number of Days in which Birth Weight Doubles
Human	5%	180
Horse	11 %	60
Cow	15%	47
Goat	17%	19
Dog	30%	8
Cat	40%	7
Rat	49%	4

The chart above shows variation in protein content in the milk of various species. Note the correlation between protein content and the number of days required for the offspring to double its birth weight. The slower-growing the species, the lower the percentage of calories provided as protein.

Nutritional Profile of Cow's Milk

So, does cow's milk provide humans with nutrition? As the following table shows, cow's milk does offer nutrients such as fat, carbohydrates, protein, and calcium. However, there is no essential nutritional factor in cow's milk that humans cannot readily obtain from a healthful food that is better suited to our well-being.

Nutrients Found in Whole Milk

Calcium	Magnesium	Protein	Vitamin A	Vitamin D (added)
Cholesterol	Phosphorus	Riboflavin	Vitamin B_{12}	
Fat	Potassium	Sodium	Vitamin B_6	

The primary justification for promoting cow's milk is the abundance of calcium it contains. But cow's milk does not have a corner on the calcium market. As we will see in Chapter Nine, there is a multitude of healthful foods from which we can derive the calcium our bodies need. Indeed, few people are aware that humans can absorb a greater portion of the calcium found in a cup of kale, broccoli, or fortified orange juice than that in a cup of cow's milk.[3] As you can see in the following table, humans absorb only 32 percent of the calcium in a glass of milk.

Calcium Absorption of Selected Foods[4]

One Cup	Brussels Sprouts	Kale	Broccoli	Turnip Greens	Mustard Greens	Orange Juice	Whole Milk	Skim Milk
Gross Calcium	19mg	94mg	83mg	106mg	128mg	350mg	291mg	302mg
Calcium Absorption	63.8 %	40.9 %	52.6 %	51.6 %	57.8%	37 %	32.1 %	32.1 %
Calories	60	42	48	28	25	120	150	86

Moreover, neither kale nor broccoli contains the cholesterol or saturated fat found in cow's milk. Both saturated fat and cholesterol are recognized as promoters of heart disease, high blood pressure, and increased risk of stroke. And unlike cow's milk, kale and broccoli are not treated with potentially dangerous hormones such as the infamous rBGH (recombinant bovine growth hormone), a genetically-engineered hormone chemical injected into cows to boost their milk yields.

As the table on page 26 shows, cow's milk also has three times the protein found in mother's milk. Apparently, nature determined that at the time of our most rapid growth, infancy, we need only 5 percent of our calories as protein. As we will see in Chapter Seven, excess dietary protein, another misunderstood and overrated nutrient, is one of the top reasons so many Americans' bones are being robbed of their calcium around the clock.

However, while a comparison of calcium content and absorption rates and protein content is important, these are just a few of the factors that need be observed to make intelligent decisions about the foods that will best nourish our bodies. Strong bones are not formed and kept strong simply because of adequate calcium intake. In the end, calcium, regardless of the source, may not be the key to bone health we've been lead to believe. Numerous other nutrients, as well as lifestyle choices, are critical to the formation and integrity of bone. For example, it has been found the body uses dietary calcium best when the diet also includes a balanced source of magnesium. Some have questioned how effectively our bodies can use the calcium found in cow's milk because it is disproportionate to the magnesium (by a factor of about eight to one).[5] In Chapter Seven, we'll look at all of the other nutrients required for lasting bone health. In the next few chapters, we'll look in detail at some of the host of health problems correlated to the consumption of cow's milk. These problems includes diarrhea,[6] iron-deficiency anemia,[7] gas, eczema,[8] arthritis,[9] bloating,[10] migraine headaches,[11] asthma,[12] runny nose, lower I.Q.,[13] sudden infant death syndrome (SIDS),[14] Type I diabetes, acne,[15] fatigue, breast, prostate, and ovarian cancer,[16] growth retardation,[17] psychological disturbances,[18] constipation,[19] and an elevated risk of osteoporosis.[20] Some of these health problems are caused by the lactose found in milk, while others are the result of food allergies caused by ingesting bovine proteins. Others may be due to chronic exposure to hormones and all-too-frequent contaminants found in a glass of milk or a wedge of cheese — including residues of antibiotics and other drugs[21] and pesticides and herbicides, some of which have been linked to blood diseases, cancer, and death in humans.[22] Let's look more closely at some of these diseases and how the consumption of cow's milk may increase the risk of developing them.

Four

Cow's Milk and Human Disease

The most damaging foods are dairy products.
— Nathan Pritikin, nutritionist and longevity researcher

"Contrary to the catchy milk-mustache campaign" says Dr. Walter Willett, Chair of the Department of Nutrition at Harvard's School of Public Health, "dairy products aren't the best way to get plenty of calcium."[1] If drinking the milk of a cow is not the best way to get our dietary calcium and can't guarantee us strong bones or protection against bone fracture, then, from a public health standpoint, we need to look carefully at the risks posed to those who live under this misconception. However great or small each of those risks might be, consumers deserve to know, so they can make truly informed decisions about what's right for them. This chapter examines how cow's milk might contribute to several human diseases and negative health effects.

Acne

Stay up late any night of the week and watch a bit of cable television and you're bound to see one of the ubiquitous infomercials for the latest solution to acne, a problem that affects at least forty million Americans.[2] Anger, fear, shame, anxiety, depression, embarrassment, bullying, feelings of insecurity and inferiority, limited employment opportunities, and even

31

suicidal ideation have been widely reported as possible outcomes from acne.[3] Between dermatological appointments and the spectrum of special creams, lotions, and prescription medications now marketed as treatments, Americans are spending $2 billion a year in an attempt to rid themselves of these blemishes. Conventional treatments include both topical and oral antibiotics, salicylic acid, sulfur preparations, azelaic acid, and birth control pills. Yet some of the current medications have unwanted side effects. For example, some people cannot tolerate benzoyl peroxide, the active ingredient in most over-the-counter products; their skin becomes bright red and blotchy and may become excessively dry and begin to peel after using products containing it. Prescription antibiotics, another course taken by many, are very helpful in eliminating the bacteria that grows in blemishes, but also indiscriminately kill off healthful bacteria in the intestines, bacteria that are critical to the proper assimilation of foods and their nutrients, including those that protect against cancer, and that help keep intestinal yeasts in check. When good bacteria are diminished, bad opportunistic bacteria such as Pseudomonas, Clostridium, and Klebsiella take their place and, it has been proposed, may increase the risk of cancer.[4] Antibiotic use may also result in anaphylaxis, vaginal yeast infections, allergic reactions, and diarrhea, and may contribute to antibiotic resistance.

There are other non-antimicrobial drugs shown to be helpful for acne yet they too have side effects, which are sometimes quite severe. One of the best known, isotretinoin (marketed under the brand name Roaccutane), used for severe acne, has FDA warnings as it has been known to increase the user's risk of depression, violent and aggressive behaviors, and even birth defects.[5]

To begin with, a genetic predisposition certainly plays a role in one's risk of developing acne. So does stress and excessive sweating. Use of certain medications, such as corticosteroids and oral contraceptives, exposure to dioxin (a regular contaminant of dairy products), or Cushing's syndrome or polycystic ovary syndrome may cause or exacerbate the condition. As with many of the chronic degenerative diseases that plague the West, acne, the scourge of up to 85 percent of adolescents (and many adults) is not nearly as common in parts of the world where the Western diet has not taken hold. While people have made anecdotal associations with certain foods, including dairy products, for years, one dermatologist took the connection more seriously. Dr. Jerome K. Fisher of Southern California spent a decade studying 1,088 of his own patients in an attempt to determine what stimulated their acne. His conclusion, which he presented to the American Dermatological Association in 1965 in a paper entitled *Acne Vulgaris: A Study of One Thousand Cases,* was that it was the milk in their diet.[6] Dr. Fisher found that as their milk consumption increased, so did the severity of his patient's acne; conversely, as they cut back on their intake of dairy, their condition improved. Compared to the general population, those suffering from acne drank up to four times the amount of milk, as much as four quarts per day. Although some physicians have cited the natural change in an adolescent's hormones as a cause of acne, Dr. Fisher came to believe that the greater influence was the effect of drinking cow's milk. The reason is that cow's milk is loaded with naturally-occurring hormones and growth factors.

In the milk sold in America, these levels are even more exaggerated. This is due to the practice of artificially inseminating dairy cows just days after they have given birth, so as to keep their milk production high. The result is that cows are milked during the period when they are releasing the highest levels of hormones into their milk. (Later in this chapter, Dr. Ganmaa Davaasambuu of Harvard University shares her concern that this practice may also be increasing risk for hormone-driven cancers in Americans.) One of these compounds, the female hormone progesterone, is broken down into the male hormone androgen. Androgen activates the production of sebum, a wax-like product secreted by the sebaceous glands on the face. When the sebum hardens it blocks the pilosebaceous canal and appears as a blackhead on the surface of the skin. It is the body's effort to rid itself of this hardened sebum that leads to inflammation and the dreaded red blemishes on the skin. These blemishes then fill with blood and lymph fluids, creating an ideal environment for bacteria to flourish.

Insulin-like growth factor (IGF-1), one of nearly 60 different hormones and growth factors found in a glass of cow's milk, may also be a concern for acne. Some researchers believe that IGF-1 and testosterone may work together to promote acne. (Later in this chapter we'll look at the link researchers have found between high levels of IGF-1 and risk of breast and prostate cancer.) Natural levels of IGF-1 peak at age fifteen in girls and eighteen in boys. Yet for decades, American dairy farmers have been breeding for cows that produce the most IGF-1 levels, because this leads them to produce more milk. Adding to the mix is the fact that the genetically-engineered hormone rBGH causes dairy cows to produce even higher levels of IGF-1, which ends up in their milk.

Dr. Bill Danby, a New Hampshire dermatologist with a practice in Manchester and a professor at Dartmouth Medical School, also suspected that the hormones in dairy products were playing a role in acne. He contacted the Harvard School of Public Health to enlist the help of researchers, including Dr. Walter Willett and colleagues, who were working on the famous Nurses Study. Using previously collected data from over 47,000 women, they found that those women who drank the most total milk and skim milk were more likely to have been physician-diagnosed with severe acne as teenagers.[7] In another study, researchers examined the diets of 6,094 girls aged nine to fifteen. The girls reported their dietary intake in three questionnaires from 1996 to 1998. In 1999, the presence and severity of their acne was assessed by another questionnaire. The researchers reported that the girls who drank the most cow's milk suffered the worst acne.[8]

Clear proof of causation is not yet available. For that, more research will be required. However, the anecdotal evidence coupled with the careful studies cited here support a simple, free, and safe experiment at home. If you or anyone you know is suffering from acne, a complete break from dairy products for several months would certainly be worth trying. These products may be causing or contributing to an ailment that teens and adults find to be embarrassing at best, and psychosocially devastating at worst, and which has the potential to permanently scar their appearance.

Addiction

Addictions are considered diseases because they are out of our control, often so much so that they lead us to behave in ways that are dangerous to our health. In its most basic definition, an addiction occurs when we are physiologically or psychologically dependent upon a habit-forming substance or behavior, to the point where its elimination from our life may result in trauma or suffering. Caffeine, nicotine, and alcohol are commonly accepted to be addictive substances. Many people would concur with that designation because of firsthand experience with such substances.

Designating a widely consumed and well-loved food as having addictive potential might seem a stretch. However, recent research has begun to shed light on the potential for addiction to certain foods, and indicates that the in-jest declaration that we are "addicted to" a particular food may be closer to the truth than we imagine.

While a number of foods, including chocolate, show potential for addiction due to a biologically active agent, one food in particular reigns supreme when it comes to addictive potential: cheese. In one recent year alone, Americans gobbled up $40 billion worth of locally-produced cheese.[9] I have heard more people declare that they could "never give up cheese" than I can remember. The determination in their faces when they assert this never ceases to amaze me.

One article describes how a woman with a genetic propensity for heart disease is working to minimize her risk. She exercises, takes her hypertension medication, and has cut back on dietary fat. Unfortunately, she laments, "I have slipped up with my addiction to cheese."[10] In a web posting for people making dietary changes, another person confesses that in spite of all the progress she has made, "I'm convinced that I possess a severe addiction to cheese, complete with withdrawals, secretive cheese binges, etc."[11] In the newsletter of Ampersand, the Learning Institute for Health Professionals, the subject of addiction to drugs, alcohol, gambling, and yes, even cheese, is discussed. "A young woman," says this article, "was struggling with her addiction to cheese. She couldn't keep cheese in the house without eating every crumb, and would even get out of bed in the middle of the night and buy cheese from an all-night store, bring it home and demolish it."[12]

Do these stories sound vaguely familiar to you? Perform a search on the Internet and you may be surprised by how many people describe their relationship with cheese as an addiction.

Surprisingly, research has shown detectable amounts of compounds identical to the narcotic opiate morphine in cow's milk. Study of the morphine found in milk has confirmed it has identical chemical and biological properties to the morphine used as an analgesic.[13] A plausible assumption is that all mammals produce this opiate compound to make sure their offspring return to the breast to acquire essential nutrients and to bond with their mother.

An additional source of opiate compounds (called exorphins) is the milk protein casein. Casein is normally broken down in the digestive process into individual amino acids. However, in some individuals, possibly due to an enzyme deficiency or other digestive defect, the protein is not completely broken down and instead remains in smaller fragments called peptides. Some of these casein-derived peptides have opiate qualities as well. Because of the reduction of water, lactose, and whey, and the concentration of casein (and fat) in the cheese-making process, casein is more abundant in cheese than in a glass of milk. This may go some way to explaining why so many of us find cheese so compelling. There may be a compounding problem that presents itself with regard to excessive exposure to the casein-derived opiates in predisposed children who develop autism. We'll look more closely at this matter in Chapter Six.

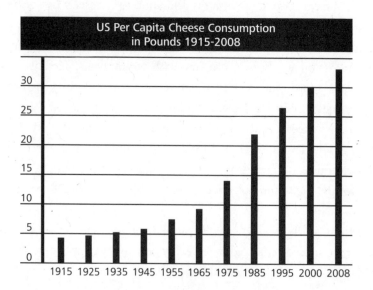

Allergy

Ever wonder about that headache that arrives each day, like clockwork? Still contending with childhood acne as an adult? Do you wish you could digest your meals more peacefully? Has it occurred to you that the cold you can't seem to get over may not be a cold at all? Have you ever suspected these symptoms might have something to do with a food you are eating? If you are like most people, the thought may never have crossed your mind. "People may suffer from chronic aching joints or a bloated stomach for years," says Jonathan Brostoff, M.D., a leading authority on food allergies at King's College London, England. "But when they cut milk out of their diet and feel a million times better, they realize that, *that* is what is normal."[14]

Dr. James Breneman, past president of the American Academy of Allergy, Asthma and Immunology, has estimated that up to 60 percent of Americans have some form of food allergy or intolerance that goes unrecognized by their health-care practitioner. Most people tell me their physicians have never spoken to them about food allergies. Indeed, the authors of a study of allergy to cow's milk published in the medical journal *Lancet* caution that the condition is "greatly under diagnosed."[15]

Many doctors lack the training to properly recognize and treat allergy, and this may be why it is so underreported. Some exceptional physicians, however, are well informed about the role of foods in disease, and are watchful for symptoms typical of food allergies. The following table shows some of the symptoms food allergies can cause.

A conservative estimate of the number of Americans with an authentic allergy to cow's milk involving the immune system is about twenty-one million people, or 7.5 percent of the population.[16] Dr. Stephen Astor, a Harvard graduate and certified allergist, is convinced that more than a third of the population suffers from some form of food allergy.[17]

Cow's milk — and the products made from it — is one of the most common food allergens.[18] This is particularly true for children.[19] According to the medical journal *Pediatric Annals*, "Cow's milk allergy is the most common food sensitivity issue confronting pediatricians today."[20] Alan Gaby, M.D., past-president of the American Holistic Medical Association, observed: "In my experience and in the experience of many of my colleagues, dairy products rank with wheat as the two most common symptom-evoking foods in allergic adults."[21] Dr. Gaby also stated that he has seen cow's milk allergy function as a causal factor in inflammatory bowel disease, irritable bowel syndrome, Crohn's disease, chronic nasal congestion, fatigue, depression, migraine headache, and symptoms of arthritis.[22]

Common Symptoms of Food Allergy

General	Respiratory	Cardiovascular	Neurologic
Chronic fatigue	Rapid breathing	Chest pain	Blurred vision
Excessive sweating	Coughing	Tachycardia	Dizziness
Frequent urination		Palpitations	Headache/Migraine
Sleep disturbances			Poor concentration

Behavioral	Gastrointestinal	Muscular	Dermatologic
Anxiety	Bloating	Cramps	Eczema
Irritability	Diarrhea	Myalgia	Hives
Nervousness	Dry mouth	Muscle spasm	
Emotional instability	Intestinal obstruction		
	Nausea/Vomiting		

What Is Cow's Milk Allergy?

Knowledge of the role of cow's milk in causing allergic reactions in humans is not new. Indeed, the Greek physician Hippocrates (460–375 B.C.E.) observed that cow's milk could cause skin rash and gastric problems.[23] Yet it was not until 1901 in Germany, and 1916 in America, that scientists began formally documenting these reactions.[24] In 1950 researchers performed the first blind, placebo-controlled study of milk allergy.[25] By 1956, using microscopes, scientists were able to view how cow's milk proteins, and those from other foods, can induce an immune system response.

Allergic reactions are triggered when immune factors called *mast cells* come into contact with an antigen (in this case, a bovine protein found in milk). This stimulates them to degranulate, or release, a variety of mediators such as heparin, histamine, prostaglandins, leukotriens, and tryotic enzymes. These elements, in turn, stimulate mucus production, muscle contraction, and inflammation.

It is important to understand the distinction between a true allergy and lactose intolerance or other adverse reactions to foods. While allergy involves an immune response, non-allergic sensitivities do not. This fact, however, does not minimize their seriousness; in fact, non-allergic reactions can involve constriction of the blood vessels or lungs and can even lead to death. Likewise, intolerances to a food, although not involving the immune system, can be very disturbing and uncomfortable, involving an array of physiological and psychological effects.

Lactose intolerance, as we will see later in this chapter, pertains specifically to an inability to break down the milk sugar called lactose. It is caused by the absence of the enzyme *lactase*. Lactase is normally no longer produced by the human body from around age four, as nature deems it of no use once an infant is weaned from the breast.[26]

An allergy to cow's milk, in contrast, is caused by the proteins in cow's milk, not by the lactose. The immune response distinguishes a true allergy from intolerance. With an allergy to cow's milk, symptoms persist even when lactose is removed. That is why people who have been improperly diagnosed as "lactose intolerant" may seek out "lactose-free" or reduced-lactose dairy products and then become frustrated when their symptoms persist.

Cow's milk contains at least thirty proteins that can elicit an allergic response; the most common include casein, B-lactaglobulin (BLG), a-lactalbumin (ALA), bovine y-globulin (BGG), and bovine serum albumin (BSA).[27] When they are ingested, allergenic proteins may cause the production of local and circulating antibodies. Reactions can be immediate (manifesting in minutes or a few hours)[28] or delayed (24 to 72 hours). Symptoms can last from several days to several weeks.[29]

Food allergy symptoms can include skin rash, hives, swelling, wheezing, congestion, diarrhea, constipation, vomiting, nausea, watery eyes, runny nose, buildup of mucus, earaches and ear infections, headaches, skin discoloration, joint swelling, asthma, ulcerative colitis, inability to focus, colic, chronic fatigue, swelling of the throat, intestinal bleeding, anaphylactic shock, and death.[30] In children, the most common symptoms include irritability, skin rash or eczema, asthma, and earaches.

The delayed onset of the symptoms makes diagnosing food allergies challenging. It also explains why people often don't attribute their condition to the foods they have eaten.

Since cow's milk is so ubiquitous in the American diet, even individuals who suspect they have a food allergy are unlikely to consider it as the culprit. After all, there is nothing exotic about cow's milk. In one form or another, most of the American population is consuming it.

In a less common scenario,[31] it seems some people can grow up free of food allergies and then suddenly develop them to certain foods at any point later in life. Identifying the allergen can be very perplexing for an unsuspecting individual who has eaten a food for fifteen or twenty years and never experienced symptoms.[32]

In one such case, a twenty-five-year-old woman who was exercising at a gym suddenly had an anaphylactic reaction that included swollen eyes, sneezing, and swelling of the tongue, lips, and cheeks.[33] She was given emergency care that included injection of steroids and antihistamines. It turned out that she had eaten a salad with a dressing containing cow's milk about twenty minutes beforehand. She had also had a history of bloating, nausea, and diarrhea when she ate dairy products over the previous twelve months; prior to that period, she had had no such symptoms. After performing a battery of tests, doctors determined that she was highly allergic to cow's milk.

In another case, a twenty-nine-year-old male was admitted to the hospital with severe bronchitis. In addition to acute bronchial spasms, he had been suffering from a dry cough, a transient sensation of breathlessness, and periodic asthma attacks that had sent him to the emergency room on several occasions.[34] After he returned to a symptom-free state, a challenge was performed in which he was given a glass of milk to drink. Some twenty minutes later, he again experienced severe bronchial spasms. Until his twenty-ninth year, the man had been able to eat any food he desired and remain symptom-free.

However, most people who are reactive to cow's milk begin showing signs very early in life. Although some health practitioners are fond of advising parents that their children will "grow out of" their allergy, often this is not the case.

Cow's milk proteins are used in numerous other products and processes that can also confer exposure. As an example of how unusual such an exposure can be, a thirty-three-year-old woman who was artificially inseminated using the sperm of her husband went into anaphylactic reaction during the procedure. Five minutes after the insemination, her symptoms included asthma, vomiting, itching, hives, and swelling of the eyelids and lips. It was determined that she had reacted to the sperm-processing medium, which included a common cow's milk protein, a frequent allergen.[35] A similar case was reported in the journal *Contact Dermatitis*.[36] Again, the protein eliciting the reaction was bovine serum albumin (BSA). Both women had no allergic reaction when a medium free of milk protein was used in a later procedure.

In a case reported in *Pediatric Annals*, a seven-year-old boy with asthma and severe cow's milk allergy was admitted to hospital. He was served a chicken broth, on the assumption that it would be perfectly fine for him to consume. The server was focused on the broth containing no lactose; unfortunately, it had been fortified with casein, the predominant protein in cow's milk. After just two spoonfuls, the boy pulled off his oxygen tube and began clawing and scratching at his chest. He had obvious difficulty breathing, his facial skin turned blue, his heart rate became bradycardic (dropped to less than fifty beats per minute), and his upper arm stiffened. A cardiac team was rushed to his bed, administered CPR, and was able to improve his respiration and heart rate. While the boy survived, he has suffered from some neurological difficulties since the episode.[37]

Allergy, Headache, and Back Pain

If no one suspects an allergy to cow's milk, patients can suffer unnecessarily for years, and can in some cases undergo inappropriate treatments.

In a case reported in the journal *Allergy*, a seventeen-year-old girl with severe headaches arrived at a hospital seeking help.[38] This young woman had a ten-year history of debilitating headaches, usually with one to two major episodes a week — many lasting hours, and some as long as an entire day. After neurological examinations, an electroencephalogram, and a CAT scan of her brain showed her to be physically normal, her doctors decided to place her on antidepressant drugs.

The drugs were of no help, so her doctors decided to cauterize her turbinates (coiled bones in the nasal cavity) because of the suspicious difficulty she had in breathing through her nose. After surgery, her condition worsened. Finally, frustrated by her lack of improvement, her doctors referred her to an allergy clinic, where she was diagnosed with severe allergy to cow's milk, among other foods.

Consider the medical radiation (from x-rays), the surgery, the inappropriate medications (antidepressants), the financial burden, and the years of misery this woman had to endure, simply because it had not occurred to her health practitioners that their patient might be suffering from an allergic reaction to cow's milk. Cases such as this one make us wonder how many patients are misdiagnosed, or fail to get relief from their symptoms, because the physicians they consult do not consider food allergy as a possible causal factor.

In one study of patients who suffered from migraine headaches and asthma, 33 of 44 patients showed significant improvement after removing all cow's milk from their diets.[39] In another study reported in the journal *Lancet*, 93 percent of the patients examined were able to free themselves of migraine headaches by eliminating cow's milk from their diets.[40]

After successfully working with numerous patients who suffered from chronic headaches and back pain, Dr. Daniel A. Twogood, who runs a chiropractic clinic in Apple Valley, California, wrote a book about his findings at his practice. "Most patients who come to see me complain of back pain, neck pain, or headaches," he wrote. "In more than 90 percent of these cases, when dairy products are eliminated from the diet, back pain and headaches stop. When these patients begin ingesting dairy products again, their symptoms return."[41]

While back pain and headaches can be caused by numerous factors, including bone structural problems, the doctor's observations are nonetheless important to consider. Eliminating cow's milk from the diet is free, while visits to medical specialists can be costly.

Arthritis and Joint Pain

Millions of Americans suffer the misery of swelling and pain in the joints, and few are able to obtain much relief from their symptoms without taking expensive and risky prescription drugs. Even with the aid of such powerful drugs, many people continue to suffer from disabling pain.

Many health professionals see arthritis as a mystery that has no specific cause. Some claim that it is inevitable — that with age, the joints eventually succumb to years of wear. Others take a different approach and ask what could be triggering the pain arthritics experience.

By now, you have probably guessed that cow's milk may have something to do with it. Although this is certainly not always the case, evidence indicates that allergy to cow's milk can be an important component with some people.[42]

Some medical authorities have scoffed at the idea that a food could trigger such a painful condition. Yet people who have found relief from their previously debilitating condition tell a different tale. There are wonderfully uplifting stories in which men, women, and children have been relieved of their crippling pain simply by removing all cow's milk from their diets.[43]

In a case described in the *British Medical Journal*, a thirty-eight-year-old mother of three was experiencing severe arthritis.[44] Her doctor had followed conventional treatment protocol, to no avail. The woman had been suffering for eleven years and was taking numerous prescription drugs (some to mitigate the side effects of others), yet none was having any lasting effect on her symptoms.

The physician she consulted shared her case with some colleagues, who then examined her medical history. They noted she had a strong affinity for cheese, and regularly ate up to a pound a day. This raised a red flag. Her physician then recommended she eliminate all cow's milk and related products from her diet. Within two weeks of doing so, her symptoms began to clear, and her grip strength began to return.

In follow-up visits over the next few months, the patient's morning stiffness completely disappeared and her general arthritis condition was almost completely resolved. She was eventually taken off all prescription drugs. As an allergy challenge, her doctor asked her to reintroduce cheese into her diet. Within 24 hours of doing so, her arthritis returned, her grip strength weakened, and the swelling in her fingers increased her ring size by two sizes. Once again, these symptoms disappeared after she eliminated cheese from her diet.

Obviously, not all cases of arthritis are caused by food allergy. However, it would seem judicious for physicians to investigate the possibility of dietary factors before subjecting a patient to surgery, risky drugs,[45] and other therapies that might prove to be irrelevant, not to mention costly and traumatic.

Lactose Intolerance

As we saw earlier, many people are incapable of properly digesting cow's milk beyond infancy, because they lack a digestive enzyme called lactase. The body needs lactase to break down the disaccharide (complex) sugar in milk called lactose.

When it is present, lactase resides in the upper gastrointestinal tract, concentrating in the jejunum, a part of the small intestine. It acts by breaking lactose down into two monosaccharide (simple) sugars, glucose and galactose. When lactase is not present, the undigested lactose moves on to the large intestine, where it is attacked by bacteria that convert it to gas and lactic acid. This can lead to subtle abdominal cramping, gas, nausea, bloating or distention, and chronic diarrhea. People who suffer from chronic diarrhea are at risk because their ability to absorb essential nutrients from their food is sharply reduced and they are at elevated risk for dehydration.

Normally the body gradually stops manufacturing lactase by age four, although it may continue to produce it in small amounts. People who are able to digest lactose are referred to as "lactase persistent," and those who are no longer able to digest the sugar are said to have "adult hypolactasia."[46]

Researchers first identified lactose as a problem in the digestion of cow's milk back in 1901. Current estimates are that fifty million Americans do not produce the lactase enzyme and thus are unable to properly digest cow's milk and related products.[47] Worldwide, it is estimated that three-quarters of the population does not produce lactase after childhood. Race is a major factor, with the highest prevalence of lactose intolerance among Asians, with an incidence of 90 percent. Nearly 75 percent of people of African descent and over 50 percent of Mexican-Americans also suffer from lactose intolerance. The following table quotes some estimates for finer population breakdowns.

Incidence of Lactose Intolerance[48]

Vietnamese	100 percent	Native Americans	50 percent
Thais	90 percent	French	32 percent
Greek	85 percent	American whites	25 percent
Japanese	85 percent	Austrian	20 percent
Arabs	78 percent	Northern European	7 percent
African Americans	70 percent		
Israeli Jews	58 percent		
Northern Italian	50 percent		

Despite the pervasiveness of lactose intolerance, few people make the association between their symptoms and the foods they have eaten.[49] Consequently, they will continue to experience these symptoms throughout their lives — unless, of course, they consult a health-care practitioner who suspects lactose intolerance.

In addition to developing reduced-lactose products and special lactase pills so consumers who are lactose intolerant can still attempt to drink milk, scientists are considering an extreme measure: genetically engineering dairy cows with rat genes so that they will produce lactose-free milk.[50]

Cataracts

A cataract is a progressive disease that results in the loss of transparency in the eye. A gray-white cloud gradually makes the eye more opaque behind the pupil. Over time, vision becomes more blurred and distorted, and sometimes doubled; eventually, if the cataract is left untreated, blindness sets in. Cataracts are the leading cause of blindness worldwide.[51]

While cataracts have been accepted as another inevitable accompaniment of greater age, their causes are not entirely unknown. For instance, experts are increasingly cautioning that heightened exposure to ultraviolet radiation, from worsening ozone depletion, is a contributing factor.[52] Smoking, too, can play a big role; it has been estimated that a person who smokes more than a pack of cigarettes a day has three times the risk of developing cataracts.[53]

A lesser-known player in some cases may be the consumption of cow's milk.[54] In *galactosemia*, a deficiency of the enzyme *galactoskinase* leads to galactose (one of the breakdown products of the milk's lactose) being converted to galactitol (an alcohol) instead of glucose. The galactitol is thought to accumulate in the lens of the eye, where it does its damage.[55]

Heart Disease

You may recall the notorious Sippy Diet. Prescribed by Dr. Bertram Welton Sippy, it was used to treat the initial stages of peptic ulcers. Followers were instructed to consume milk and cream every hour or two in an effort to neutralize gastric acid. In 1915, Dr. Sippy published a paper about this treatment in the then *Journal of the American Medical Association* (JAMA) titled *"Gastric and duodenal ulcer; medical cure by an efficient removal of gastric juice corrosion."* The diet fell out of favor after it was shown to be of no use. However, important insight was gained by studying those who followed the diet and comparing them with ulcer sufferers who did not. Ulcer patients who followed the Sippy diet died from heart attacks six times more often than ulcer patients who did not use the diet.[56] In the following pages we'll learn why.

Heart disease is the number one killer in America, taking more lives annually than all forms of cancer combined. The average American has a one in two chance of developing heart disease.

Two of the better-known risk factors for heart disease are the excessive intake of dietary saturated fat and cholesterol. Cow's milk contains both. The Food and Drug Administration (FDA), for example, stated in its "Eating for a Healthy Heart" brochure: "Some fats are more likely to cause heart disease. These fats are usually found in foods from animals, such as meat, milk, cheese and butter."[57]

Most people are aware that higher cholesterol levels are associated with an elevated risk of heart attack and stroke. However, fewer people realize that saturated fat stimulates the liver to produce cholesterol in the body, and that over 60 percent of the fat in cow's milk is of the saturated variety. Thus cow's milk packs a "double whammy" wallop when it comes to the risk of heart disease.

Mike Rayner, a nutrition expert at Oxford University who focuses on heart health, says, "As far as cardiovascular disease and strokes are concerned, the very top of the danger hierarchy is saturated dairy fat, including the stuff that's made its way back into the food chain."[58] Walter C. Willett cautions, "There is a major campaign being planned to try to get adults to drink three glasses of milk every day. That's what the milk mustache campaign wants to do. If we do that, we'll increase saturated fat consumption in adults. That inevitably will increase heart attack rates."[59]

A study involving seven countries, published in the *International Journal of Cardiology*, showed that as the milk supply grew, so did the incidence of death from heart disease.[60] Another study, this one involving thirty-two countries, also examined the relationship between milk intake and the risk of heart disease, and showed a strong link. Milk was found to have the highest statistical association with heart-disease risk of any food.[61] Cited as possible causal factors were the excess calcium and its potential to calcify the arterial lining, the fat, and something referred to as the xanthine oxidase (X.O.) factor (more on this a little later).

Research in the journal *Lancet*, comparing food intake and death from heart disease, again showed the highest correlation with milk. The study reported: "Changes in milk-protein consumption, up or down, accurately predicted changes in coronary deaths four to seven years later."[62]

In an effort to stem the epidemic of heart disease, the American Heart Association promotes "heart-healthy" standards for eating, which include consuming 30 percent of our calories as fat. Oddly, no scientific evidence exists that indicates this level of fat intake will protect us from heart disease, and there is considerable evidence it will not.

In fact, a landmark study clearly showed that people with established heart disease who elected to follow the AHA guidelines experienced a progression of their illness, rather than improvement[63] Further, the National Academy of Sciences 1982 report on nutrition and disease stated: "The scientific data do not provide a strong basis for establishing fat intake at precisely 30 percent of total calories. Indeed, the data could be used to justify an even greater reduction."[64] Evidence suggests that the standard should be far lower — perhaps in the area of 15 to 20 percent of calories as fat, or less.

Nearly half of the calories in whole milk are from fat. Even "low-fat" milk gets about 38 percent of its calories from fat. Many people erroneously believe that "2%" milk is 2 percent fat. Unfortunately, this is not the case. Milk labeled "2%" is 98 percent fat-free by weight only; it still gets 34 percent of its calories from fat — more than the (already-inflated) federal guideline for people's overall diet of 30 percent. Low-fat cow's milk does have less fat, but it's still fat nobody needs, and the quantity of artery-clogging cholesterol is just the same.

Attempting to meet these dubious federal guidelines for a healthy heart is a considerable challenge if dairy products make up much of a person's diet. As an illustration, examine the percentage of calories as fat in the

Fat's Share of Calories in Dairy Products

American Cheese	74% calories as fat
Butter	100% calories as fat
Cottage Cheese (4% fat)	38% calories as fat
Cream	97% calories as fat
Cream Cheese	74% calories as fat
Ice Cream	48% calories as fat
Sour Cream	88% calories as fat
Whole Milk	48% calories as fat
"2% Milk"	34% calories as fat*

*Note the labeling of 2% milk is misleading, as it is a calculation by the weight of the product.

dairy products listed in the table above. Clearly, these products should not be part of a heart-healthy diet.

Some ice creams are exceptionally rich in artery-clogging fat. Take a scoop of Ben & Jerry's Chunky Monkey ice cream, served in a waffle cone dipped in chocolate. To some, this might sound like a relatively harmless Sunday-afternoon indulgence. However, this snack packs more saturated fat than a pound of spare ribs. Similarly, a Haagen-Dazs Mint Chip Dazzler sundae has as much fat as a T-bone steak, Caesar salad, and baked potato with sour cream, combined.[65]

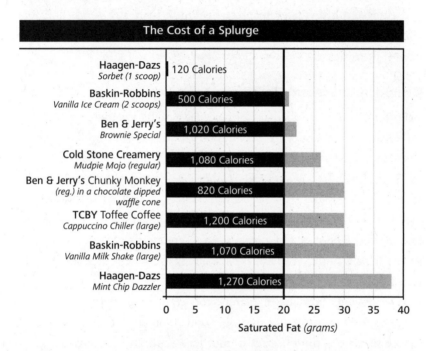

The Cost of a Splurge

Product	Calories
Haagen-Dazs *Sorbet (1 scoop)*	120 Calories
Baskin-Robbins *Vanilla Ice Cream (2 scoops)*	500 Calories
Ben & Jerry's *Brownie Special*	1,020 Calories
Cold Stone Creamery *Mudpie Mojo (regular)*	1,080 Calories
Ben & Jerry's Chunky Monkey *(reg.) in a chocolate dipped waffle cone*	820 Calories
TCBY Toffee Coffee *Cappuccino Chiller (large)*	1,200 Calories
Baskin-Robbins *Vanilla Milk Shake (large)*	1,070 Calories
Haagen-Dazs *Mint Chip Dazzler*	1,270 Calories

Saturated Fat *(grams)* — 0 5 10 15 20 25 30 35 40

While the artery-clogging potential of fat and cholesterol is well known, there are other, less-discussed factors specific to milk that may increase the risk of heart disease. Kurt Oster, M.D., chief of cardiology at Park City Hospital in Bridgeport, Connecticut, is a strong proponent of "the X.O. factor" as an underlying cause of heart disease. It seems that bovine *xanthine oxidase*, an enzyme present in homogenized milk, can be absorbed through the human gut and enter the bloodstream, where it may promote the growth of atherosclerotic (artery-clogging) lesions.[66]

Normally, this enzyme would not be able to enter the bloodstream. However, Dr. Oster believes that the milk homogenization process, which shrinks fat molecules, may then envelop the xanthine oxidase enzymes, thereby enabling them to pass through the intestinal lining and into the blood. Antibodies to bovine xanthine oxidase have been detected in the blood, and the enzyme itself has been found in arterial plaque samples taken from people with heart disease.[67]

One thing is certain: when dairy products make up a large part of the diet, they not only contribute a good deal of artery-clogging saturated fat and cholesterol; they also displace healthful, fiber-rich foods and foods containing important antioxidants and phytochemicals, which protect against heart disease, cancer, and cataracts.[68]

Overweightness and Obesity

According to the National Center for Health Statistics, there are fifty-eight million overweight, seventy-two million obese, and three million morbidly obese individuals living in America today. In the five-year period between 1998 and 2002, bariatric surgery (otherwise known as stomach stapling) increased four-fold.[69] This procedure reduces stomach size and bypasses a portion of the intestines in an attempt to reduce the intake and absorption of food. The state of Louisiana has offered to pay for state employees' gastric bypass surgeries in hopes of reducing the state's burgeoning health-care costs.[70]

The obvious burdens of being overweight or obese include limited range of motion, difficulty finding clothes that fit, difficulty fitting into airline seats, and the like. Yet it's not just adults who are challenged by their weight. A *Pediatrics* study revealed that, with the doubling of rates of obesity in children aged two to five over the last three decades, it is increasingly difficult for the parents of some 280,000 children ages one to six to find child car seats that can accommodate their oversized children.[71] As a person's weight rises, so do the risks of numerous illnesses, including hypertension, heart disease, stroke, diabetes, urinary incontinence,[72] and a generally shorter life span.[73] According to the International Agency for Research on Cancer, people who are overweight have a greater risk for several forms of cancer, including breast, colon, kidney, esophageal, and uterine cancers.[74]

Our crisis with overweight Americans has even become a national security issue, as for the first time in its history, the military is discharging thousands of soldiers who are unable to keep their weight under control. At the same time, the pool of potential recruits is shrinking. Forty-three percent of women and 18 percent of men seeking a position in the military today are simply too overweight to qualify for admittance.[75]

When people ask me how to lose weight, the first thing I recommend is that they eliminate cow's milk from their diets. As I indicated earlier, cow's milk is formulated to double a calf's birth weight in a mere 47 days, and grow it to an awesome 300-pound animal in just 12 months. This tendency to encourage weight gain can be a real burden for people trying to manage their own weight.

Contrary to the messages in the milk advertisements of the last several years, people who consume cow's milk are more likely to have weight problems.[76] And the more they consume, the greater the problems. This shouldn't be a surprise, given that three eight-ounce servings of milk add 450 calories and 24 grams of fat to the diet.[77]

Since 2003, the National Dairy Council has spent $200 million on its "Healthy Weight with Dairy" campaign, broadcasting the message that cow's milk helps people lose weight.[78] You couldn't miss the ads, because they appeared in thirty different magazines and newspapers and cited only a single study. According to the Center for Science in the Public Interest, that single published study (involving a mere eleven participants) was funded by the dairy industry and authored by an individual holding a patent on the claim that dairy products help with weight loss.[79]

Independent studies with no suspect funding, such as one published in the *American Journal of Clinical Nutrition*, refuted this claim, citing no weight-loss benefit.[80] A subsequent study published in the journal Obesity Research also failed to demonstrate any weight-loss benefit from dairy supplementation.[81] Yet more research has been published that failed to support the claim that dairy foods promote weight loss. The authors of another study, published in the *American Journal of Clinical Nutrition*, concluded that the data "do not support the hypothesis that an increase in calcium intake or dairy consumption is associated with lower long-term weight gain in men."[82]

The largest study of its kind, published in the *Archives of Pediatrics & Adolescent Medicine,* looked at more than twelve thousand children aged nine to fourteen from every state in the nation. It found that the more milk they drank, the heavier they were.[83] Contrary to expectations, the children who gained the most weight did so by consuming low-fat milk. The researchers postulate that another element, such as the growth hormones or the bovine proteins themselves, may have been the influential factor.

"The take-home message," said Harvard Medical School's Catherine Berkey, lead author of the study, is "children should not be drinking milk as a means of losing weight or trying to control weight." The study's authors further noted: "Given the high prevalence of lactose intolerance, the energy (calorie) content and saturated fat in milk, and evidence that dairy products may promote both male (prostate) and female (ovarian) cancers, we should not assume that high intakes are beneficial. Furthermore, these cancers may be linked to consumption during adolescence."[84]

In an overview written for the symposium "Dairy Product Components and Weight Regulation" and published in the *Journal of Nutrition,* the authors conclude, "Clearly, calcium intake or dairy products are not a 'magic bullet,' and energy balance remains the underlying cause of obesity and the metabolic syndrome."[85]

From a purely anecdotal perspective, it has been my experience in working with people trying to lose weight, that those who choose to eliminate cow's milk (in all its forms) from their diets invariably enjoy a drop in body weight.

Crohn's Disease

Crohn's disease, along with a similar condition known as ulcerative colitis, fall under the heading of chronic inflammatory bowel disease (IBD). First described in 1932 by American physician Burrill Crohn, it is a condition in which inflammation and lesions in the gastrointestinal tract result in bloody diarrhea. This results in significant morbidity that can be caused by vitamin and mineral deficiency, protein loss, anorexia, anemia, dehydration, and electrolyte imbalances, and progresses intermittently with remissions and relapses. Crohn's strikes those people aged fifteen to twenty-four. There can be a dramatic psychosocial impact brought about by the stigma of the disease and the manner in which it physically and emotionally restricts one from pursuing a normal life. Presently, there is no cure.

Technically, Crohn's disease is an autoimmune disease, in which the immune system attacks the body's own tissues. The standard treatment involves immunosuppressive and anti-inflammatory drugs, both of which have very serious potential side effects that can lead to secondary diseases, including cancer.

In addition to chronic pain in the gut, most people who suffer from Crohn's disease are plagued by an unpredictable urgency to use the bathroom. Richard Driscoll, director of the National Association for Crohn's and Colitis, says, "The best way to describe the condition to non-sufferers is to tell them to think of the worst tummy bug they have ever had on holiday and then try to imagine living that every day."[86] It is not uncommon for sufferers to undergo surgery in which a portion of their digestive tract is removed, leaving them with a stoma or colostomy for the rest of their lives.*

About half a million Americans presently suffer from Crohn's disease and historically, about three thousand new cases were diagnosed every year. However, it has been reported that rates of Crohn's and other autoimmune diseases have doubled in just the last four decades.[87]

Until recently, other than a hypothesis that it may be instigated in some people by measles vaccinations, little was known about the cause of Crohn's disease. However, there is very persuasive evidence that it may be sourced back to a contaminant found in cow's milk. In Britain and other countries, this idea has made the front pages of newspapers. The British government

---

* A stoma is an opening in the gut wall through which an external bag that collects stool is attached to the body.

has even conducted surveys of retail milk supplies. Yet in America, the mainstream media have shown scant interest, so few people have heard of the association.

First described over ninety years ago in Germany, paratuberculosis (also called Johne's disease) is a disease found in cattle. It is caused by infection by a mycobacterium (*Mycobacterium avium* subspecies *paratuberculosis,* or *MAP*) similar to the ones that cause tuberculosis and leprosy. It produces the same symptoms in cattle as Crohn's disease in humans, including weight loss and chronic diarrhea. Like Crohn's, it is also intermittent with relapse and remission.

In 1996, a National Animal Health Monitoring System study reported that 22 percent of America's dairy herds were infected with MAP; the most recent survey made available by the USDA raises that number to 68.1.[88] In the United Kingdom, the herd infection rate is estimated at 42.5 percent.[89] In the US, losses due to infected cows now cost $1.5 billion a year.[90]

Michael Collins, a University of Wisconsin veterinarian and president of the International Association for Paratuberculosis, says that most cows become infected as calves, when they are exposed to the diarrhea of infected adult cows.[91] The infected cow sheds bacteria in its milk,[92] and these can survive the pasteurization process.[93] It has thus been proposed that people who drink cow's milk may unwittingly consume the bacteria and thereby greatly increase their chance of developing the human form of the disease.

In late 2003, the *Journal of Microbiology* reported that scientists at St. George's Hospital in London, led by surgeon John Hermon-Taylor, had detected the mycobacterium in 92 percent of the intestinal tissue samples removed from patients with Crohn's disease.[94] Only 26 percent of patients in a control group had the bacterium. Based upon what he has seen thus far, Dr. Hermon-Taylor speaks plainly, saying the cow's milk–Crohn's link "constitutes a public health disaster of tragic proportions."[95]

In Ireland, research by Dr. Irene Grant of Queen's University Belfast revealed that DNA from MAP was detectable in 20 percent of several hundred cow's milk samples, and that living bacteria could be successfully grown from those samples. And what of the British milk survey? The Ministry of Agriculture findings were not encouraging: three out of every hundred cartons of milk sampled off the store shelf grew live MAP bacteria![96]

Live MAP bacteria have also been found in milk sold in Wisconsin, California, and Minnesota.[97] In tests conducted at the University of Zurich in Switzerland, nearly 20 percent of 1,384 tanks of milk from across the country were found to contain the paratuberculosis bug. The mycobacterium has even been found in 2 percent of retail milk samples in the Czech Republic.[98] Although these rates are alarming enough, they may well be higher, since MAP is notoriously difficult to grow in culture.

Dr. Walter R. Thayer of Rhode Island Hospital points out that Crohn's disease is not distributed evenly around the world, but is instead more prevalent in areas where a great deal of cow's milk is consumed, including Australia, New Zealand, Europe, Canada, and the United States. In Denmark, a country with a fervor for dairy products, the incidence of Crohn's disease has risen six-fold over the last twenty-five years.[99] In Scotland, the incidence of Crohn's in adolescents between the ages of twelve and sixteen doubled in a recent fifteen-year period.[100]

While researchers are not yet absolutely certain that the disease is transmitted by way of cow's milk, the evidence supporting this theory is very compelling. We know that MAP causes Johne's disease in dairy cattle, and Johne's disease shows the same symptoms as Crohn's. We also know that infected cows secrete the mycobacterium into their milk,[101] and that current pasteurization methods (which heat milk to 161 degrees for fifteen seconds) do not kill them, as clearly shown by both the Queen's University Belfast research and the British Ministry of Agriculture survey.[102] The only way to confirm that a dairy cow is infected is to perform a lengthy and inaccurate test, the results of which may take months. It is also worth noting that as the incidence of Johne's disease in dairy cattle rises in a region, so does the incidence of Crohn's disease in humans.[103]

Dr. Hermon-Taylor seems confident about the link, cautioning, "What I can say now categorically, from both our own work and work from the United States, and China, and Germany, and Australia ... is that MAP is present ... in humans with Crohn's disease, and it's probably causing about 90 percent of Crohn's disease."[104] If MAP is indeed the source by which

Crohn's is acquired, obviously many people remain somehow protected. It has been suggested that extracellular exposure to MAP, say through one's occupation as a farmer, may confer immunity to Crohn's.[105] So there must be some inherited or acquired susceptibility to the bacterium. Yet how does one determine one's susceptibility? Those who ignore the evidence thus far will not be getting a medal for bravery!

Cancer

The incidence of cancer in its various forms is growing toward epidemic levels.[106] In recent years, it has become clearer and clearer that dietary choices are important in lowering the risk for numerous forms of cancer. More specifically, we now know that consuming certain foods increases the risk for developing certain forms of cancer.[107]

The evidence of dietary fat's role in cancer risk is quite compelling. So much so that the US National Research Council stated in its landmark report, *Diet, Nutrition and Cancer:* "Of all the dietary compounds studied, the combined epidemiological and experimental evidence is most suggestive for a causal relationship between fat intake and the occurrence of cancer."[108]

There are several possible explanations for this relationship. First, when we eat fatty foods, these tend to displace the foods known to be protective against cancer. These beneficial foods are rich in fiber, vitamins, antioxidants, minerals, and various plant compounds known as phytochemicals, which studies have shown protect against cancer in a variety of ways.

The link between cow's milk consumption and cancer risk is not new. Cow's milk may exert its influence through a variety of mechanisms. It boosts intake of calories, saturated fat, and protein, and exposes the individual to a host of both naturally occurring and synthetic hormones and growth factors that would not otherwise be consumed. Finally, milk drinkers are exposed to potentially carcinogenic contaminants such as pesticides and other industrial chemicals that tend to accumulate in animal fat and thus show up concentrated in milk.

Another factor may be casein. T. Colin Campbell, Ph.D. is a proponent of moderate protein consumption — with an emphasis on protein derived from plant sources — as a means for lowering cancer risk. Originally inspired by a 1968 study published in *Archives of Pathology*[109], Dr. Campbell's research has for decades included studies of casein. He has found that as casein intake increases, so does the likelihood of developing cancer.

Researchers exposed laboratory animals briefly to a known liver carcinogen, aflatoxin. Then they exposed them to casein. Animals exposed to the cow's milk protein were more likely to develop liver cancer. Eventually, Dr. Campbell said, researchers were able to regulate growth of the cancer — turning it on or turning it off — by modifying the amount of casein to which the animals were exposed.

Let's look at a few specific forms of cancer and their possible relationship to cow's milk.

Breast Cancer

Breast cancer now strikes one in eight women in their lifetime. According to the American Cancer Society, 142,000 new cases are diagnosed each year and 46,000 women die from the disease.

The *Journal of the National Cancer Institute* published a study from Brigham and Women's Hospital in Boston and Harvard Medical School on breast-cancer risk and diet among 90,000 pre-menopausal women. The study showed a cancer link to fatty foods. In addition to meat, it specified whole milk, cream, ice cream, butter, cream cheese, and other cheeses as food culprits.[110] Head researcher Eunyoung Cho reported, "When we compared the women in the highest fat intake group with women in the lowest intake group, those with the highest intake had a 33 percent greater risk of invasive breast cancer."

There are several possible ways that cow's milk may be contributing to heightened risk of breast cancer. In full-fat form, cow's milk contains substantial amounts of fat. We know that as a woman's fat intake rises, her levels of the hormone estrogen rise as well. We also know that much, although not all, of the breast cancer we see today is hormone-dependent; it is encouraged by estrogen. While estrogen does not cause breast cancer, it can be thought of as the fertilizer that supports the cancer's cascade. Indeed, when reviewing all of the conventionally accepted risk factors for breast cancer, most point back to cumulative lifetime exposure to estrogen as the primary yardstick in determining a woman's risk.*

A woman's lifetime exposure to estrogen is increased by factors such as early menarche (first menstruation), late or no full-term pregnancy, not breastfeeding, late menopause, use of estrogen replacement therapy, and alcohol consumption. Dietary fat, which also boosts levels of the hormone, is one additional factor that a woman can readily control.

For decades, epidemiological studies have supported the theory of a dietary fat–breast cancer link.[111] In October 2004, researchers from Harvard Medical School reported findings from a study that examined 100,000 women between ages twenty-six and forty-six. It found that the women who ate the most meat and dairy products had a risk of breast cancer one-third higher than the women who ate the least.[112]

All foods derived from animals — such as beef, chicken, pork, milk, and butter, and ice cream — are devoid of fiber. We hear a great deal about dietary fiber's role in reducing the risks of colon cancer and heart disease, but little about its likely role in reducing the risk of breast cancer. Dietary fiber plays a critical role in binding with the hormones our body no longer needs and in escorting them out of the body via defecation. However, when the diet does not contain enough fiber — a common occurrence given the typical American diet — hormones that would and should have been excreted may be instead reabsorbed into the system. This boosts hormones to levels that may be unhealthful.[113]

When we consume more calories than our body needs, especially in the form of fat, we begin to accumulate body fat. In women, this body fat converts the male sex hormones (*androgens*) into estrogens, with the help of an enzyme called *aromatase*.[114] As body fat levels go up, so too do levels of aromatase.[115]

In addition to the fat, casein — the cow's milk protein mentioned earlier as a potential cancer promoter — may play a specific role in breast

---

* Breast cancer is a multifactorial disease. For an in-depth look at the primary risk factors for breast cancer, as well as a powerful lifestyle *risk*-reduction program, see Dr. Joseph Keon's *The Truth About Breast Cancer: A Seven-Step Prevention Plan* (Mill Valley, CA: Parissound, 1999).

cancer risk. Like T. Colin Campbell, E. J. Hawrylewicz, a biochemist and research director at Mercy Hospital and Medical Center in Chicago, found that casein intake increased the likelihood of developing cancer. Through a series of experiments, Hawrylewicz found that laboratory animals were more likely to develop breast cancer when given casein than when they consumed soy protein.[116]

The Hormone Link

Bioactive hormones from cow's milk present another possible cancer risk factor. A glass of milk contains a variety of hormones and growth factors — as many as fifty-nine, including as many as eight pituitary hormones, seven hypothalamic hormones, seven steroid hormones, six thyroid hormones, and eleven different growth factors. Among these are the steroid hormones *estradiol, estriol, progesterone*, and *testosterone*.[117] How these components might promote the growth of breast or prostate cancer is uncertain, but the potential link surely warrants caution. Since cancer is essentially the unregulated growth of cells, it would seem prudent to eliminate any unnecessary exposure to growth-promoting compounds. Ganmaa Davaasambuu, a physician with a Ph.D. in environmental health, a working scientist at Harvard University and a fellow of the Radcliffe Institute for Advanced Study said, "Among the routes of exposure to estrogens, we are mostly concerned about cow's milk," the source of between 60 and 80 percent of all estrogens consumed.[118] She points out that estrogen levels in milk are so high because of the modern practice of milking cows throughout their pregnancy, when estrogen levels increase significantly. Milk derived from a cow in late-stage pregnancy can contain as much as thirty-three times more estrogen (estrone sulfate) than milk from a cow that is not pregnant.

It is enough of a concern that cow's milk is a cocktail laden with hormones and growth factors; but the administration to cows of an additional synthetic hormone, rBGH — and the subsequent rise in IGF-1 levels that this causes — makes the situation even more troubling.

In 1998, Jane Plant, CBE, the winner of the Lord Lloyd of Kilgerran Prize (the United Kingdom's most prestigious science honor) and one of Britain's most distinguished scientists, made an astonishing discovery. Professor Plant had been diagnosed with breast cancer. Naturally inquisitive, she was looking at all aspects of her lifestyle to determine what might have caused or be promoting the condition. Some of her research prompted her to eliminate cow's milk from her diet. After a few days, she noticed a large secondary tumor (an offshoot from her breast cancer) beginning to shrink. Six weeks later, it had shrunk so much that she could no longer locate it.[119] Was it the casein, the naturally occurring hormones, the pesticide residues, or some other factor in the cow's milk that made such a difference? It is impossible to know for sure, but the most recent findings on the relationship between cow's milk consumption and risk of breast cancer do give some direction. Professor Plant's personal story is recounted in her inspiring book, *Your Life in Your Own Hands*.

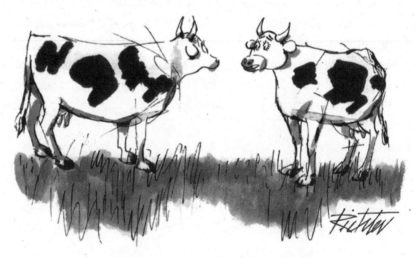

"I said no to drugs, but the F.D.A. said yes."

rBGH and Breast Cancer Risk

Most of us have heard of the genetically engineered hormone rBGH (recombinant bovine growth hormone), also called bovine somatotropin or BST, which is used to boost a cow's milk yields. Literature from the dairy industry says that BST "does not harm the animal"... and ... "is safe to be used in foods for human consumption."[120]

Many medical experts share an urgent concern over this bioengineered drug's unknown effects on humans. There has been little research into the synergistic effect that rBGH may have when combined with the other hormones used to accelerate animal growth. Despite this, Americans have been lapping up rBGH-treated milk — mostly unwittingly — as though it had been proven safe for human consumption. In another section, we will look more generally at the risks posed to both cows and humans from consuming this hormone. For now, however, we'll focus on a growing body of research that has focused specifically on the potential link between rBGH and breast cancer.[121]

By 1999, studies had shown that rBGH induces cancer in mice. Dr. Samuel Epstein — professor of environmental toxicology at the University of Illinois, Chicago, and a world authority on cancer — said: "All women will now be exposed to an additional breast-cancer risk due to milk from cows treated with recombinant bovine growth hormone."[122] This assertion has been bolstered by a number of more recent studies suggesting that milk from rBGH-tainted cows may be a risk factor for breast cancer.[123] When two award-winning American journalists, both twenty-year veterans, prepared a story that would report this publicly, they were abruptly fired from their jobs.[124]

IGF-1 and Breast Cancer

Insulin-like Growth Factor One (usually abbreviated as IGF-1) is a natural hormone found in humans and cows. It is a *mitogenic* compound, which means that it stimulates cell division. This hormone is active, for instance, during the growth of breast tissue in girls during puberty, when it acts on IGF-1 receptor sites on breast tissue cells. IGF-1 levels are naturally highest in the rapid period of growth during puberty. As we age, our levels of IGF-1 decrease.

What do rBGH and IGF-1 have to do with one another? IGF-1 occurs in cows at higher levels than in humans. However, when cows are injected with rBGH, their levels of IGF-1 increase further. Eventually, a dairy cow's IGF-1 passes into her milk, which is then consumed by humans. Here is where the problem may begin.

The concern is that IGF-1 from cow's milk may survive digestion and pass into our bloodstream.[125] What risk might this pose to consumers? Could it boost undesirable cell division and growth in our bodies, and thereby cause or promote a cancerous tumor? We are not certain. Since rBGH went on the market, in 1994, researchers have been hard at work trying to answer that question. Their findings, thus far, are less than encouraging.

A study reported in the medical journal *Lancet,* based upon the work of researchers at Brigham Women's Hospital and Harvard Medical School, is one example. The authors estimated that the post-menopausal women in the study with the highest levels of IGF-1 in their blood had three times the risk of breast cancer than the women with the lowest IGF-1 levels; in pre-menopausal women, the highest IGF-1 group had seven times more risk of breast cancer. "[T]here is substantial indirect evidence of a relation between IGF-1 and risk of breast cancer,"[126] the authors concluded. Other research has shown that the consumption of both whole and nonfat milk raises IGF-1 levels in adults;[127] in adolescent females, as little as a pint of milk a day can boost IGF-1 levels by 10 percent. It takes about three glasses (one and a half pints) of nonfat milk a day to achieve the same result in adult women.[128]

Research has established that IGF-1 is required for tumor formation, and clearly accelerates malignant cell growth and the ability of cancer cells to spread to other organs (a process known as *metastasis*). The more IGF-1 present, the more aggressive tumors seem to be. This may be due not only to the fact that IGF-1 is *mitogenic* (stimulates cell division) but also that it is *anti-apoptotic*, meaning it prevents programmed cell death — a characteristic that is the central theme of cancer.

Dr. Epstein has expressed his concern that, in addition to elevating the risk of breast cancer, rBGH may also contribute to premature growth in infants and inappropriate development of breasts (*gynecomastia*) in male children.* Some researchers also point out that the breast cells of fetuses

---

* It is worth noting that more than 14,000 American men seek breast reduction surgery annually, according to the American Society of Plastic Surgeons.

and infants are highly vulnerable to hormonal influences, and exposure to higher-than-normal levels of IGF-1, through cow's milk, may create an imprinting that raises the future risk of breast cancer. They express concern that early exposure to high levels of IGF-1 may also heighten sensitivity of the breast cells to future assaults, such as from ionizing radiation used in mammography or from hormone-mimicking pesticides.[129]

Based upon the findings thus far, it is a wonder that any woman wishing to prevent breast cancer would unnecessarily expose herself to such a risk. Dr. Epstein rightly points out that, "with the active complicity of the FDA, the entire nation is currently being subjected to an experiment involving large-scale adulteration of an age-old dietary staple by a poorly characterized and unlabeled biotechnology product. Disturbingly, this experiment benefits only a very small segment of the agrochemical industry while providing no matching benefits to consumers. Even more disturbingly, it poses major potential public health risks for the entire US population."[130]

Although some dairy farmers have elected to stop administering rBGH to their cows,* Elanco, a division of Eli Lilly, which currently markets the product under the brand name Posilac, says that "approximately 8,000 dairies are currently taking advantage of the benefits offered by Posilac."[131] Citing concerns over human safety and animal welfare, rBGH remains banned in more than twenty-five countries, including Canada, Australia, New Zealand, Japan, and the entire European Union.

In December 2009 the American Public Health Association (APHA), the oldest and largest association of public health professionals in the world, announced its opposition to the use of rBGH in dairy cattle. Whether

---

* The Posilac insert cautions that use of the drug in dairy cows may result in a number of undesirable side effects, including reduced pregnancy rates, increases in cystic ovaries and disorders of the uterus, retained placenta, increased risk for clinical mastitis and subclinical mastitis, increases in the need for medications, increased body temperature, increases in digestive disorders, increases in enlarged hocks and lesions (e.g. lacerations, enlargements, calluses) of the knee, disorders of the foot region, and permanent swelling up to four inches in diameter at the injection site.

it is the proteins, the animal fat, the naturally occurring hormones, the bioengineered bovine growth hormone (rBGH), or the synergy of these factors, the evidence again clearly suggests that the prudent thing to do is to avoid cow's milk in all its forms.

Ovarian Cancer

Ovarian cancer is the fifth most common cancer in women. By now, it probably won't surprise you to learn that some, though not all, studies show the same result: women who consume the most dairy products have a higher risk for the disease. Researchers at the Harvard School of Public Health found an increased risk of ovarian cancer in women who drink skim or low-fat milk, compared to those who do not. In the study, women who drank two or more glasses of milk a day showed a 44 percent increase in the risk of developing ovarian cancer in general, and a 66 percent increase in the risk of developing *serous tumor cancer* — the most common type of ovarian cancer to strike American women.[132] Another Harvard University study, involving twenty-seven countries and published in the *American Journal of Epidemiology*, found a strong correlation between per capita consumption of cow's milk and the incidence of ovarian cancer.[133] The Iowa Women's Health Study, involving twenty-nine thousand post-menopausal women, showed — among other things — that women who consumed the most lactose (the sugar found in milk) had a 60 percent higher risk of ovarian cancer when compared to those who consumed the least.[134] A more recent Swedish study, published in the *American Journal of Clinical Nutrition*, followed sixty thousand women for thirteen and a half years. It found that a woman who drinks more than one glass of milk a day (full-fat, reduced, or skimmed) may double her risk of ovarian cancer.[135]

In *The Milk Letter: A Message to My Patients*, Robert Kradjian, former chief of breast surgery at Seton Medical Center, describes a study of female workers at the Roswell Park Cancer Institute in Buffalo, New York. The women who drank one glass of whole milk a day (or the equivalent) were found to have three times the risk of ovarian cancer when compared to those who drank no milk.[136] Another study, a meta-analysis* of twenty-one studies on the subject, found that for women who consume dairy products every day, each 10 grams of lactose (milk sugar) they ingest raises their risk of ovarian cancer by 13 percent.[137]

Gynecologist Dr. Daniel W. Cramer points out that, in addition to other factors that may be playing a role, this correlation holds for women who are able to digest lactose, and that again, the culprit may be galactose, the breakdown product of lactose. While the women may be able to break down the lactose into its two monosaccharide sugars (galactose and glucose), they may not be able to further metabolize the galactose properly.

Dr. Cramer believes that the unmetabolized galactose may damage ovarian egg cells, or perhaps even interfere with cell *apoptosis* (programmed cell death), eventually leading to ovarian failure.[138] Premature ovarian failure is a harbinger of ovarian cancer.

The enzyme needed to break down galactose, called GALT, may be limited, or produced in a less active form (called N314D), in approximately twenty million American women. Galactose occurs in greatest abundance in yogurt, cheese, and other forms of fermented cow's milk. Here it is worth noting that Denmark, Sweden, and Switzerland have the highest rates of ovarian cancer in the world, and the highest percentages of women who can still digest lactose (lactose persistence); their per-capita milk supply is also among the highest in the world. [139]

While the correlation has yet to prove a causal role for cow's milk in ovarian cancer, the findings and proposed theory are certainly worth considering — particularly if there is a history of ovarian cancer in your family.

Prostate Cancer

The concern over IGF-1 levels and breast-cancer risk also applies to the risk of prostate cancer. Today, if you are an American male, you have a one in six chance of being diagnosed with prostate cancer in your lifetime.[140] With odds like that, it obviously would behoove men to adopt any healthful strategy that might lower the risk. However, like women concerned

---

* A meta-analysis is a statistical process that involves pooling findings from a collection of past studies. The process creates one large study in which important findings, not discovered in smaller individual studies, may be revealed.

about breast cancer who are simply told to get annual mammograms, men wishing to lower their risk of prostate cancer are given little useful information about how to do so. Instead, they are told to get a prostate-specific antigen (PSA) test, which — like a mammogram — does nothing to prevent the disease.

Researchers have called the association between dairy products and prostate cancer "one of the most consistent dietary predictors for prostate cancer in the published literature."[141] There are now at least twenty published studies demonstrating a link between prostate cancer and consumption of cow's milk.[142] As with breast cancer, a positive association has been found between elevated IGF-1 levels and prostate cancer risk."[143] A Harvard University study found that men with elevated levels of IGF-1 were up to four times more likely to develop prostate cancer than men with normal levels.[144] For men in their sixties, the risk was even greater; they were eight times more likely to develop the disease than the men in their age group with the lowest levels!

The *International Journal of Cancer* published a controlled study comparing 320 men suffering from prostate cancer with 240 men who were cancer-free; it found that cow's milk and related products were positively associated with an increased risk of their condition.[145] Yet another study, published in the journal *Cancer*, analyzed the diets of 371 men suffering from prostate cancer. Those who drank three or more glasses of whole milk a day faced a risk 2.49 times higher than men who reported drinking no milk at all.[146]

The Health Professionals Follow-up Study, which did not focus on IGF-1 levels, examined forty-three thousand men. It found that men who consumed the most milk and dairy products were up to 70 percent more likely to develop prostate cancer. The study also noted that men who took calcium supplements as well faced an even higher risk. The men whose calcium intake exceeded 2,000 mg daily had a risk of developing metastatic prostate cancer up to four times higher than did men with moderate calcium intake.[147]

In another study that looked at diet and the incidence of prostate and testicular cancer in forty-two countries, the strongest dietary link for prostate cancer was milk consumption; for testicular cancer, it was cheese consumption.[148] A meta-analysis by Japanese researchers that looked at eleven controlled studies from eight countries also confirmed a strong correlation between milk consumption and risk of prostate cancer.[149]

It is unclear if this link is caused by the fat, the IGF-1, the calcium, or a combination of all three, or by another factor, such as the cow's-milk protein casein, which might promote the abnormal growth of prostate cells. One of the authors of the Health Professionals study, Harvard professor of nutrition and epidemiology Edward Giovannucci, has proposed that excess calcium may be a contributing factor because, in abundance, it depletes vitamin D stores, which protect against cancer.[150]

But we do know that people with elevated concentrations of IGF-1 have higher risks of cancer. *Acromelagy*, a condition in which growth hormone stimulates high levels of IGF-1 production, is associated with elevated risk of breast, prostate, and colorectal cancers. We also know that we can lower the risk of cancer in animals by restricting calories; this caloric restriction lowers the levels of circulating IGF-1. As stated earlier, IGF-1 might increase cancer risk by preventing the programmed death of cells that have become malignant — that is, preventing a normal process through which the body interrupts, and therefore delays, the cancer cascade.

Multiple Sclerosis

Nearly half a million Americans suffer from multiple sclerosis, or MS. This disease affects the central nervous system (CNS), including the brain, spinal cord, and optic nerves. Symptoms may involve varying degrees of numbness in the limbs, loss of vision, and paralysis.

All nerves are coated with a protective sheath called *myelin*. Myelin is essential to a nerve's ability to transmit electrical impulses to and from the brain. MS involves the gradual loss of myelin from the nerve; what remains is scar tissue, called sclerosis. The vulnerable nerve fibers may then be damaged or even broken.

MS can strike in various forms. One involves a progressive worsening over time, with little relief. In another form, called relapse-remit, the

disease alternates between flare-ups and states of remission in which a suf-
ferer may partially or totally recover their neurological functions.

While experts agree that MS has both a genetic and an environmental component, most conventional treatments — which ignore the role of
dietary influences — produce little improvement for sufferers. Less known,
but well supported, is research that shows a correlation between dairy consumption and the incidence of MS worldwide.

Early research had already shown that people who consume a high level
of saturated fat are at elevated risk of developing MS. In 1974, the *Lancet*
published a study that found MS was more prevalent in regions where
cow's milk formed a significant part of the diet. In 1993, a worldwide epidemiological study that surveyed twenty-seven countries found that as a
population's intake of cow's milk went up, so did the prevalence of MS.[151]
The role cow's milk might play in the onset of MS is still not certain, but
recent research again supports the theory that offending bovine proteins
cross the gut wall and trigger an autoimmune response in susceptible individuals. Portions of dairy proteins appear very similar to portions of myelin
proteins. If the body mounts an ongoing attack against antigenic cow's milk

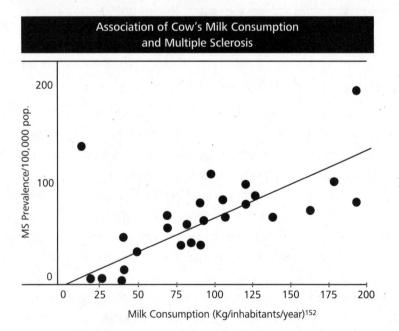

Association of Cow's Milk Consumption and Multiple Sclerosis

MS Prevalence/100,000 pop.

Milk Consumption (Kg/inhabitants/year)[152]

proteins that also results in attacks to myelin proteins, the result may be the destruction of the nerves' myelin sheaths over time.[153]

Comparing milk consumption internationally, MS is more prevalent in dairy-consuming populations and rare in areas where dairy is not a dietary staple, such as Africa and South America.

Parkinson's Disease

Named after British physician James Parkinson, Parkinson's disease is a chronic condition that involves the degeneration of the central nervous system — specifically, the destruction of dopamine-producing brain cells in the region known as the substantia nigra. The disease is marked by its effect on memory and thought, and by the presence of hand tremors, loss of facial expression, and an uncoordinated gait. One million Americans are currently suffering from this disease. Well-known individuals with the condition include actor Michael J. Fox, former Attorney General Janet Reno, and former heavyweight boxing champion Muhammad Ali. It is likely that an unknown gene or combination of genes predisposes people to the illness, by making them more susceptible to assaults from environmental toxins. MPTP (1-methyl-4-phenyl-1,2,3,6-tetrahydropyridine), a known neurotoxin that has at times been a contaminant in the illicit recreational opioid drug MMMP, causes rapid onset (within 3 days) and permanent symptoms of Parkinson's disease. Autopsies on exposed individuals have confirmed the destruction of their dopamine-producing brain cells.

Harvard School of Public Health researchers published a report that suggested that cow's milk consumption may be involved in the development of Parkinson's disease. They found men who consumed the most lactose, calcium from dairy, Vitamin D from dairy, and dairy protein had a 50 to 80 percent higher risk of developing Parkinson's than men who consumed the least amount of these nutrients.[154] In another study of 7,500 men, a significant association was found between milk consumption and risk of Parkinson's disease. Compared to men who drank no milk, the men who consumed more than sixteen ounces (two glasses) a day had twice the incidence of the disease.[155] Most recently, researchers at the National Institute of Environmental Health Sciences examined the relationship between Parkinson's disease and dairy consumption; their nine-year study, published in the *American Journal of Epidemiology*, included fifty-seven thousand men and seventy-three thousand women. They found a striking correlation for men but not for women, and while all dairy products were shown to increase risk, the association was strongest for milk. The men who drank the most milk (three to four glasses a day) had 60 percent higher risk of developing Parkinson's than the men who drank the least.[156] The reason for this link is unclear, and it may have nothing to do with the nutrients in the milk. Instead, these may simply be markers for another element commonly found in dairy products. At the top of the list of possible players are the neurodegenerative pesticides and polychlorinated biphenyls (PCBs) that frequently contaminate cow's milk and foods made from it. A number of studies, using both animal models and cell cultures, have highlighted the link between pesticide and herbicide exposure and the risk of Parkinson's disease.[157] A 2006 study of 143,000 men and women published in the *Annals of Neurology* added more evidence to this relationship. Those who received "low-dose exposures," either occupationally or otherwise, had a 70-percent greater risk of developing Parkinson's disease.[158] In a 2009 study, researchers found that people who had been chronically exposed to the agricultural chemicals paraquat and maneb, due to their proximity to crops treated with these neurotoxins, also had a 70 percent greater risk of developing Parkinson's disease than the general population.[159] Given that many pesticides are formulated expressly to destroy the nervous system of "pests," it should be no wonder that these insidious compounds may be playing a role in human neurodegenerative disease.

Whether our contact is through residues in milk or other foods or through direct application of pesticides in the home or workplace, all of us should take whatever steps we can to protect ourselves from exposure to such powerfully destructive chemicals. We'll look more closely at these relationships in Chapter Five.

Infertility

As evidenced by the media's coverage of the growing number of multiple births caused by fertility drugs, infertility has become a major problem for

American men and women. Today, an astounding one in five couples is infertile.[160] While there are a variety of possible reasons for this — including significantly lower sperm counts worldwide — some intriguing studies have suggested one that may pertain to dietary choices.

A study published in the *American Journal of Epidemiology* has shown a correlation between the consumption of cow's milk and infertility in women. Specifically, researchers found that in countries where the most milk products are consumed, infertility is more prevalent and occurs earlier in life. In another study of 18,555 women over an eight-year period, the researchers found that the women who consumed more than two servings of low-fat dairy products were 85 percent more likely to be infertile due to ovulation failure than women who ate full-fat products.[161]

Some researchers have developed a hypothesis based on the clinical and experimental studies showing that galactose, the breakdown product of the milk sugar lactose, is toxic to ovarian germ cells: the risk of premature infertility may be higher in populations that consume milk and digest lactose into galactose.[162] Other experts have speculated that in susceptible women, undiagnosed cow's-milk allergy may cause the production and buildup of mucus in the fallopian tubes, thereby preventing the ovum (egg cell) from passing into the uterus for implantation.

Menstrual Cramps

Some women suffer from menstrual cramps so severe that they are unable to work. In fact, it has been estimated that some fourteen million work hours are lost annually to disabling menstrual pain in the United States alone. These women may be found in bed, or even on the floor, curled up in a fetal position. Some resort to the use of powerful painkilling drugs.

The menstrual cycle is regulated by the hormones estrogen and progesterone, as well as by hormone-like substances called *series-2 prostaglandins*, which are produced by the cells lining the uterus. These prostaglandins trigger muscle contractions and inflammation. In overabundance, they can contribute to menstrual pain; women who suffer most from menstrual pain have measurably higher levels of prostaglandins.[163] The good news is that our diet can affect our production of prostaglandins. We know that the series-2 prostaglandins are derived from the fat in dairy products, meat, and eggs. So by sharply cutting back our intake of these foods, or eliminating them entirely, we can alter the production of the compounds that promote muscle contraction.

We also know that estrogen levels affect menstrual pain. Estrogens cause the lining of the uterus to build up each month in preparation for possible implantation of an egg. Excessive estrogen levels can compound menstrual pain because they cause the body to retain salt and fluids. This can lead to congestive symptoms, such as bloating and dull pressure in the pelvic region and lower back.

As we saw earlier, estrogen levels are influenced by the foods we eat: the more fat we consume, the higher the levels; the less fat we consume, the lower the levels. A woman who cuts her fat intake in half can see a 20 percent drop in estrogen levels in just a few weeks.[164]

More aggressive cuts in fat intake can yield even greater reductions in estrogen levels. In a University of California Los Angeles (UCLA) study, women experienced a 50 percent drop in estrogen levels in just three weeks. Other studies have shown similar reductions.[165] Such dietary changes can help limit the buildup of the uterine lining, and therefore, the quantity of cells that must be shed in the menstrual flow.

As mentioned earlier, another way that diet can affect estrogen levels is by way of dietary fiber. When the body is finished with estrogens, it sends them to the digestive tract via the bile duct. The hormones then bind with dietary fiber and are escorted from the body with feces. However, in the absence of adequate fiber, the hormones may be reabsorbed into the bloodstream, thereby pushing estrogen levels higher.

Dairy products can wreak havoc on hormone and prostaglandin levels. Their fat type boosts the series-2 prostaglandins that promote muscle contraction, and their fat content contributes unnecessarily to the overall fat intake that boosts estrogen levels. When they make up a large part of the diet, they displace fiber-containing foods that are important to hormone balance.

Noted gynecologist and best-selling author Dr. Christiane Northrup cautions that, in addition to menstrual cramps, cow's milk consumption has been associated with recurrent vaginitis, fibroids, and increased pain from endometriosis.[166]

Mad Cow Disease

By now, everyone has heard of "mad cow disease," or bovine spongiform encephalopathy (BSE). This is a brain-wasting disease that kills cattle. The human equivalent is called Creutzfeldt-Jakob disease, or CJD for short, and scientists believe people contract it by consuming the meat of infected cattle. The infectious agent is believed to be a sort of prion, a malformed or twisted protein.

In cattle, BSE is almost certainly a result of feeding "rendered" animal parts to cows who are, by nature, herbivores. While Britain has suffered the most devastating and long-lived episode of mad cow disease and its human crossover, with 146 people dead from CJD to date,[167] experts on the disease had predicted that it would be only a matter of time before it surfaced elsewhere. The last place anyone suspected it would strike was the United States — except Howard Lyman, the "Mad Cowboy," who ignited a firestorm of criticism and a subsequent lawsuit when he predicted BSE's arrival on these shores.

But it did indeed surface here. The first case was found in a dairy cow in Mabton, Washington, in 2003.[168] Canada has confirmed five cases of BSE since that date, the latest in a dairy cow in April 2006.[169] Losses since the first animal was identified are estimated at $2 billion to farmers, and it now appears no country is safe from this deadly disease.

Until recently, it was unclear whether prions were found in milk derived from a mad cow and whether they could pass on the disease. A Swiss biotech firm named Alicon reported that, using their cutting-edge analytical technology, they have confirmed the presence of prions in both pasteurized and homogenized milk purchased from supermarkets. Whether or not these were disease-inducing prions was unclear. "In the case of the prion proteins detected, it is highly likely that they were of a normal variety posing no danger to health," noted Dr. Ralph Zahn, Alicon's head of research. But he also cautioned, "So far there has been no scientific basis for assuming that only 'healthy prion' proteins were present in milk and those causing disease were not."[170] The presence of healthy prions certainly gives credence to the possibility that unhealthy prions could make it into milk as well.

Tuberculosis

Earlier, we looked at the relationship between Johne's disease in dairy cows and Crohn's disease in humans. Johne's is caused by a bacterium called MAP which is related to the tuberculosis organism. Tuberculosis (TB) (not Johne's disease) occurs in various forms, including the human form and a bovine form caused by *Mycobacterium bovis*. The bovine form is found in dairy and beef herds in the United States and other parts of the world, including Great Britain and India. Bovine tuberculosis is a chronic, infectious disease that is difficult to detect in its early stages. However, as it advances, it results in emaciation, lethargy, anorexia, fever, and pneumonia. In the US, it is a major and costly disease in dairy cattle that is little known to consumers.[171] Yet efforts to eradicate tuberculosis in dairy herds began back in 1917.[172]

Tuberculosis can be transferred to humans by way of unpasteurized infected cow's milk and cheese, and is an occupational hazard to dairy farmers.[173] In Great Britain, more than nineteen thousand dairy cattle have been slaughtered in recent years in an effort to stem a TB outbreak that continues to spread and infects about forty people a year.[174]

In October of 2000, Secretary of Agriculture Dan Glickman declared an emergency and requested special funding of $44 million to combat the TB outbreak in US dairy herds.[175] Due to financial constraints, the USDA has historically tested only animals exhibiting obvious symptoms. In 1995, four thousand animals were tested, but by 1999, a mere nine hundred were tested. Estimates to properly assess the incidence of the disease in US dairy herds require that ten thousand cows be tested annually.

Yet even with adequate funding, the test does not always detect the disease, according to Dr. Oliver Williams, epidemiologist for the USDA's Animal and Plant Health Inspection Services.[176] Although random testing has occurred for years, it has only been partly successful, as it is voluntary. For these reasons, Dr. Williams says, when inspectors suspect bovine tuberculosis, they prefer to "depopulate" the herd — a euphemism for slaughtering large numbers of cows, regardless of proof of their infection.

Susan McAvoy, a USDA spokesperson, says that the millions of dollars currently designated for the tuberculosis eradication program are used primarily for indemnity payments — meaning, to buy entire herds from farmers. In recent years, dairy farmers in El Paso, Texas, received $25 million in buy-out payments, and in Michigan, farmers received some $7 to $8 million. In the indemnity program, if the dairy farmer wishes to restart a dairy business, he is required to move to a new location; otherwise, he must find a new source of income not involving dairy cows.

In 2002, the USDA reported that ten cattle herds were infected with bovine TB in the states of Michigan, New Mexico, and California (home to the largest dairy-cattle population in the nation). Five of those herds were "depopulated," at a cost of $11 million to US taxpayers.[177] In 2008, another 4,800 dairy cattle were slaughtered at three California dairies after tuberculosis was found in the herds. In India, bovine tuberculosis was recently reported to be ravaging the dairy herds in the state of Dharamsalah, with 60 percent of their dairy-cattle population infected with the disease. Local health experts say the disease is being passed to humans who unwittingly drink the unpasteurized milk of infected cows.[178]

In this chapter, we have seen substantial evidence linking cow's milk consumption with numerous chronic, degenerative diseases. A number of these diseases are now occurring in epidemic proportions. Yet for many of the conditions presented, the link between milk consumption and risk of the diseases is rarely discussed openly. Little has been done to inform the public of the risks we may face, however small they may be. Milk buyers remain poorly informed about the choices they make.

In the next chapter, we will look at more disconcerting evidence confirming consumption of cow's milk by humans is indeed risky business.

Five

The Contamination of Cow's Milk

There is one thing dairy products have more than any other
food I can think of: contamination.

— John McDougall, M.D.

Hindu worshippers show penance and gratitude in a ritual carried out annually at the Taipusam festival north of Kuala Lumpur, Malaysia. The ritual involves self-flagellation, meditation, and a drink of milk from the sacred cow. The milk, it is maintained, is a purifier.[1] After reading this chapter, you may come to agree that the milk we buy off the supermarket shelf is the antithesis of a purifying medium.

An article in the *New York Times* was titled "More Buyers Asking: Got Milk Without Chemicals?"[2] More often than not, the answer to this question is a resounding "No!" Cow's milk and its related products are the source of numerous contaminants, some of which pose serious threats to human health. In fact, as you will see in this chapter, cow's milk — along with beef, chicken, and fish — is where the bulk of dietary contaminants are found.[3]

Numerous news reports have revealed how serious chemical contamination of our food has become. Some of the contaminants are known or suspected carcinogens while others have been shown to wreak havoc on the economy of human thyroid hormone production. Others may be playing a role in our society's plague of behavioral and learning disorders.

Using blood the American Red Cross obtained from umbilical cord samples, researchers discovered a level of chemical exposure previously unimagined. The average sample contained 287 different contaminants, including pesticides, flame retardants, the Teflon chemical PFOA, and mercury. In their accounting of these substances, the authors reported, "Of the 287 chemicals we detected ... we know that 180 cause cancer in humans or animals, 217 are toxic to the brain and nervous system, and 208 cause birth defects or abnormal development in animal tests."[4]

Where is this enormous array of contaminants coming from? While some chemicals reach us through the air we breathe, the water we drink, and our work and home environments, the majority are delivered to us through the foods we eat. As the American Red Cross study indicated, much of the chemical burden in a mother's body will be passed on to her immensely vulnerable baby before it is born. Clearly, one of the most important protective actions we can take to reduce our own exposure — as well as the contaminant legacy we pass on to the next generation — is to wisely choose which foods we ingest.

As food contamination climbs, more Americans are asking for more stringent standards to protect consumers. Despite claims of authorities taking action, the overall message remains clear: the responsibility for protecting our health falls on nobody but ourselves. It has become abundantly clear that the manufacturers of chemical contaminants will not protect us, and the federal government has chosen not to devote the necessary resources to protect us either.

If you still falsely assume that the federal government will somehow protect us from consuming contaminated food, do a brief Internet search or peruse the archives of a major newspaper such as the *New York Times* using the key words "food recall." Reading through the enormous number of recalls that have been ordered in the past twelve months due to serious contamination and poisonings is a sobering experience.

The recalls are focused on cow's milk, cheese, and yogurt, and, of course, beef and chicken. Most frequently, they pertain to bacterial contamination. Yet that's just the beginning; there's much more that never reaches the headlines. Unfortunately, the federal government is well aware of many of the non-bacterial contaminants commonly found in cow's milk and related products, but rather than addressing the source of the contaminants, it sets levels of "tolerance." Tolerance levels have little meaning in the real world, since most of us are being exposed to a cocktail of numerous chemicals, all of which have the potential to interact with one another and thereby compound or multiply their toxicity. Besides, how do we establish a level of "tolerance" for a chemical for which there is no documented safe level of exposure — how do we know how much will cause harm in the long term?

Often, what ends up in milk is determined by what ends up in cows. Cows receive certain substances through injection or implantation, and others are added to their feed. Because of the ubiquitous contaminants in the environment, they are also exposed to toxic substances which enter the food chain (and water) and are concentrated in animal fat (and thus milk). This process of concentration is called *biomagnification*.

Chemicals released into the environment — through industrial emissions, agricultural chemicals sprayed on crops, and even waste dumping — enter the water, air and soil. Over time, feed crops absorb these contaminants, and cattle eat the crops. Cows also ingest more contaminants directly from the air and drinking water. Many of these chemical compounds are *lipophilic*, or "fat-friendly," meaning they migrate to, and form deposits in, the fat tissue of animals, and then move on to humans that eat the animals or their products.

The human body takes years to break down and excrete most of these chemicals. Their half-lives — the time it takes for the body to eliminate 50 percent of a substance — range from ten to forty years. There is one exception, however: mammals, including humans, mobilize fat stores to produce milk for their offspring. This is why it has been found that nursing is an effective way to reduce the chemical burden held by the body.[5] Unfortunately, the milk thus produced is tainted with a variety of contaminants that get passed on to the offspring — or, in the case of commercially produced cow's milk, to human consumers. Let's focus on the contaminants that may be found in the cow's milk you buy at the supermarket.

Rocket Fuel

The latest contaminant to be found in cow's milk is, oddly enough, rocket fuel.[6] But don't worry — folks are working hard to determine a "permissible level" for this newly detected poison. As a result, *perchlorate* — the explosive ingredient in the fuel that propels missiles, rockets, and fireworks, which is also used in automobile airbag inflation systems[7] — will not be removed from cow's milk or drinking water, but instead only regulated.

Perchlorate was probably the last thing the California Department of Food and Agriculture expected to find while testing the sensitivity of new, cutting-edge detection technology. Strangely, however, the department elected not to share its findings with other state public health agencies. The agency defended its inaction by maintaining that its test was performed simply to "validate" new technology and not to assess a public health risk.[8]

It was only months later, after the nonprofit Environmental Working Group obtained the state documents, that the public learned of their risk of exposure. The documents revealed that perchlorate had been found in 31 of 32 milk samples tested in California.[9] State-detected levels were as high as 10 ppb (parts per billion), and averaged 5.8 ppb.[10] And it is not just California's milk that is tainted. A FDA report disclosed that perchlorate has been detected in 217 of 232 samples of milk derived from supermarkets in fifteen states, including Arizona, California, Georgia, Kansas, Louisiana, Maryland, Missouri, North Carolina, Pennsylvania, South Carolina, Texas, Virginia, and Washington state.[11]

Although we do not know all of the long-term threats posed by this chemical, evidence indicates it damages the hormone-producing ability of the thyroid gland.[12] This means perchlorate exposure may contribute to motor-skill defects, I.Q. deficit, and mental retardation in children, and may cause cancer.[13] Subtle changes in thyroid function during pregnancy can have devastating, lifelong consequences for a child. According to Dr. Thomas Zoeller of the University of Massachusetts, these may include a predisposition to a future of Attention Deficit Disorder (ADD).[14] Other studies have also indicated this risk.[15] Even after birth, children remain at high risk since their proper growth and development require three times more iodine than non-pregnant adults require.

People with lower levels of iodine (about 36 percent of American women) are at particular risk because perchlorate blocks the uptake of iodine by the thyroid gland. The thyroid gland needs iodine to manufacture the hormone thyroxine, which is involved with regulating metabolism and levels of thyroid-stimulating hormone (TSH). Researchers who studied 2,299 men and women aged twelve and older found an association between levels of perchlorate in the body and a decrease in thyroid function. Exposures of just 5 micrograms of perchlorate per day produced a 16-percent change in thyroid hormone levels. The Environmental Working Group's computer-assisted analysis of current levels of perchlorate contamination suggests that just by drinking contaminated milk, 7 percent of women of children-bearing age, 35 percent of children aged six to eleven, and 50 percent of children aged one to five will exceed the exposure level the EPA deems safe.[16]

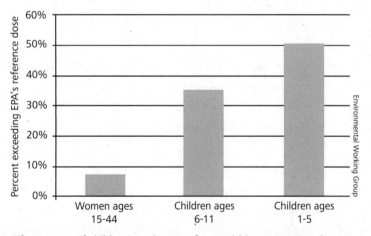

Fifty percent of children aged one to five could be consuming, by way of milk, more perchlorate a day than the EPA deems safe.

Perchlorate has also been identified in 329 drinking-water sources in twenty states, thus far, as well as in foods grown with contaminated irrigation water. The rocket propellant is leaking from hundreds of military bases and defense contractors' facilities, and has concentrated in the Colorado River. Perchlorate contamination apparently began when producers and authorities allowed the substance to leech into the Colorado River, which

California, Arizona, and Nevada all rely heavily upon for both drinking water and irrigation. Arizona has a particular problem with contamination, as it is home to at least six facilities that use or manufacture perchlorate.

When contaminated water is used to grow alfalfa and other cattle feed, the animals eating the food concentrate the perchlorate in their bodies, and then pass it on to us in their milk.

Flame Retardant

A shocking case reported in the *American Journal of Public Health* told of a flame retardant called *polybrominated biphenyls* (PBB) that was accidentally shipped to a dairy farm, where it was used in place of a dairy-cattle feed additive called magnesium oxide. The milk from the cows was distributed to Michigan residents. Five years after unwittingly ingesting the chemical, 97 percent of the people tested still showed measurable levels of it in their bodies.[17]

This kind of mix-up is admittedly rare. But sadly, we can now be exposed to flame retardants through our food even without such flagrant errors. *Polybrominated diphenyl ethers*, or PBDEs — another form of flame retardant — have now been found in milk. This is not due to a specific accident, but because of the substance's pervasiveness in the environment and its entrance into our food chain.[18]

Pesticides

Along with antibiotics, pesticides are probably the most frequently detected contaminant in cow's milk.[19] Pesticides are designed to kill living things. Today, there are sixteen thousand different pesticide compounds registered for use in the United States,[20] and one billion pounds of these chemicals are dispersed over our food crops, forests, schoolyards, homes, and parks each year.[21]

Most of us consume pesticides in our food with no immediate symptoms, so we might assume that they pose little, if any, overt risk. Yet the short- and long-term risks these chemicals pose to human health are being better and better documented. Individually, many pesticides have been linked to infertility, birth defects, weakening of the immune system, hormone disruption,[22] and childhood[23] and adult cancers.[24] The effects of exposure to combinations of pesticides (one or more at a time) are not well understood, but new research is beginning to shed light here as well.

At this point you may be wondering, am I exposed to pesticides? Based on the latest research, it's guaranteed. A study by the Centers for Disease Control and Prevention found pesticides in every single person tested.[25] These insidious chemicals are now found in our amniotic fluid, blood, breast milk, fat tissue, infant *meconium* (first stool), and umbilical cord blood.[26] They are even detected in fog![27] The average American now consumes about 156 micrograms of pesticides *every day* through his or her diet.[28]

As previously stated, animal products are the primary sources of pesticide residues in our diet. This is because these chemicals work their way up the food chain and *bio-accumulate* —concentrate over time — in the flesh of animals. Eventually, when humans eat animals and foods made from them, we take in all of the chemical residues that have been concentrating in the animals' bodies over their lifetimes.

A sobering example of the persistence of these chemicals is the pesticide DDT. Although DDT was banned in 1971 in the United States, it remained the most commonly detected contaminant in milk samples tested between 1984 and 1991.[29] Its metabolite, DDE, routinely shows up in Arizona's milk supply, more than three decades later.[30]

Finding a conventionally produced dairy product that is free of pesticide residues is a real challenge today. Residues of suspected cancer-causing pesticides — including BHC, chlordane, dieldrin, DDT, heptachlor, HCB, and lindane — have been found in cow's milk. The FDA's Total Diet Study found pesticides in 70 percent of cheese samples tested; thirty-two of the compounds detected (including vinclozolin, a known endocrine-disrupting* chemical) were also found in sixteen samples of

---

* Endocrine disruptors are chemicals that either behave like natural hormones found in our bodies, or block those hormones. The presence of endocrine disruptors in our environment has alarmed many scientists, who see substantial evidence that these compounds contribute to the escalating rates of breast and prostate cancers, as well as various types of birth defects.

fruit-flavored yogurt.[31] Another FDA survey of milk samples from supermarkets across the country found 73 percent contained pesticide residues.
In its own survey, the Center for Science in the Public Interest found over
half the dairy products it tested contained pesticide residues. In another
survey published in *Consumer Reports*, investigators found pesticide residues in 21 of 25 milk samples derived from five milk-producing states.[32] In
2006, the latest results from the FDA's Pesticide Data Program, an eighteen-
year running study, revealed that all 739 milk samples examined contained
pesticide residues; the average sample contained 2.88 different residues.[33]
The pesticides detected included diphenylamine, DDE, dieldrin, endo-
sulfan, permethrin, and seven others. In 2008, the Bush administration
abruptly terminated the USDA pesticide-testing program, saying that the
$8 million-a-year cost was too expensive.[34]

These surveys suggest that when an American consumer puts milk,
yogurt, cheese, butter, cream, or ice cream in their market basket, he or she
now has roughly a one-in-two chance of bringing home a product tainted
with a pesticide.

What threat do pesticides pose to human health? The medical literature contains studies that implicate common pesticides in the development
of leukemia and lymphoma, as well as breast, brain, ovary, and testicular cancers. Fifty-three of the pesticides presently registered for use on
major American crops are classified as carcinogenic. The Environmental
Protection Agency (EPA) classifies another 165 as "potential carcinogens."
In addition, over seventy supposedly "inert ingredients" used in pesticide
mixtures are confirmed to cause cancer in humans and animals. Others
may suppress immune-system function. Still others damage the nervous
system, or alter the production of thyroid hormone.

As we saw earlier, research suggests that there may also be a relationship
between some pesticides and Parkinson's disease.* This relationship has

---

* As mentioned earlier, Parkinson's disease is an incurable condition; it results in the progressive
destruction of dopamine-producing brain cells. Although cell damage may occur over many
years, it only becomes evident once about 60 to 80 percent of the cells are dead. For more information about Parkinson's disease symptoms and their consequences, see Chapter Five.

been further substantiated by the work of researcher Deborah Cory-Slechta and her colleagues at the University of Rochester School of Medicine and Dentistry. They found when two of the most common pesticides used in agriculture, maneb and paraquat, are administered to mice, the rodents suffer from precisely the same pattern of brain damage seen in human Parkinson's patients.[35] Again, since many pesticides are *designed* to destroy the nervous systems of various forms of life, such findings should not be surprising.

We know that people who live in farm areas and rely upon wells for drinking water are more likely to develop Parkinson's disease. This may be due to pesticide exposure through contaminated drinking water. Autopsies of people who have died with Parkinson's have also shown that they tend to have higher concentrations of pesticides in their brain tissue than the general population.[36]

One of the better-known cases of acute pesticide exposure through cow's milk occurred in Hawaii. In 1993, a famous large pineapple plantation sprayed its crops with copious amounts of the pesticide heptachlor.[37] Heptachlor use had been severely restricted in the United States in 1978, because the compound was already known to have multiple harmful effects: it compromises the immune system, promotes birth defects and cancer,[38] and increases the body's absorption of other toxic chemicals. Despite this data, regulators set a standard of tolerance for heptachlor at 0.3 ppm (parts per million).

The Hawaiian milk supply was significantly contaminated with the chemical.[39] The leaves left after processing the pineapple plant, which had been treated with heptachlor, were also chopped up and fed to the dairy cattle as food — or "green chop." The chemical then accumulated in the cows' flesh and was released in their milk. Tests revealed that the 0.3 ppm standard was exceeded tenfold! Yet, as so often is the case, these test results were not disclosed until after many unsuspecting consumers had purchased and consumed the contaminated milk.

Like many other pesticides, heptachlor is lipophilic, or fat-friendly, so it accumulates in fat. One prime storage area is breast tissue, until the fat tissue is mobilized to create mother's milk. Thus women who had consumed the tainted milk and were also breastfeeding were found to have hepta-chlor in their breast milk at an astounding 400 ppm! From plant, to cow, to mother, to baby, the chemical legacy was passed on.

Many pesticides are able to pass through the placenta and reach the fetus, and may cause permanent damage if exposure occurs during a critical window in pregnancy.[40]

Pesticides and Endocrine Disruption

As mentioned earlier, researchers have shown that some pesticides actually mimic the natural hormones produced by our bodies. Hormones can be considered as keys that unlock special locks or receptors on cells through-out the body, thus initiating a myriad of processes. One example would be cell proliferation. Hormones are also critical in controlling how an embryo develops genitalia, ovaries, and other sexual traits.

Some pesticides can masquerade as a hormone the body recognizes, and can thereby gain access to a cell's DNA. In so doing, these "hormone mimics" may initiate processes that might not otherwise be desirable, or simply block receptors so that naturally occurring hormones cannot acti-vate desirable processes.

Some scientists believe certain of these hormone-mimicking chemi-cals can "superactivate" a process, producing much stronger effects than natural hormones. Also, while naturally produced hormones are metabo-lized normally and excreted from the body after use, hormone mimics can interfere with the enzymes that facilitate natural hormone excretion. This causes hormone levels to climb to levels higher than desired, for extended periods of time.

A prime example of a pesticide having a hormonal influence on the body is the previously mentioned chemical vinclozolin. This fungicide, which is commonly used on fruits and vegetables, interferes with male hormones. If male mice are exposed to it during their embryonic develop-ment, their male offspring are born without penises or with *hypospadias*, a severe deformity of the penis.[41]

The incidence of hormone-dependent cancers — breast, uterine, and prostate — has been increasing at startling rates. So has the incidence of sexual deformities (including un-descended testicles and malformed genitalia) in both humans and animals. This has led many researchers to believe that research on hormone-mimicking chemicals should become a top priority. Until it does, each of us would be well advised to minimize exposure to them.

Pesticides, Learning Disabilities, Attention Deficit, and Aggression

Many of us are painfully aware of the sharp rise in the number of children diagnosed with learning, developmental, and behavioral disorders. The Census Bureau tells us that an astonishing twelve million American children under the age of eighteen now suffer from such conditions. Half — six million of them — are contending with Attention Deficit Hyperactivity Disorder (ADHD).

The impact of these conditions can be enormous, affecting social, educational, psychological, and other aspects of a person's life, well into adulthood. Many schoolteachers report having to alter their teaching style to accommodate the ongoing decline in the attention span of their students.

In the hope of controlling their children's inattention, overactivity, and impulsiveness, millions of American parents, feeling helpless, have consented to the use of powerful prescription drugs on their children. Some of these drugs have been reported to carry serious risks, including liver failure and, in some cases, sudden death.[42] Others have been recalled because of "superpotency" (up to three times the indicated potency) or "subpotency" problems.[43]

Medications are end-point responses that treat symptoms. They also carry risks of side effects. So it seems worth looking into what may be contributing to the rise of cognitive and behavioral disorders in our society.

Some experts have long suspected that toxic pesticides are playing a role in these disabilities. *In Harm's Way*, a groundbreaking report published in 2000 by Physicians for Social Responsibility, looks closely at the relationship between exposure to toxic chemicals and children's developmental disabilities. It quotes National Academy of Sciences' (NAS) findings that conclude, "[T]he emerging data suggests that neurotoxic and behavioral effects may result from low-level chronic exposure to some pesticides."[44]

These NAS's findings have been bolstered by the University of Wisconsin's Dr. Warren Porter who, among other areas of study, has been examining the effects of pesticides and other agricultural contaminants on animal health. Dr. Porter has demonstrated that when pesticides cause elevated thyroid hormone production in otherwise docile animals, the result can be heightened levels of aggression and irritability, and an inability to concentrate — precisely the problems we are witnessing with increasing frequency in children and adults across America.[45]

While much of the concern about pesticide exposure has centered on the developing child, Dr. Porter has delved even deeper into this alarming subject to show that damage may be occurring in the unborn. He reminds us that balanced thyroid hormone levels during pregnancy are critical for proper brain development. To illustrate, Dr. Porter says, "If you've got a pregnant woman, for example, in day 20 when the fetus's neural tube is closing and she gets exposed (to a pesticide) ... her thyroid level goes up or down, the hormone crosses the placenta and can permanently alter the developmental pattern of the fetus's brain .... Mom doesn't even know she is pregnant, and you may have an offspring that is neurologically compromised and wonder, 'How did this happen?'"[46]

Dr. Porter points out that while the toxicity of pesticides is now measured in the parts-per-trillion range, fetuses are affected at parts-per-quadrillion. In other words, it only takes a tiny amount of these compounds to wreak havoc.

Other researchers may have given us a window into what that havoc may look like in the first years of life. Elizabeth Guillette and her colleagues published an important comparative study that evaluated the health of two groups of four- and five-year-old children in Sonora, Mexico.[47] The first group consisted of Yaqui children living in a valley region where pesticide use in farming is embraced. The second group of children lived in the foothills, where pesticide use is rejected. The researchers noted that the genetic backgrounds, diets, water mineral content, cultural patterns, and even social behaviors were similar between the two populations. Among other findings, children living in the pesticide-exposed area were found to have much less stamina, poor gross motor skills, poor fine eye-hand

Pesticides and Other Industrial Chemicals Present in Select Dairy Foods

FDA Total Diet Study, June 2003.
Summary of food residues found by food market baskets 91-3 – 01-4.

Whole milk	Benzene; chloroform; DDE, p,p''; dieldrin, endosulfan sulfate; heptachlor epoxide; methoxychlor, p,p-; permethrin, cis; permethrin, trans; styrene; tetrachloroethylene; toluene.
Low-fat (2% fat) milk, fluid	DDE, p,p''; dieldrin, endosulfan sulfate; methoxychlor, p,p''.
American processed cheese	1,1,1-trichloroethane; 1,2,4-trimethylbenzene; benzene, bromodichloromethane; chlorobenzene, chloroform; DDE, p,p''; dichlorobenzene, p-; dieldrin, diphenyl 2-ethylhexyl phosphate; endosulfan sulfate; ethyl benzene; heptachlor epoxide; hexachlorobenzene; lindane; styrene, tetrachloroethylene; toluene; trichloroethylene; xylene,o.
Cheddar cheese	1,1,1-trichloroethane; 1,2,4-trimethylbenzene; 1,2-dichloroethene, trans; azinphos-methyl; benzene; chlordane, trans; chlorobenzene; chloroform; DDE, p,'; dichlorobenzene, p; dieldrin; diphenyl 2-ethylhexyl phosphate; endosulfan sulfate; ethyl benzene; heptachlor epoxide; hexachlorobenzene; methoxychlor, p,p''; octachlor epoxide; permethrin, cis; permeethrin, trans; styrene; tetrachloroethylene; xylene, m-and/or p-.
Butter	1,1,1-trichloroethane; 1,2,2-trimethylbenzene; benzene; BHC, alpha; butylbenzene, n-; chlordane; chloroform; cumene (isopropyl benzene); DDE, p,p''; DDT, p,p''; dichlorobenzene, p-; dieldrin; diphenyl 2-ethylhexyl phosphate; endosulfan sulfate; ethyl benzene; heptachlor epoxide; hexachlorobenzene; lambda-cyhalothrin; lindane; methoxychlor, p,p''; nonachlor, trans; octachlor epoxide; permethrin, cis; permethrin, trans; polychlorinated biphenyls; propylbenzene, n-; styrene, tetrachloroethylene; toluene; trichloroethylene; xylene, m- and/or p-; xylene,o-.
Half & half cream	Chloroform; DDE, p,p''; dieldrin; heptachlor epoxide; hexachlorobenzene; methoxychlor, p,p''-; octachlor epoxide; permethrin, trans; xylene, m- and/or p-.

Pesticides and Other Industrial Chemicals cont...

Swiss cheese	1,1,1-trichloroethane; 1,2,4-trimethylbenzene; 1,2-dichloroethene, trans; benzene; BHC, alpha; bromodichloromethane; chlorobenzene; chloroform; chlorotoluene, 0-; DDE, p,p''; dieldrin; heptachlor epoxide; hexachlorobenzene; lindane; methoxychlor, p,p''-; octachlor epoxide; permethrin, cis; permethrin, trans; styrene; tetrachloroethylene; toluene; trichloroethylene; xylene, m- and/or p-; xylene, o-.
Vanilla ice cream	1,1,1-trichoroethane; 1,2,4-trimethylbenzene; benzene; bromodichloromethane; butylbenzene, p-; chloroform; DDE, p,p''; dichlorobenzene, p-; dieldrin; endosulfan sulfate; heptachlor epoxide; hexachlorobenzene; permethrin, cis; permethrin, trans; styrene; tetrachloroethylene; toluene; trichloroethylene; xylene, m- and/or p-.

Detected in Cow's Milk and Related Products

Chemical Contaminant	Health Effect
Aldrin, Dieldrin, Endrin	Probable human carcinogen Immune system suppression Nervous system disorders Reproductive damage Liver damage Birth defects Kidney damage Suspected endocrine disruptor Developmental toxin
Chlordane and Heptachlor	Probable human carcinogen Immune system suppression Blood disorders Liver damage Central nervous system disorders Suspected endocrine disruption Developmental disorders
DDT, DDE	Probable human carcinogen Reproductive failure in wildlife Liver damage Central nervous system disorder

Detected in Cow's Milk and Related Products cont...

Chemical Contaminant	Health Effect
DDT, DDE	Known endocrine disrupter Developmental disorders Shortened lactation in nursing women
Dioxins	Known human carcinogen Altered immune function Central nervous system disorder Liver and kidney function disruption Reduced fertility Endometriosis Known endocrine disruption Developmental disorders

Agency for Toxic Substances and Disease Registry, *Toxicity Profiles*;
International Agency for Research on Cancer (IARC), 1997; Orris, et al., 2000;
US EPA Integrated Risk Information System and Office of Pesticide Program's List of Chemicals
Evaluated for Carcinogenic Potential, Aug. 26, 1999, as reported in *Nowhere to Hide*,
Pesticide Action Network, North America, 2001, and *Commonwealth*, Nov. 2000.

coordination, poor memory, and — most shocking of all — a profound inability to draw a simple stick figure of a human being. Even while looking directly at a model, the exposed children were incapable of producing anything remotely suggestive of a person.

Because of their smaller size and their limited ability to metabolize, detoxify, and excrete these chemicals, children may be far more vulnerable than adults to pesticide exposure through food and the environment. In

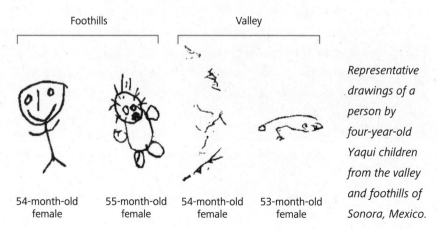

Foothills   Valley

54-month-old   55-month-old   54-month-old   53-month-old
female   female   female   female

Representative drawings of a person by four-year-old Yaqui children from the valley and foothills of Sonora, Mexico.

addition, because of the accelerated rate at which their cells are dividing, children may be exceptionally vulnerable to carcinogenic pesticides.

A big step in minimizing pesticide exposure for you or your children is to simply avoid foods where these toxins are known to concentrate. A second step is to choose organically produced foods at the market, whenever possible. A further step is to avoid the use of pesticides (both self-applied and professionally applied) in the home and garden. A final important step is to filter your tap water, which for many Americans is a significant source of pesticide exposure.[48]

Antibiotics

When antibiotics first became widely available in the 1940s, they were hailed as miracle drugs. They effectively controlled infections that only a few years before had been untreatable. Moreover, they did so with what seemed to be minimal risk to the patient. Over the last fifty years, the United States has gone from producing about two million pounds of antibiotics a year to in excess of fifty million pounds. With such production, we might expect that all the dangerous bacteria would be under control. Unfortunately, this is far from the case. Today, physicians are faced with the terrifying reality that many previously indispensable drugs have lost their effectiveness, and pharmaceutical companies are faced with the daunting task of developing ever more powerful and toxic drugs to take their place. The problem is drug resistance.

As an example, many strains of the bacterium *S. aureus,* acquired most frequently during stays in the hospital, are now resistant to all antibiotics except vancomycin. Three other bacterial species (*Enterococcus faecalis, Mycobacterium tuberculosis,* and *Pseudomonas aeruginosa*) are now untreatable with current antibiotics. This means they are resistant to over a hundred drugs! The Centers for Disease Control and Prevention have reported that thousands of patients are now dying in American hospitals annually because their bacterial infections are resistant to the antibiotics doctors use.[49]

How did things get so bad? There are a number of factors contributing to drug resistance, including health professionals prescribing antibiotics for conditions unaffected by them, such as the common cold. Antibiotics are effective at killing or limiting the growth of bacteria. Yet patients may demand a prescription for a virally induced condition, and all too often, they are given that prescription. It has been estimated that only one in ten antibiotic prescriptions is actually appropriate — physicians succumb to the expectations of their patients.[50]

Another contributing factor is that many patients do not complete their full course of antibiotics when they suddenly feel better. Yet another is the way patients stockpile partially used prescription drugs and share those drugs informally.

Of course, natural selection also plays a role. Stronger bacteria cells survive and replicate, creating larger colonies of "superbugs," and cellular mutations periodically create new strains of resistant bacteria, which also replicate. And gene exchange, in which resistant bacteria share their resistance predisposition by handing over a gene to a weaker bacterial cell, is also a factor.

However, there is another challenge to the effectiveness of antibiotics — one an increasing number of experts feel is the primary culprit in drug resistance. Antibiotics are routinely given to farm animals. An estimated twelve thousand tons of antibiotics are used non-therapeutically every year in the United States. That is, they are administered to healthy animals.

According to Congress's Government Accountability Office (GAO), the FDA has approved eighty different antibiotic drugs for use on factory farms, of which thirty are for use on dairy cows alone.[51] Unfortunately, the milk supply is tested for only four common antibiotics.[52] While some antibiotics are used to treat ill animals, the majority are given as feed additives to promote growth, even though virtually nobody can yet explain how that process works.

The most costly, and one of the most common, health problems the dairy industry faces is *mastitis*, or the infection of a cow's udders.[53] In a USDA report, US dairies cited mastitis as the primary reason for premature slaughter of dairy cows, and the second-most common cause of death.[54] Mastitis is most frequently caused by exposure to the bacteria

Staphylococcus aureus or E. coli. The condition can result in the loss of up to 522 kilograms of milk output from a single cow during its lactation period.[55] The prevailing method for treating it is the use of antibiotics. The USDA reports that in 2007, a full 85 percent of dairy operations were using antibiotics (including cephalosporin and lincosamide) to treat cows with mastitis.[56]

It seems that, as humans receive chronic exposure to these antibiotic residues through foods, these drugs lose their effectiveness in controlling illnesses that truly require them. Even the American Medical Association has declared, "The spread of bacterial resistance arises not only from unnecessary clinical use in human medicine, but also from massive use in animal agriculture, with increasing evidence that resistance developed in animals is spreading to human pathogens."[57]

Simply put, when the bacteria in cow's milk develop resistance to an antibiotic, they can transfer that resistance to the bacteria in a person's intestinal tracts. Later, when the person develops an illness, the resistance can be transferred yet again to the bacteria that caused the illness, threatening the potential for curing the illness.

As far back as 1983, three hundred scientists saw the disaster on the horizon. By petition, they urged the FDA to take control of the abuse of antibiotics in farm animals, which they felt was a chief cause of the enormous surge in antibiotic-resistant infections.[58] Yet, as we can see, the warning was not heeded.

The dangers of antibiotics extend beyond the promotion of drug resistance. Some people are highly allergic to antibiotics, and may unwittingly expose themselves to them by drinking cow's milk or eating milk products. This can result in any number of allergic reactions.[59]

Research published in the *Journal of the American Medical Association* (JAMA) has shown a link between breast-cancer risk and exposure to all types of prescription antibiotics.[60] Women who received the most prescriptions were found to have twice the risk of breast cancer compared to women who received none. The researchers emphasized that this finding may be a result of antibiotics suppressing the body's natural immune system, thus rendering the user more susceptible to cancer. Or the women's risk might have been increased by the very diseases that they are treating with drugs.

But it also may be that, while antibiotics eradicate "bad bacteria," they also wipe out the healthy microflora, or "good bacteria," in our gut. We need these bacteria to properly break down foods and access those foods' vital anticancer nutrients, commonly called *phytochemicals*. While more research is surely needed, including a replication of the study mentioned above, these are important findings that have forced us to look more closely at the potential ramifications of the use and abuse of antibiotics.

In addition to the sub-therapeutic doses of antibiotics added to animal feed, other antibiotics are administered *prophylactically* — meaning, in the hope that they will prevent sickness in livestock. Yet more antibiotics are sprayed on crops in aerosol form, as a sort of pesticide.[61]

Even with the growing evidence that the widespread use of antibiotics in farming is undercutting our ability to treat human conditions, the Union of Concerned Scientists reports that more antibiotics are being used now than ever before.[62]

What happens to the drugs that are fed to animals? The following reports are telling. The *Wall Street Journal* conducted an independent investigation of milk safety, which found antibiotic-drug residues in 38 percent of fifty retail milk samples taken from ten major American cities.[63] The Center for Science in the Public Interest conducted its own analysis of twenty milk samples from metropolitan Washington, D.C., and found that 20 percent contained sulfa drugs. New York television station WCBS also conducted its own investigation, and found that 80 percent of the fifty milk samples they tested from the New York metropolitan area contained antibiotic residues.[64] An FDA survey found antibiotics in 51 percent of seventy milk samples from fourteen cities.

As the problems associated with antibiotic use and abuse become more apparent, we might hope better control would be exercised in order to protect consumers. Unfortunately, this does not seem to be the case. In the *FDA Journal*, investigators reported finding residues of sixteen illegal drugs in the cows at an Oregon dairy farm, including streptomycin, neomycin, and gentamicin. The same journal reported that two Arkansas companies were fined for allowing cow's milk contaminated with penicillin, tetracycline, and sulfa drugs — including a suspected cancer-causing drug known as sulfamethazine[65] — to be sold to consumers.[66] It is not reassuring that the FDA only tests for a handful of the eighty antibiotic drugs currently in use. The organization simply lacks the personnel and resources to adequately test every dairy, annually. There are some 145,000 dairy farms in America; testing just 50 percent of them would require the FDA to inspect 1,394 farms a week — a challenge that is close to humanly impossible!

Inspections or not, the use and abuse of antibiotics in farm animals persists. Humans will continue to suffer exposure, unless, of course, we simply avoid the products altogether.

The good news is the evidence that, if the US government were willing to take action and enforce regulations to reduce rampant antibiotic abuse, much could be achieved. This has been demonstrated by Denmark, which instated a voluntary ban on the drugs' use in animals in 1998. The level of drug use dropped by 54 percent. This was followed by a dramatic reduction in the extent of drug-resistant bacteria found in Danish livestock. Prior to the ban, drug-resistant bacteria was found in 80 percent of livestock; today it has fallen to a mere 5 percent![67]

The questionable news is that biotechnology researchers have developed an antibiotic *transgene*: they have used recombinant DNA technology to grow Jersey cows that produce an antimicrobial protein, called *lysostaphin*, which wards off the bacterium that most frequently causes mastitis.[68] This could reduce the need for antibiotics in dairy cattle. While the transgenic cows have proven sharply resistant to developing mastitis, they are resistant because the altered, gene-induced protein lysostaphin is expressed in their milk — something consumers may or may not welcome.

Other Drugs

Synthetic hormones and antibiotics may not be the only drugs being administered to farm animals. Six years after it had been banned, residues of an arthritis drug, called *phenylbutazone*, were still found in meat sampled from dairy cow carcasses. Even if you suffer from arthritis yourself, there is good reason why you won't want to consume this drug unwittingly. Originally designed for humans, phenylbutazone was found to cause toxic reactions in some people, including blood disorders such as plastic anemia — and was even fatal to a few people.[69]

Radioactive Substances

In his seminal work *The Politics of Cancer*, the distinguished epidemiologist Samuel Epstein, M.D., wrote, "Milk is a prime route by which consumers are exposed to radioactive contaminants released by nuclear plants." Most Americans cannot begin to imagine the degree to which our environment has been contaminated with radioactive materials.[70] Few have been informed of the very real threat exposure to these materials poses to our health. Further, our ignorance is only allowing the problem to steadily worsen. The most recent assessment of the issue is grim. According to a report by the National Research Council, "At many sites, radiological ... hazardous wastes will remain, posing risks to humans and the environment for tens or even hundreds of thousands of years." The report continues, "Complete elimination of unacceptable risks to humans and the environment will not be achieved, now or in the foreseeable future."[71]

In the mid-1950s, a naïve zeal to develop new variants of "The Bomb" led the American military to detonate nuclear bombs in the open (atmospheric testing) — an example other countries followed. The result is that parts of the United States were highly contaminated with radioactive fallout. Radioactive isotopes rained down upon crops, lakes, and rivers, and like most other contaminants humans produce, eventually entered the food chain.[72] Milk, it was found, is the primary route of dietary exposure to radioactive fallout.

Since atmospheric testing of nuclear bombs has been banned, today our greatest risk of exposure to radioactive isotopes comes from nuclear power plants and nuclear research facilities. However, we need not necessarily live in close proximity to them to be subject to exposure. After the 1986 catastrophic meltdown of the Chernobyl nuclear reactor occurred in the Ukraine, its radioactive fallout was detected in the milk supply in

Minnesota nearly six thousand miles away. Moreover, a meltdown isn't required for the release of radioactive material into the environment. As a matter of course nuclear power plants release radioactive substances into the environment and — albeit with less regularity — research facilities are also prone to such releases. For example, Idaho National Labs research facility (now called INL) released radioactive isotopes into the surrounding environment on eight occasions between 1990 and 1999. The facility blamed "filter failures" for these releases. The Sandia research facility in New Mexico has reported releases of plutonium-239, cobalt-60, and cesium-137 over a period of many years. Radioactive fallout that has settled into the environment decades ago can be remobilized into the air and carried long distances by events such as forest fires.

As cows drink water and eat plant food that is contaminated with radioactive particles, they concentrate the radioactive matter in their body. Eventually these isotopes are released into their milk.[73]

The most common radioactive elements released from nuclear power plants include strontium-90, iodine-131, and cesium-137, as well as gases that can transform into radioactive solids. Strontium-90, a carcinogen with a half-life* of twenty-eight years, is absorbed through the bowel wall after ingestion. Because its chemical structure is similar to that of calcium, it concentrates and remains in our bones and teeth, continually emitting cancer-causing radiation. Iodine-131, which has an 8-day half life, concentrates in the thyroid gland.[74] Cesium-137 has a half-life of thirty years and concentrates in human muscle tissue. Once these deadly elements are lodged in the body, irradiating surrounding tissues, ultimately, they may stimulate a cancer. Due to the latent period of carcinogenesis, the cancer could appear anywhere from five to fifty years later. In addition, such radioactive particles can cause stillbirths, birth defects, and other genetic damage that may appear in future generations.

A report on women with strontium-90 in their bodies noted the radioactive contaminant "came chiefly from milk," and, to a lesser degree, from

---

* The term *half-life* relates to the time it takes for half of a specific quantity of an isotope to undergo radioactive decay.

other foods they consumed.[75] In 1957, Britain experienced a major nuclear accident at its Windscale nuclear facility (since renamed Sellafield) that released a massive radioactive cloud, which soon descended upon agricultural fields. The government monitored contamination levels, and it discovered that the local milk supply was tainted with radioactive fallout. It ordered thousands of gallons to be poured into the sea.

Writing about exposure to radioactive elements from releases at the Hanford facility in Washington state, Genevieve Roessler, Ph.D., said: "The highest estimated doses were received by people living downwind of Hanford who drank milk from cows grazing on fresh pasture that was contaminated with Iodine-131 from air releases."[76] Some research has shown that areas where high levels of strontium-90 have been detected in the food chain show a correspondingly high incidence of breast cancer.[77] Writing in *The Politics of Cancer*, Sam Epstein M.D. notes, "Milk is associated with increased risk for breast cancer, and the combination of pesticides and radiation have been proposed as one possible explanation."

Cold war atmospheric testing of nuclear bombs left a tragic legacy of broadspread contamination and related disease, but the ongoing reliance upon nuclear power and the low level releases of radioactive materials inherent in this manner of producing electricity create a continuing risk of contamination of the environment and of our food supply. Writing in the July 1989 issue of the *Journal of Dairy Science* in the article "Recent research involving the transfer of radionuclides to milk," Gerald M. Ward said, "Large-scale human radiation assessment studies are underway, all of which consider the dairy food chain as a critical component." Given the history in which the public has been deprived of news about radioactive releases for days, weeks, and even years after the fact, one can only wonder how the dairy industry goes about protecting its products from contamination.

Aluminum

Aluminum poisoning has been associated with memory loss, dementia, Parkinson's disease, ALS (amyotrophic lateral sclerosis — also known as Lou Gehrig's disease), and Alzheimer's disease.[78] Aluminum may also play a role in bone disease, because it interferes with the body's bone-repair process.

Frequently, Alzheimer's patients who die from that disease are found to have greater amounts of aluminum accumulated in their brain tissue than those who die from other causes.[79] Research has shown that the aluminum from some pans gradually migrates into the food cooked in them, raising their aluminum content significantly.[80] This has led to consumer interest in non-aluminum pots and pans for cooking. Although there are some quality brand pans that only have aluminum cores, some famous brands of pots and pans are still made with aluminum outer layers that come in contact with food.

Aluminum is also detected in cow's milk, and therefore its products, including cheese and cream.[81] A study published in the *Journal of Pediatric Gastroenterology and Nutrition* found dangerously high aluminum levels in samples of cow's milk.[82] Baby milk formulas can also be high in aluminum, depending on the formulation or brand. For example, the average fortified version may contain as many as 160 micrograms of aluminum, whereas the average casein hydrolysate formula could contain as much as 773 micrograms.[83]

Rabies

Rabies infection in humans usually occurs after a bite from an infected animal. The virus attacks the central nervous system and is potentially fatal. With advance preparation, the infection can be prevented using a series of specific immunoglobulin shots, at a cost of between $2,500 and $4,000. The disease has a long incubation period of three to twelve weeks, often making it difficult to determine visually if an animal is infected.

The Centers for Disease Control and Prevention in Atlanta reported two incidents in which humans were exposed to rabies through unpasteurized milk from infected cows.[84] In the first case, an infected cow was milked twelve times in the week preceding its death in 1998. That milk was pooled with other milk and distributed to stores without being pasteurized, a process that would have killed the virus. Public health officials were able to identify sixty-six people who had consumed this milk; all were treated with post-exposure prophylaxis (PEP). How many others may have been missed is unknown.

In another case an infected cow was milked the week prior to her death, and the milk was consumed by fourteen people. All were treated with PEP. In late 2005, at least forty-five people had to undergo the costly post-exposure treatments after raw milk from a rabid cow (which later died) was combined with the milk of up to seventy other cows, then sold to consumers.[85]

Dioxin

Dioxin refers to a class of chemicals (dioxins and furans) that includes seventeen different variants. The most toxic and widely reported of them is 2,3,7,8-TCDD. A contaminant in the Agent Orange used in the Vietnam War, it is considered one of the most powerful carcinogens known, and is an established endocrine disruptor.

Dr. Arnold Schecter, a medical expert on dioxin and an advisor to the World Health Organization (WHO), has said even tiny amounts of dioxin have been shown to result in nervous system and liver damage.[86] Other research has emphasized the link between prenatal (fetal) exposure to dioxin and the ufltimate strength of the developing immune system. A pending EPA report says people who consume the most dioxin-containing foods (fatty foods including dairy products) may have a significantly elevated cancer risk.[87] Robert Lawrence, M.D., professor of preventive medicine at Johns Hopkins Bloomberg School of Public Health, and an expert on dioxin, stresses that both the developing fetus and infants are uniquely vulnerable to dioxin and may develop varying degrees of neurological damage that may manifest itself in developmental delays or other dysfunctions of the central nervous system (CNS).

Dioxin is a byproduct released into the environment during certain manufacturing processes. These include the production of certain pesticides, chlorine-containing chemicals, pharmaceuticals, plastics, and the chlorine bleaching of wood pulp to make paper products. Other major sources of dioxin are waste incinerators that burn plastic, paper, and chlorine-containing medical waste. According to the EPA, the highest levels of dioxin ever recorded were produced from the collapse and incineration of the World Trade Center towers at Ground Zero in New York City.[88]

However dioxin is produced, it enters the air and ultimately returns to Earth in rain and fog, where it is then absorbed by plants which are then consumed by animals. After its entry into the food chain, dioxin builds up, or biomagnifies, in the flesh of exposed animals, until they are either slaughtered or their milk is extracted for human consumption. After it enters the human body, it can continue to build up in our own tissues.

It was not until August 2000 that consumers became aware that dioxin is a regular contaminant in cow's milk, and thus all dairy products.[89] At the Dioxin 2000 conference, a sample serving of Ben & Jerry's "World's Best Vanilla" ice cream was revealed to contain 2,200 times the amount of dioxin legally permitted to be discharged into the San Francisco Bay by the nearby Tosco Oil refinery.[90]

In France, sixteen dairy farms were forbidden from selling their milk after tests showed that samples contained an "unacceptable" level of dioxin.[91]

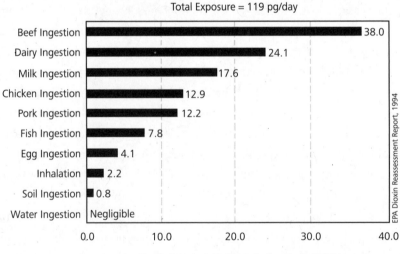

Estimated Total Daily Exposure to Dioxin and Sources

Total Exposure = 119 pg/day

North American Daily Intake (pg/day) of TEQ*

EPA Dioxin Reassessment Report, 1994

* TEQ refers to dioxin Toxic Equivalent, which is determined by considering all dioxins and furans and comparing them to the most toxic dioxin, 2,3,7,8-TCDD. Thus some dioxins or furans may be calculated as half a TEQ if they are determined to be half as toxic as 2,3,7,8-TCDD.

Investigators believed the dioxin was coming from nearby waste incinerators. Since the incinerators were not shut down and dioxin contamination
from them continues, we can only assume that the problem persists.

Because dioxin has a strong affinity for fat tissue, the majority of human
exposure to this toxin is through the foods we eat. The more fat a food contains, the higher its accumulated burden of dioxin tends to be. Therefore,
animal products such as cow's milk and meat pose a higher risk than fruits
and vegetables. The EPA has reported that Americans will receive 95 percent of their dioxin exposure from meat, fish, and dairy products,[92] and
that dairy products alone account for 30 percent of dioxin exposure in
adults and 50 percent of exposure in children.[93]

In its *Nutrition Action Health Letter,* the Center for Science in the Public
Interest advised: "Clearly, one way to minimize your exposure to dioxin is
to avoid animal foods, including dairy products."[94]

Hormones

In an advertisement for the Promised Land brand of flavored cow's milk,
the manufacturer touts its product as "all natural milk, free of hormones."[95]
The truth may shock even the most conscientious of mothers.

As we learned in Chapter Five, even a glass of organic milk, which is
free of introduced hormones, contains a variety of other naturally occurring bioactive hormones and growth factors — as many as fifty-nine.[96]
According to the research of Pennsylvania State University endocrinologist Clark Grosvenor, this may include eight pituitary hormones, seven
hypothalamic hormones, seven steroid hormones, six thyroid hormones,
and eleven different growth factors. What role are these naturally occurring bovine hormones playing in human disease? There are no studies to
tell us definitively, but many experts have expressed concern, particularly
since much of the surge in cancer we see these days is in the varieties fueled
by hormones: breast, prostate, uterine, and cervical cancers.

The human body strives to keep its hormone economy in a delicate
balance. Hormones themselves are extremely powerful, and exert their
various effects at astonishingly miniscule doses — at parts-per-trillion.
To illustrate this ratio, Dr. Theo Colborn, a leading expert on endocrine

disruption, asks us to "imagine a quantity so infinitesimally small by thinking of a drop of gin in a train of tank cars full of tonic. One drop in 660 tank
cars would be one part in a trillion; such a train would be six miles long."[97]
No wonder there is such deep concern in the medical community over the
introduction of hormone substances into foods consumed by humans.

When the genetically engineered milk hormone rBGH (recombinant
bovine growth hormone; see Chapter Five) was introduced in 1993, there
was a great deal of publicity in connection with breast cancer. Also known
as BST (bovine somatotropin), rBGH was developed to make dairy cows
produce more milk. This might seem a needless goal, considering the enormous surplus of dairy products produced in the United States annually.*

But rBGH appears not only to increase milk yields, but to also increase
the risk of serious disease in both cows and humans. Dr. Richard Burroughs
is a Cornell University–trained veterinarian who has spent half his thir-
teen-year career working for the Food and Drug Administration, studying
the effects of the synthetic hormone use in cows. He has said: "The very
first data I saw ... showed that it [rBGH] increased reproductive and udder
infections in cows." Use of rBGH in cows has also been associated with
ovarian cysts, disorders of the uterus, an 18-percent increase in infertility,
and a 50-percent increase in lameness. Cows that develop mastitis — and
as many as 79 percent of cows treated with rBGH develop the condition
— are routinely treated with antibiotics.[98] These drugs may end up in their
milk, and eventually pass on to the consumer.

Despite enormous pressure from the United States to adopt the use of
the synthetic hormone, the Canadian government decided rBGH "presents
an unacceptable threat to the safety of dairy cows" and banned its use.[99]

In November 2004, the FDA approved the use of another milk produc-
tion-enhancing product. Rumensin, produced by Elanco Animal Health,
is a supplement intended to "increase milk production efficiency ... by
delivering more milk per pound of feed." The FDA maintains that this food

---

* Fifty years ago, an average dairy cow produced two thousand pounds of milk per year. Through
the administration of hormones, feed additives, bulking diets, and selective breeding practices,
one cow may now produce as much as fifty thousand pounds per year!

additive poses no threat to humans, as long as it is administered "according to the approved labeling."[100]

Dry-Cleaning Solvent

The reality is that there is nothing "dry" about dry-cleaning. The process uses an extremely toxic solvent known as *perchloroethylene,* or "perc." Today, some twenty-five thousand dry-cleaning establishments in America use this compound on our favorite garments. Beyond toxic exposure through direct contact (absorption through the skin), and through dispersion from clothes hanging in our closets, perc is now ubiquitous in our environment.[101] Consequently, like other toxins, it has made its way into the food chain.

Environmental Health Perspectives' Fifth Annual Report on Carcinogens reported that perc is now appearing in cow's milk, and there is evidence that it causes cancer. Perc is a central nervous system depressant, and in experimental models, it has been shown to induce leukemia and cancers of the kidney and liver.[102]

While perc will be phased out entirely by 2023, until then, it will continue to be present in the environment, and thereby, likely enter the food chain.

Cow Cancer — Bovine Leukemia Virus (BLV)

Studies regarding the leukosis virus in dairy cows have been published in at least three prestigious journals: *British Medical Journal, Science,* and *AIDS Research and Human Retrovirus.* These articles have described how Bovine Leukosis Virus, a retrovirus, is believed to be the precursor to leukemia in dairy and beef cattle. Dairy farmers are concerned with the cost of replacing an infected cow, the loss of income from the carcasses of infected cows that happen to be identified, and the inevitable reduction in fertility and milk production in infected cows. I'm concerned about risks presented to humans.

An estimated 40 percent of the American beef herds, and 89 percent of American dairy herds, may be infected with bovine leukemia.[103] A 2007 National Animal Health Monitoring System (NAHMS) survey found a prevalence rate of at least 70 to 80 percent in Michigan herds alone.[104] This is the most common fatal malignancy in dairy cows. The disease is thought to be spread through common needles, the sharing of blood contaminated-syringes between cows, cross-placental transmissions, rectal palpations, and the use of gouging dehorning devices that become bloodied. Once a cow is infected, the viral cells navigate through its blood, tainting both meat and milk; they are also found in the host's saliva and semen.

Can bovine leukemia infect humans? We don't know. However, BLV has been shown to infect human cells in test-tube experiments.[105] Evidence indicates BLV can cross species barriers under natural conditions; this has been successfully demonstrated in experiments with sheep, goats, and chimpanzees,[106] all of which developed leukemia when exposed to the bovine form of the disease. Some researchers have cautioned that infections transferred to chimpanzees often transfer easily to humans. Given that humans share 97 percent of their genetic makeup with chimpanzees, this should not be surprising.

Conventional wisdom holds that the pasteurization process would inactivate any leukemic virus in cow's milk. However, some people prefer to drink unpasteurized or "raw" milk. And unpasteurized milk has at times been mistakenly introduced into pasteurized milk, contaminating the entire supply. This was the cause of an outbreak of salmonella poisoning in Chicago in 1985 which affected 150,000 people.[107] Chicago suffered a second outbreak in 1996, and another occurred in Massachusetts in 1998.[108] There is a growing trend of consuming raw milk, which some people believe is more healthful than pasteurized and homogenized milk. It is estimated that half a million Americans drink raw milk.[109]

In one study, bovine leukemia virus was recovered from two-thirds of randomly collected raw milk samples.[110] This raises the question of whether any of the consumers involved in the accidents mentioned were exposed to a live leukemic virus. This is nearly impossible to determine, because the population has not been tracked and the virus can take many years to manifest its effects. Further, if and when cases of leukemia develop in this population, it seems unlikely that the individuals would make the association between their illness and milk they drank years earlier.

While it remains unclear whether bovine leukemic virus can infect humans, researchers at the University of California, Berkeley, demonstrate that humans are exposed to the virus at an alarming rate. By measuring the presence of antibodies to BLV in a sampling of Berkeley residents, the researchers found that 74 percent of participants had the antibodies. This means they had been exposed to either living or dead viruses.[111] If this rate of exposure holds consistent in the general population, it is reasonable to assume that millions of Americans have been exposed to the virus.[112]

We know dairy farmers are one population that suffers from an elevated rate of leukemia.[113] It is also disconcerting to note that in the general population, we find a statistically significant increase in (human) acute lymphatic leukemia rates in regions where there is a high incidence of bovine leukemia in dairy herds.[114] These clusters of human leukemia also occur most predominantly in children, who consume especially high amounts of cow's milk. In another disturbing study, BLV was detected in the breast tissue of ten out of twenty-three breast cancer patients.[115]

"The epidemic of bovine leukemia virus is increasing with lightning speed," according to dairy manufacturing expert Virgil Hulse, M.D., M.P.H. "Cows are giving off the bovine leukemia virus in their milk, and America's men, women and children are drinking milk every day with this retrovirus."[116]

Given that current research does not exclude the potential for human infection through unpasteurized cow's milk, and the fact that unpasteurized milk does accidentally make it into milk supplies marketed as pasteurized, it would seem reasonable to inform consumers of the potential risk.

Suffice it to say, we don't need leukemia retroviruses, inactivated through pasteurization or not, on our corn flakes. Instead, why not choose an alternative like organic soy milk, hemp milk, rice milk, oat milk, almond milk, or hazelnut milk?

Bacterial Contamination

One of the worst bacterial contamination outbreaks in history occurred in Japan in 2001. This tragedy, which involved Snow Brand Milk Products Company, infected more than thirteen thousand people and led to the forced closure of thirty factories across the nation and the resignation of the company's CEO. The cause was staphylococcus, or "staph," bacteria that flourished around some of the processing equipment.[117]

Processing, storing, and transporting cow's milk to market are inherently difficult tasks. There are many opportunities for bacterial contamination. Never before in history have we seen the frequency and seriousness of outbreaks we see today. In the United States, over a five-year period, more dairy products were recalled due to contamination — chiefly by bacterial agents — than any other food.[118] Let's look closely at the most frequently detected bacterial offenders.

Salmonella

Infection from food tainted by salmonella bacteria (which is named after the veterinarian-pathologist David Salmon) is characterized by abdominal pain, fever, bloody diarrhea, nausea, and vomiting. These symptoms can last from two to five days, with the exception of the fever, which can last up to two weeks. Research has shown that, like Lyme disease, salmonella poisoning can instigate a form of arthritis in about 15 percent of those exposed.[119] The arthritis condition may last for years.

Salmonella poisoning has become all too common, and more often than not, the poisonings involve cow's milk products.

In 1980, nearly 340 cases of salmonella poisoning in Colorado were linked to cheddar cheese sold in the state.[120] A 1982 outbreak in Canada was also attributed to cheese. In April 1985, an enormous outbreak of salmonella from cow's milk poisoned 180,000 people in Chicago.[121] In 1989, Minnesota and Wisconsin suffered an outbreak from mozzarella cheese.[122] In 1994, 200,000 people across the United States were poisoned. This time, the source was ice cream contaminated by raw eggs.[123]

Such outbreaks aren't constrained to the United States and Canada. In Scotland, there were twenty-one outbreaks of salmonella in milk between 1980 and 1982. A total of 1,090 people became sick and eight died, two of them children.[124]

Listeria

Listeria (named after the English surgeon Joseph Lister) can cause very serious and potentially fatal infections, particularly in young children, pregnant women, and the elderly. People who consume listeria-tainted food are at risk of abdominal pain, diarrhea, nausea, fever, miscarriage, and even death.

Listeria contamination of cow's milk is far more common than most people realize. In a case reported by the Associated Press on February 17, 1999, a milk-processing plant in the US attempted to recall 400,000 gallons of listeria-tainted milk that had been distributed across the country. Luckily, the word got out before too many people were infected. In May 1999, a Missouri dairy recalled hundreds of pounds of cheese because federal inspectors discovered it was contaminated with listeria.[125] In the same month, listeria-tainted milk was served to children in a school cafeteria in Santo Domingo, Dominican Republic. More than a thousand students were sickened, and fifty were hospitalized with vomiting, headaches, and diarrhea. In January of 2008 the Boston Globe reported the sickening of five people and the death of three elderly men who drank pasteurized milk tainted with Listeria. In September of 2010 the FDA reported a regulatory sampling at a Missouri dairy lead to a nationwide recall of 68,957 pounds of cheese due to Listeria contamination.

Pus

It seems some people will eat or drink just about anything, as long as it tastes good to them. They'll even eat pus, more politely referred to as somatic cells.

Webster's Dictionary defines pus as "a thick, yellowish-white fluid formed in infected tissue that contains bacteria, white blood cells, and tissue debris." The presence of white blood cells is an indication the immune system is working to fight an infection; a lower count is an indication of less infection and, presumably, better health.

Somatic cell count (SCC) is the measurement of white blood cells per milliliter of milk. Currently, the upper limit is 750,000 per milliliter. Somatic cell counts have even been used to bestow health honors on dairy herds. Consider the Green County Dairy Herd Improvement Farmer Appreciation Luncheon, an event sponsored by the Green County Milk Quality Council of Wisconsin.[126] At their March 2005 event, top honors went to a herd that had an SCC of 70,000 per milliliter, and second place went to a herd with an SCC of 98,000 per milliliter. It is perfectly legal to sell milk from sick cows, as long as its SCC does not exceed the 750,000 limit.[127] Thus, you can legally enjoy an eight-ounce glass of milk containing tens of millions of white blood cells.*

Consumers Union reported that with the administration of the synthetic hormone rBGH, infections of cows' udders increase. Consequently, the milk is likely to contain even more pus than that from a cow that has not been drugged.[128]

Vitamin D and Vitamin A

How can vitamin D be considered a contaminant? After all, it is a vitamin, and vitamins are essential to our good health.

The answer is that when vitamins occur in their natural form — in whole, unrefined foods — they are the most healthful for us, because they are available in a balanced chemistry designed by nature. When we begin fortifying foods with vitamins, things get tricky, for two reasons. The first is that there is no way to be certain of a particular person's diet. Thus, there is little standardization regarding the total amount of a specific vitamin we are getting from all the fortified foods we are eating. The second, and perhaps even more disconcerting, reason is excessive vitamin fortification.

Vitamin D was first added to milk in the 1940s, to prevent the disease rickets from occurring in children. Rickets is extremely rare today, and usually only occurs in areas where children receive very little sunlight. Vitamin D is actually a hormone produced in the body when ultraviolet light reaches the skin surface. Normally, people have no problem producing all the vitamin D they need, unless they are confined indoors or live in a climate with little sun. There are other conditions that may inhibit vitamin D production that we'll examine shortly.

People are surprised to learn about the variations in the amount of vitamin D added to cow's milk.[129] In a survey of forty-two milk samples, only 12 percent came close to the content reported on the carton label. Some cow's-milk–based infant formulas have been found to have as much

---

* 750,000 x 240 milliliters (8 ounces per glass of milk) = 180,000,000 white blood cells.

as four times the amount stated on the label.[130] In a case reported in the *New England Journal of Medicine,* the vitamin D content of milk samples varied from zero to 232,565 I.U. (international units) per quart of milk. That upper measurement is 581 times the Reference Daily Intake (RDA) of 400 I.U., the legal limit allowable per quart! This same study found that of the ten infant formula samples tested, seven contained more than twice the amount of vitamin D stated on their labels. One contained more than four times the stated amount.

In another case, an Ohio dairy attempted to recall chocolate milk in what it called a "manufacturing error." The milk had been sent to market containing not only 4,000 I.U. of vitamin D, but also 44,000 I.U. of vitamin A. This was twenty-two times the 2,000–3,000 I.U. of vitamin A that the milk should have contained. While these levels of vitamin A can cause liver problems for anyone, consumption by infants or pregnant women can lead to brain damage and birth defects. Unfortunately, this particular recall was made after the milk had been on store shelves for thirteen days![131]

Vitamin over-fortification is a serious problem, because vitamin D, like vitamin A, is toxic in excessive dosages.[132] The side effects of excess vitamin D include kidney stones, hypercholesterolemia, hypercalcemia, mental retardation, and damage to the eyes, heart and circulatory system.[133] Since added vitamin D is an artificial means of promoting calcium deposition, and since some people consume ample quantities of milk and other dairy products, there is a risk of calcium depositing in parts of the body where it is not desirable, such as soft tissues. Over time, calcium may accumulate in the kidneys, making the organs less and less permeable until the inevitable happens: the calcium crystallizes into kidney stones.[134]

Vitamin D is essential to bone health. It promotes calcium absorption, helps maintain proper serum levels of calcium, and enables bone growth and the bone remodeling process performed by osteoclast and osteoblast cells. The good news is we don't need cow's milk to meet our daily needs; normally, people get all the vitamin D they need from the sun.[135] However, there are exceptions that need to be considered, particularly now that recent surveys are showing moderate levels of vitamin D deficiency. If you live in northern latitudes, are homebound, or have a job that limits your sun exposure, you may not get adequate sun to produce the vitamin D you need. Likewise, if you have liver disease, Crohn's disease, or cystic fibrosis, you may have problems synthesizing enough of the vitamin. If you cover up your skin and use sun screen when outside, you may be at greater risk of deficiency. The easiest way to assure adequate vitamin D is to take a supplement.

In the face of such sobering evidence of milk's contamination, it is important to remember that humans have no need whatsoever for the milk of a cow or any other animal. If cow's milk does not assure us the bone health we seek, and calcium is readily available in many other healthy foods, where is the justification in exposing oneself to all the contaminants?

In the next chapter, we'll explore how milk consumption may adversely affect children.

Six

Cow's Milk and Children's Health

The difference in my son from the day we took him off dairy has been spectacular, astonishing, and unmistakable.

— Karen Seroussi, author of *Unraveling the Mystery of Autism*

Today, more than ever before, there is a concerted effort to get children to drink cow's milk. It comes in the form of vast advertising campaigns, literature in parents' magazines, "educational" materials distributed to school teachers, and, more recently, milk vending machines appearing in the halls of public schools around America. Then there are the array of new milk beverages hitting the market; one of the most recent, called Refreshing Power Milk and aimed at children who favor soft drinks, has been carbonated, and comes in chocolate and cappuccino flavors.[1] A study by the National Dairy Council is leading to a milk-packaging revolution for schools. It found when producers replaced traditional paper cartons with plastic bottles, children consumed 18 percent more milk at school.[2] Is all this effort really for the betterment of children's health?

We have already reviewed the extensive array of contaminants that may be found in a glass of milk, and we know any toxin poses a greater threat to a child's body than to an adult's. Moreover, no child should be exposed to the hormones found in milk. Yet putting these issues aside, let's focus on the primary reason milk is promoted to children: the supposedly essential role it plays in promoting their bone health.

An important study examining this issue was published in the journal *Pediatrics* in March 2005. It reviewed fifty-eight already-published studies of varying types, and the conclusion was hardly inspiring. The authors found that "in clinical, longitudinal, retrospective, and cross-sectional studies, neither increased consumption of dairy products, specifically, nor total dietary calcium consumption has shown even a modestly consistent benefit for child or young adult bone health."[3] A year later, another meta-analysis was published, this time in the *British Medical Journal*. This study examined the effect of calcium supplements in children, and its conclusion was no more inspiring. The minimal effect seen from supplementation was considered "unlikely to reduce the risk of fracture, either in childhood or later life to a degree of major public health importance."[4] Since the primary motive for drinking milk, we are told, is to maintain bone health, this news is discouraging. Milk's apparent failure to support children's bone health becomes even more disconcerting when we study the host of children's health problems which reliance on milk may cause or contribute to. This is the focus of this chapter.

Adding flavors or carbonation to milk doesn't solve the serious health risks milk may pose to infants and children. Most of the conditions presented here are believed to be related to either an allergic response to a protein found in cow's milk, or in some cases, an inability to digest lactose, the sugar in milk. However, there may be other, more complex paths by which milk in the diet presents risk to a child, as we will see when we examine the link between milk and autism.

Allergy to cow's milk is grossly underdiagnosed. In cases where it is recognized, parents often hear the refrain, "Don't worry, she'll grow out of it." However, studies indicate that while symptoms may change in type and severity, many children do not grow out of their allergy to cow's milk, and are still reactive years later.[5] In fact, many who demonstrated allergy symptoms as toddlers show reactions well into their adult years — only the number and types of allergens grow or change.

The following is a personal story about a little girl named Rhiannon. Her parents, Nigel and Janet, have shared their account of raising a child with a severe allergy to cow's milk.[6]

When Rhiannon was nine weeks old, her parents decided to try feeding her formula. Although Rhiannon had been breastfed from birth, her parents wanted to know whether she could tolerate formula. They never expected what followed.

Within half an hour of Rhiannon's first encounter with formula, she began wheezing, and a blotchy red rash appeared over her body. She then began projectile vomiting. Because of the delay in their daughter's response, at first Rhiannon's parents did not make an association with the formula she had ingested and her ill health. A week later, they fed her another bottle of formula. Within one hour, the family was in the emergency room of their local hospital. In addition to the projectile vomiting, the young girl's breathing had become labored, and she repeatedly choked and gagged on an abundance of mucus that had formed in her throat.

When Rhiannon was fourteen months old, her parents brought her back to the hospital to have her tested for a suspected allergy to cow's milk. Again, her reaction was violent and included projectile vomiting. Rhiannon's father commented after this episode: "I think the nurses eventually understood when we said she got *very sick* from milk." At age seven, after numerous tests, Rhiannon had not outgrown her allergy to milk.

Although the severity of Rhiannon's reaction is uncommon, the projectile vomiting, skin rash, and labored breathing are but a few of the symptoms that can occur in a child allergic to cow's milk. Most symptoms are more subtle; others are extreme, even life-threatening. Take, for example, the heartbreaking case of five-month-old Thomas Egan. In April of 2009 while at a nursery, he was accidentally fed a breakfast cereal for babies that contained cow's milk proteins. He had an allergic reaction to the protein and died a few hours later.[7] The important point for parents to keep in mind, however, is that their child's negative reaction to cow's milk may begin long before the child is directly fed the substance.

The subject of food allergy is complex. Specialists continue to debate the accuracy of various diagnostic tests. True allergy involves the immune system. However, non-immune-mediated reactions (often referred to as *intolerances* or *sensitivities*) are valid and deserve serious attention. For this reason, I often tell people to rely upon their personal experience. You don't need a medical degree to eliminate a food from your own or your child's diet, and then see if certain symptoms improve or are alleviated. If removing cow's milk provides these benefits, it doesn't really matter what the "experts" say. As you will see, even the best-informed and best-credentialed practitioners do not fully understand the complicated mechanisms involved in food allergy. Remember, you don't need a doctor's prescription to stop eating a food that may be causing you ill health!

Allergic responses to cow's milk can include immediate symptoms (those that occur within minutes after consumption or exposure) or delayed symptoms (those that occur hours or even days after consumption). Immediate reactions make diagnosing allergy substantially easier. But when symptoms are delayed, diagnosis becomes difficult, and chronic disease may continue indefinitely without medical intervention.

In Chapter Five, we made the distinction between lactose intolerance and allergy to cow's milk. This distinction remains confusing for some people, including well-meaning doctors. Lactose intolerance is the inability to digest the naturally occurring sugar (lactose) in milk; to do so properly requires the enzyme lactase, which the body usually stops producing around age four. Allergy to cow's milk, on the other hand, is a response to the various proteins found in the milk. This is why patients who are truly having an allergic reaction, but are prescribed lactase pills or instructed to consume "lactose-free" or "lactaid-fixed" products, invariably do not see an improvement in their symptoms. The only way they will obtain relief is by totally eliminating the milk that contains the offending proteins.

Dairy Products, Pregnancy, and Infancy

Women are urged by their physicians and the media to drink plenty of milk and eat other dairy products both during pregnancy and while nursing their babies. As old and mainstream as this advice is, there is no scientific basis to support it. As you have seen in earlier discussions, the research indicates that a mother who avoids dairy products — before, during, and after pregnancy — will not only improve her own health, but can also reduce the risk of a number of undesirable side effects for her developing child. Successfully protecting children from exposure to dairy products begins during pregnancy, and continues long after they have stopped nursing. The risks of juvenile diabetes, ear infections, skin rashes, colic and iron deficiency may all be reduced by the avoidance of cow's milk-based formulas and other dairy products.[8, 9]

In the medical journal *Annals of Pediatrics*, pediatrician Robert H. Schwartz wrote: "Cow's-milk allergy is the most common food sensitivity issue confronting pediatricians today."[10] Unfortunately, too often, people do not recognize the association between milk and certain symptoms until after considerable interventions — such as medications and even surgeries — have been attempted to eliminate symptoms. Sometimes the association is never recognized, and individuals grow up suffering unnecessarily for their entire lives.

Over forty-five years ago, Dr. Benjamin Spock, world-famous authority on children's health, wrote the all-time bestselling book on raising healthy children, *Baby and Child Care*. Worldwide sales of his book remain second only to those of the Bible. In his final revision to his book, Dr. Spock stated cow's milk "causes intestinal blood loss, allergies, indigestion, and contributes to some cases of childhood diabetes." He also wrote: "Cow's milk in the past has always been oversold as the perfect food, but we are now seeing that it isn't the perfect food at all and the government really shouldn't be behind any efforts to promote it as such."[11]

Just as for adults, the chief problem for children may be allergy to one or more of the many proteins found in cow's milk. An important study offered some hope when it showed that if women eliminated all dairy products from their diet just six months before pregnancy, their babies had significantly lower levels of antibodies to nonhuman milk and, during the twelve-month follow-up period after birth, far fewer allergic reactions than babies whose mothers had continued to consume dairy products throughout pregnancy.[12]

Furtive propaganda is used to coerce parents and teachers into believing they would be doing children a grave disservice were they to discourage consumption of cow's milk. Yet many of the health problems from which adults suffer may well be a consequence of how foods like cow's milk were introduced into their diet as children. Many daycare centers and elementary schools require that cow's milk be served to children. Schools that do not include milk in every menu may be deprived of their meal-cost reimbursement from the federal government's National School Lunch Program.[13] Recall the letter sent to childcare providers by the Contra Costa Child Care Council Food Program, described in Chapter Two. It is a sad indication of how children may be manipulated into drinking milk.

In another case, renowned pediatrician Charles R. Attwood, M.D., told how a seven-year-old's mother was given a note from the boy's school dietician. The note described the dietician's great concern over the child's avoidance of milk at lunchtime. Heavily underlined in the letter was this sentence: "Milk is absolutely necessary for calcium and protein!"

From the wording of the dietician's letter, it seems she was unaware of two things. First, no human child of any age at any time requires the milk of another species in order to meet nutritional needs.[14] Second, in this case, the young boy had been instructed to eliminate cow's milk from his diet by his pediatrician, Charles Attwood. Dr. Attwood had made the recommendation because cow's milk clearly worsened the boy's asthma.

The policy of pushing milk upon children in inner-city schools is particularly problematic when we take race into account. African-American children have a lactose intolerance rate of about 75 percent. Many such children may be subject to intestinal cramping, gas, and diarrhea when they are coerced into drinking a fluid never intended for human consumption, and particularly problematic for children of color.[15]

Worse, children who have made the healthful transition to beverages made from rice, soy, or almonds are out of luck when they get to school. That's because any public school in America that attempts to serve these beverages in place of cow's milk will lose its federal support.[16] This is unfortunate because, when given the option, schoolchildren — particularly those who are more likely to suffer from lactose consumption — will embrace alternative beverages. In a study published in the *Journal of the*

American Dietetic Association, after just four weeks, nearly 25 percent of children in three ethnically diverse elementary schools chose soy milk over cow's milk.[17] Noting that cow's milk is also the single largest contributor of saturated fat to a child's diet, the research authors were encouraged by the acceptability of soy milk to elementary school children.

In the first year of an infant's life, the ideal food is mother's milk. Human milk has been formulated by nature to contain the right constituents in the proper balance for the developing child. Unfortunately, most of us are introduced to cow's milk shortly after (if not during) infancy. This is when a host of health problems may begin. Cow's milk is terribly deficient in the essential fatty acids (EFA) that are required for human health. Mother's milk has up to ten times the amount of essential fatty acids that cow's milk contains! Consider that during infancy — the most critical time in human development, when the body is growing more rapidly than it will ever grow again — mother's milk provides 5 percent of its calories as protein. Cow's milk, as we saw in Chapter Four, contains three times this share — far more protein than nature intended for a human infant. The levels of sodium, calcium, and phosphorus in cow's milk are also excessive for an infant.

Nutrient Comparison (nutrients per 3.5 ounces)

	Human Milk	Cow's Milk
Protein (g)	1.1	4
Fat (g)	4	3.5
Carbohydrate (g)	9	4.9
Phosphorus (mg)	18	97
Sodium (mg)	16	50
Calcium (mg)	33	118

Beyond its nutritional profile, cow's milk also contains many different proteins that can elicit allergic reactions in children. As many as 50 percent of children today are allergic to cow's milk, according to some estimates, yet most of their allergies take their ravaging toll on their bodies without ever being properly diagnosed.[18] Removing cow's milk from the diet of the child and the mother (if she is breastfeeding) can totally eliminate these symptoms.

Research is showing us that many conditions common in infants and young children — including asthma, colic, and earaches — may actually have roots in the child's diet. More specifically, they may be caused or exacerbated by the consumption of cow's milk and other common allergens. Let's examine a few in detail.

In one case, thirty infants were determined to be allergic to cow's milk when they were observed and tested in a hospital setting. Their symptoms included runny nose, sneezing, cough, eczema, colic, and diarrhea. When cow's milk was eliminated from their diets, twenty-one of the infants experienced a complete elimination of symptoms.[19]

Sudden Infant Death Syndrome (SIDS)

For forty years, many pediatricians and researchers have been dumbfounded about what causes Sudden Infant Death Syndrome (SIDS). While a number of associations have been identified, including a negative reaction to immunizations, some experts are convinced an allergic reaction to cow's milk may also be a primary culprit, in some cases.[20]

Some researchers believe a child fed a bottle of cow's milk or formula based on cow's milk before bed, as some children are in parents' efforts to ease them to sleep, may experience an allergic reaction shortly after falling asleep. For some infants, the reaction may be anaphylaxis, caused by the infant regurgitating the recently consumed cow's milk and then inhaling a small amount of the regurgitated milk into their lungs. Since the lungs are a major shock organ for anaphylaxis, this inhalation can lead to shock and sudden death.[21]

Writing in the journal *Clinical and Experimental Allergy*, researchers Coombs and Holgate stressed: "However gauged, the evidence for this anaphylactic sensitivity is overwhelming."[22] Some studies have shown that infants fed cow's milk are twice as likely to die of SIDS compared to those not given cow's milk.[23] Even the American Society of Microbiologists recognizes the association, which they acknowledged at their annual symposium in 1982 by reporting that "exclusively breastfed babies are far less likely to succumb to SIDS."[24] Sadly, despite this evidence and concern, few pediatricians make mothers aware of this risk.

Asthma

Asthma is a serious disease whose incidence is growing rapidly in America and other industrialized nations. It is a miserable condition for many infants and children, and can lead to death in some cases. Although a number of contributing factors have been identified — notably, the appalling air quality found in most major cities — one factor, allergy to cow's milk, is not commonly suspected. Yet as far back as 1959, it was clear that cow's milk could cause severe asthma in children.[25] It has been estimated that as many as 30 percent of people who are allergic to cow's milk will develop symptoms of asthma when exposed.

In a study published in the journal *Clinical Allergy*, twenty-five of thirty-one infants who had family histories of allergy developed asthma after receiving cow's milk.[26] As a comparison, only eight of thirty infants in the control group developed asthma after exclusive breastfeeding. We must ask why the breastfed group (the control group) had even eight cases. One possible reason is that even if an infant is exclusively breastfed, if the mother continues to consume dairy products, she will pass the offending proteins on to her infant through her breast milk. Sure enough, in this study, the authors stated: "No attempt was made to influence the diet of nursing mothers, and reduce the opportunity for any allergens [cow's milk protein] to be transferred to the infant in the breast milk."[27] Had the researchers ensured the mother's diet was dairy-free, the incidence in the control group may have been markedly lower.

A study reported in the journal *Annals of Allergy* found a significant number of infants with asthma also tested positive for allergy to cow's milk. All of the infants six months old or younger experienced relief from their symptoms once cow's milk was eliminated from their diets.[28]

In another study, fifteen of twenty-two asthmatics were placed on a dairy-free diet. Their conditions improved noticeably within two weeks, but the subjects experienced maximal relief after two to three months had passed. The improvement of eight of the patients was so great that they only needed their inhalers occasionally instead of regularly. One patient, who had been on daily doses of 30 to 40 mg of the steroid medication Prednisone, was able to slash his dose to 10 mg daily. After fourteen months, the patient still had not had an acute attack. Of the improved patients, fourteen were willing to reintroduce dairy protein into their diet. Five had severe attacks within one week of the reintroduction; one had to be hospitalized and treated with steroid therapy.[29]

Cow's milk doesn't always have to be ingested to elicit an asthmatic reaction. In a case reported in the journal *Allergy,* a female worker at a chocolate factory experienced "occupational asthma" after she inhaled dried-milk powder that she had applied to confections. After five years of suffering, it became apparent her condition was alleviated during evenings and weekends. Testing showed she was reacting to the lactalbumin protein in the dried milk at work.[30]

Autism

In 1970, autism occurred at a rate of one in ten thousand children, nationwide. Over the last couple of decades, particularly during the 1990s, there was a dramatic increase in the number of cases diagnosed.[31] In 2005, the National Institutes of Health estimated that a diagnosis of an autism spectrum disorder was as high as one in five hundred children.[32] In October 2009, the Department of Health and Human Services, the Centers for Disease Control and Prevention, and the National Institutes of Health held a press conference to announce the figure had been revised to one in a hundred children, making for an increase in incidence of over 6,000 percent since 1970. [33]

Yet this problem is not unique to America; it is also a worldwide phenomenon, seen from America to South Africa, and from Russia to India.[34] Nobody seems able to explain the enormous surge in autism cases, but some parents and physicians are witnessing the unexpected: reversals brought about by a regimen of dietary intervention, and by other therapies.

Originally thought to be a form of schizophrenia,[35] autism is the most prevalent of a range of disorders that fall under the umbrella known as *autism spectrum disorders* (ASDs). This group also includes *Asperger's*

Syndrome and *Pervasive Development Disorder — Not Otherwise Specified* (PDD–NOS).[36] Autism is typically diagnosed within the first three years of life, and it strikes boys three to four times more often than girls.

Classic symptoms of autism include introversion, or withdrawal from communication with others; self-absorption; repetitive play; and an attachment to rhythmical movements such as rocking. Autistic children often have difficulty interpreting emotional cues and facial expressions, and may also exhibit rage and self-injurious behavior. Many autistic children do not make eye contact with their parents or care providers, and some may cease to communicate verbally. One out of three autistic children will also experience epileptic seizures.[37]

The emotional, financial, and social impacts on parents of autistic children are tremendous. Reflecting on the astronomical number of cases seen today, Andy Shih of the National Alliance for Autism Research cautions, "The financial burden that this will place on our society is going to be just stunning." A Harvard Medical School study has estimated that the medical treatments, special education, and therapies possibly required for a single child with autism can cost parents up to $72,000 a year and $3.2 million over a lifetime.[38] Many insurance plans do not cover such treatments, or do so with limitations.

There is no shortage of theories about the cause of autism, and a lively debate ensues. But one theory has attracted enormous attention — spawning numerous websites and support and advocacy organizations around the world — and seems to have the most scientific evidence to support it. This theory involves both vaccines and diet. It holds that autism begins when a component of some child vaccines or other factor causes an assault to a child's gastrointestinal (GI) tract. After the GI tract has been impaired, partially broken-down proteins or protein fragments called peptides are able to cross the gut and enter the bloodstream. From the bloodstream the peptides are able to reach critical cell receptors in the brain, whereby havoc ensues.

Normally the mucosa, the lining of the intestine, acts as a barrier to different elements entering the blood.[39] It was originally believed that, due to their size, peptides never crossed the gut wall, and instead acted on hormones and cell receptor sites with which they came in contact in the gut. However, recent research has shown that in some individuals, peptides are able to cross the gut wall and enter the bloodstream, ultimately traveling to the brain, where they interfere with neurotransmission.

An infant's gut is already more permeable than an adult's, to accommodate the larger colostrum molecules that precede mother's milk. However, it is theorized that something else, possibly an assault of some kind, may increase the gut's permeability further, and for a longer period of time. This something else — whether it be a vaccine, a virus, or another factor, such as yeast overgrowth — renders the gut abnormally permeable, allowing undesirable opiate peptides to enter the bloodstream in large quantities. According to this theory, these peptides then instigate an *antigenic* or allergy response, as well as interfere with the proper functioning of the central nervous system.

It has been well documented for more than thirty years that autistic children frequently suffer from gastrointestinal problems such as diarrhea, bloating, and intestinal cramps.[40] These problems seem to be nearly synonymous with autism, as they are with other developmental disorders.[41]

One of the first to identify this was Andrew Wakefield, a British gastroenterologist who published his findings in the prestigious medical journal *Lancet*. Dr. Wakefield had found severe GI problems in all of the autistic children in his first study. In a later study, he found GI problems in forty-eight children with developmental disorders, many of whom were diagnosed with autism.[42]

It has also been reported that the GI problems typically seen in autistic children frequently appear at the same time as their symptoms of autism.[43] Upon close examination, researchers using endoscopy and biopsies have confirmed irregularities of the intestinal mucosa, referred to as *ileal nodular hyperplasia,* in these children.[44] The common term used is "leaky gut." Researchers have also confirmed that autistic children frequently have very high levels of opiate peptides in both their blood and urine.

Evidence indicates that the peptides crossing the gut wall come from none other than cow's milk, as well as certain grains. As we have seen, milk contains a protein called casein that, when broken down incompletely in the digestive tract, produces short-chain peptides with opiate-like qualities called *casomorphins*. Similarly, the protein gluten, found in wheat, rye, barley, and oats, will produce opiate-like peptides called *gliadorphins* if incompletely digested.[45] The theory linking autism to opiate compounds was first postulated in 1979 by J. A. Panksepp.[46]

Like prescribed opiate drugs, casomorphins and gliadorphins have sedative, pain-numbing, and even hallucinogenic properties. Traveling in the bloodstream, they reach the brain, then connect with opiate receptors. These are the same receptors targeted by morphine administered in a hospital setting, or by heroin used recreationally. Compounds like this affect perception, cognition, emotions, mood, and behavior, and disrupt normal neurotransmission. If you have been in the presence of patients under the influence of morphine — say, after a major surgery — you know how trying their own experience (and yours trying to interact with them) can be. Not only does their experience of pain shift, but they also may see and hear things not actually present in their room. They may experience distortions of spatial perception, or show a delay in (or absence of) response to various stimuli. Their memory of events before, during, and after the surgery may be sketchy, at best. These perceptual and hallucinogenic effects may offer some insight into the classic behaviors of autistic and schizophrenic children. Indeed, the symptoms in these two conditions are very similar.

Proof Positive

Is there evidence that food-derived opiates are accessing the brain? Having conducted research on childhood schizophrenia and autism for decades, University of Florida's J. Robert Cade, M.D., stated, "We now have proof positive that these proteins are getting into the blood and proof positive they're getting into areas of the brain involved with the symptoms of autism and schizophrenia."[47]

Although he had detected twelve different casomorphin peptides, Dr. Cade had experimented with one in particular: *beta-casomorphin-7* or BCM7. This is the casomorphin he and other researchers have found in the greatest abundance in subjects they studied, and the one he suspected of being the most potent. After injecting rats and other animals with the substance, Dr. Cade and colleagues noted behavioral changes, and then examined the animals' brains. They found BCM7 was taken up by forty-five different parts of the brain, whereas the gluten-related peptide gliadorphin (GD7) was affecting only three areas of the brain.

The animals displayed behavioral changes strikingly similar to those of autistic children. For example, they didn't respond when a bell was struck next to their cage. Normally, the experimental animals would have looked to see where the noise was coming from, but after administration of the milk-borne opiate, they seemed oblivious to the sound.[48] Parents of autistic children often describe their children as oblivious to sounds or to the calling of their names — it is as if they were deaf. "There are a whole number of behaviors," says Dr. Cade, "that the rat has after beta-casomorphin-7 that are basically the same as one sees in the human with autism or schizophrenia."[49]

Dr. Cade's research also showed that more than 80 percent of the autistic and schizophrenic children studied had sharply elevated levels of antibodies to both casein and gluten, indicating the immune system was highly stimulated and attempting to defend the body from some constituent in these compounds.

Recovering Children

Inspired by his findings in the animal studies, Dr. Cade decided to apply the theory to children. If some autistic children were indeed reacting to peptides formed from cow's-milk protein and gluten, which crossed their gut wall and wreaked havoc on their neural systems, how would they respond if the offending proteins were eliminated from their diets? Very well, Dr. Cade discovered. His team placed eighty-one confirmed autistic or schizophrenic children on the GFCF diet, a diet free of cow's milk and gluten-containing grains. In 80 percent of their autistic subjects the researchers documented remarkable improvements in eye contact, vocalization, hyperactivity, and risk of panic attack and self-mutilation, within three months. They continued to monitor the children for up to eight years. There was a 40 percent improvement in the schizophrenic children (the researchers noted that the dietary protocol was abandoned for schizophrenic children who showed no immediate signs of improvement, which could explain why a smaller percentage showed improvement).

These amazing results were published in the journal *Autism*.[50] Dr. Cade and colleagues later reported that dialysis, the artificial kidney process that filters small particles from the blood, produces the same improvements as the dietary intervention.

After using dietary interventions, a growing number of mothers and fathers are coming forward to share how they have experienced stunning recoveries or at least significant improvements in children they thought they had lost to a mysterious internal world.[51] Their heartbreaking stories are an inspiration to the many parents who are faced with dead-end outcomes from the conventional medical approaches. One parent, in particular, became quite well known after her story was published in a wonderfully hopeful book, *Unraveling the Mystery of Autism and Pervasive Developmental Disorder*.[52] The author, Karyn Seroussi, went from being a grief-stricken lay-mother to the coeditor of a major website and newsletter that provide late-breaking research, articles, and support to parents of autistic children.[53] Along the way, she also reversed her son's autism! Karyn has received more than forty thousand letters and e-mails from parents around the world who were inspired by her story, many of whom saw dramatic improvements or complete recoveries using the dietary intervention she had pioneered.[54]

At fifteen months of age, Karyn's son, Miles, suddenly understood very little and stopped using the words he knew. He stopped gesturing and failed to make eye contact with his parents. In Karyn's words, her son seemed to be "disappearing into himself." Miles's parents assumed his changes were the result of his chronic ear infections. Why else would he be exhibiting a most unusual tendency to drag his head across the floor, they wondered?

Once Miles's parents took him to a specialist for evaluation, they were given a grim prognosis: Miles would "never be able to make friends, have a meaningful conversation, learn in a regular classroom without special help, or live independently." As any parent can imagine, this was devastating. For Karyn Seroussi, however, it also provided the inspiration that would lead to intensive research. She spent hours at the research library and scouring the Internet on her home computer, seeking out and conversing with parents whose children had received a similar diagnosis.

It is not just the courage and determination of Miles's parents that makes his story so compelling, but the fact that they applied what they learned and successfully reversed their son's devastating condition. In fact, they were so successful that Miles was not only eventually "declassified" by four different specialists — but by age three, he tested eight months above his age level for social, language, self-help, and motor skills. By age six, enrolled in the first grade, he was reading at a fourth-grade level.

In another case, April and Eric Schnell of Minnesota went through many of the same challenges with their son Tim. Tim screamed incessantly through the night, to the point that his parents took turns, one sleeping at a hotel while the other watched him at home. This was the only way they could get any sleep. It was not until their son was three years old that the director of the Special Children's Center in Hudson, Wisconsin, mentioned to his parents that they might want to try a dietary intervention. A few days after they removed milk and gluten from his diet, Tim slept through the entire night for the first time in his life. Then suddenly, reported his mother April, "he became more verbal." Tim's parents added additional therapies to his regimen, and eventually he was keeping up with his classmates at school and proved to be a lively, inquisitive, and outgoing child.[55]

Some parents who have had success in improving their child's condition — or, in the case of the Seroussis, in achieving a genuine reversal — insist diet was the determining factor. Miles's recovery began when his parents removed all cow's milk, and later gluten, from his diet. "The difference in my son from the day we took him off dairy has been spectacular, astonishing, and unmistakable," said Karyn. Then there is Debbie Paulo, who noticed a dramatic improvement in her three-year-old autistic son, Bailey, after she removed milk from his diet. "It revolutionized my life .... I never thought he would say 'I love you mummy,' but the difference was just amazing," she reported.[56]

Consider James R. Laidler, M.D., whose two sons were given a diagnosis of autism. Dr. Laidler is Assistant Professor of Anesthesiology and Pain

Management at Oregon Health and Science University in Portland. While he was evaluating conventional, but admittedly unfruitful, therapies, his wife (also a physician) learned of the potential improvements from eliminating cow's milk and gluten from the diet. "Not being the confrontational sort," Dr. Laidler writes, "I held my tongue (more or less) and let her do these crazy things to our kids. My thought was that I would be able to show her that these treatments did not work and then we would go back to the therapies I was more comfortable with." In fact, Dr. Laidler reports, the dietary changes worked "spectacularly."[57]

Jill McIntosh, a New Hampshire parent, told me how she had successfully reversed her son Alex's autism by eliminating all foods containing cow's milk or gluten from his diet. By age three, he demonstrated all of the age-appropriate skills, was socially outgoing, and was invited into an early-education program because of his intellectual prowess.[58]

As stated, opiates are highly addictive substances, and in a hospital setting are used with great prudence. Perhaps this explains why some autistic children crave cow's milk, and drink enormous amounts daily. For example, Miles Seroussi was drinking up to half a gallon of milk a day prior to dietary intervention. "We got in the habit of keeping cups of milk handy at all times just to avoid the screaming," said Karyn. "On ice, in our bedroom, for at least one nighttime awakening. Three cups in the diaper bag for a two-hour trip to the mall."[59] Another parent of an autistic three-year-old reported that his son was consuming a gallon of cow's milk a day.[60] Other parents have related how their autistic children retain insatiable appetites for milk (and wheat), and how they may become infuriated if they are deprived of the substance. In other words, many autistic children seem to develop a strong affinity for the very agent that is doing them profound harm.

The Vaccination Link

Even with this highly compelling potential for altering autistic or schizophrenic children's symptoms through dietary changes, many parents and researchers come back to the question of how a child becomes susceptible. How can one child drink cow's milk and eat gluten-containing grains with abandon and seemingly experience no adverse symptoms, while another enters into what has been likened to a chronic LSD trip? This question becomes particularly intriguing when one remembers that a diagnosis of autism frequently seems to coincide with the administration of vaccinations.

The proposal that vaccinations were somehow involved in causing autism was first suggested thirty-five years ago by Dr. Bernard Rimland, in his classic book *Infantile Autism*. Dr. Rimland later asserted that the action of some vaccines leads to damage of the gut wall. "There is an enormous amount of credible evidence that vaccines can and do cause harm," he claimed.[61] More recently, Dr. Andrew Wakefield has focused his attention on the "MMR" (measles, mumps, rubella) vaccination, stating: "The measles virus resides in the intestinal tract, where it can damage the gut wall, and let viruses or toxins pass through and attack the brain."[62]

According to Karyn Seroussi, the original changes in her son Miles coincided with his MMR vaccination. His response to the injection was certainly not normal. He was admitted to a hospital shortly after the shot, with seizures and a fever of 106 degrees. Jill McIntosh also recalled her son Alex was given the MMR vaccination, at sixteen months of age. Within a week of the injection, he began to decline significantly.

Dr. Rimland believed that at least one of the damaging components of the vaccine is mercury. Historically, in addition to containing aluminum and formaldehyde, many vaccines — as well as influenza shots[63] — have been preserved with a mercury-based solution called Thimerosal. This preservative, first introduced (and approved by the FDA) in the 1930s, contains 49.5 percent ethyl mercury by weight.[64]

Mercury is a well-established neurotoxin. Therefore, many parents and health-care professionals feel it should not be injected into humans, particularly not children.[65] After thousands of parents filed federal-court lawsuits demanding restitution for damages that they believed their children had suffered due to exposure to Thimerosal, lawmakers urged vaccine manufacturers to remove the preservative from all childhood vaccines in 2002.[66] Yet in May 2004, the mother of an autistic child testified that her son had recently received an immunization containing Thimerosal.[67]

Furthermore, mercury-based Thimerosal is still used in a number of vaccines as of 2010, including seasonal and H1N1 vaccines.*

The Centers for Disease Control and Prevention now recommends at least one of these flu vaccines for both pregnant women and infants aged six to twenty-three months. Thimerosal is also present in the Rhogam injections given to Rh-negative mothers about twenty-eight weeks into their pregnancies. While a mercury-free Rhogam shot is available, few women are made aware of this option. Vaccinations sometimes also contain aluminum, which — as we have already seen — has been cited as a risk to neurological health.

Public health advocates and researchers have revealed that, because of expanded vaccine schedules, the amount of mercury infants received from injections in the United States tripled in the 1990s! If parents followed the recommended schedule of vaccines, their children could receive a whopping dose of this dangerous element. Even with mercury's widely accepted designation as a neurotoxin, the EPA considers a dose of 0.1 micrograms per kilogram per day to be acceptable exposure.

At a congressional hearing on vaccines, Representative Dan Burton (R–Indiana) revealed that his grandson had become autistic shortly after a routine vaccine. To the horror of the investigating panel, he explained that the boy had received, by way of the vaccine preservative, forty-one times the amount of mercury deemed safe for an *adult* — in one day![68]

Yet during the 1990s, if an eleven-pound infant were given all recommended vaccines at his two-month exam — and all those vaccines had contained Thimerosal — that infant would have been exposed to 62.5 micrograms of mercury. This is 125 times the EPA guideline. If parents followed the vaccine recommendations in 1992, their infant would have received mercury exposures as follows: 12.5 micrograms at birth, another 12.5 micrograms at one month, 50 micrograms at two months, 50 micrograms at four months, 62.5 micrograms at six months, and 50 micrograms at fifteen to eighteen months. The total exposure in just that period of

---

* For a listing of some of the vaccines that still contain Thimerosal, see the Institute for Vaccine Safety's table at vaccinesafety.edu/thi-table.htm

time would be 237.5 micrograms of a known neurotoxin, all given during a critical period of neuron development.

To add to the hazards, if the vial from which an injection is drawn is not shaken well, a child may receive up to ten times the normal mercury exposure, due to settling and concentration of the heavy metal.[69]

Donald Miller, M.D., a professor of surgery at the University of Michigan, points out that "autism was discovered in 1943, in American children, twelve years after ethylmercury (Thimerosal) was added to the pertussis vaccine. The disease was not seen in Europe until the 1950s, after Thimerosal was added to vaccines there."

While the Centers for Disease Control and Prevention exonerated the preservative compound, saying there was no evidence of a link to autism, others, such as the US Congress's Subcommittee on Human Rights and Wellness, have taken a different position. In its report *Mercury in Medicine,* the committee stated that "Thimerosal used as a preservative in vaccines is likely related to the autism epidemic. This epidemic in all probability may have been prevented or curtailed had the FDA not been asleep at the switch regarding injected Thimerosal and the sharp rise of infant exposure to this known neurotoxin. Our public health agencies' failure to act is indicative of institutional malfeasance for self-protection and misplaced protectionism of the pharmaceutical industry."[70] While it was naive to assume that subjecting infants to significant loads of a neuro toxic heavy metal would not have some ill effects, we must question why the number of children diagnosed with autism continues to rise, now that the mercury-based preservative has largely been phased out.

Current thinking is that even in the absence of the heavy metal, some children suffer from a genetic predisposition that leaves them very sensitive to certain assaults on their developing immune system. The burden of a triple vaccine, such as the MMR or DPT, may lead to an abnormal response from the child's developing immune system. Illnesses that follow may result in treatment with antibiotics that disrupt intestinal flora and allows candida yeasts, normally held in check, to flourish. This yeast may cause damage to the gut wall. A damaged gut may then not produce the correct enzymes at the levels needed to properly break down the proteins.

It may also become more permeable in what has been referred to as "leaky gut", a condition in which large peptides are allowed to pass into the bloodstream. The peptides can then act directly on opiate receptor sites of cells in the brain.

Many questions remain unanswered, but one thing remains clear: parents around the world who are experimenting with removing foods containing cow's milk and gluten from their children's diet are noting improvements, and in some cases what could be called miraculous results.

As further confirmation, some curious parents, such as the Seroussis, have intentionally reintroduced cow's milk after weeks or months of a dairy-free and gluten-free diet — and witnessed the rapid return of autistic symptoms in their children. Other parents have witnessed the same regression when their children accidentally consumed food containing cow's milk.

At a biomedical conference addressing developments in autism research, Dr. Bernard Rimland, who spent fifty years researching autism, said, "In 1972, I told an audience that in 15 years, when a mother takes her child to the pediatrician, the pediatrician would know to suggest that the parent put the child on a casein- and gluten-free diet. I'm embarrassed that this isn't the case today, though."[71] Karyn Seroussi told me, "There are a lot of doctors out there, especially those who are developmental pediatricians, diagnosticians, or neurologists, who over the years have told parents, 'There's nothing you can do.'" Yet even without the support of their doctor, thousands of parents are adopting that dietary protocol. If you are a parent whose child is faced with a diagnosis of autism, pervasive developmental disorder (PDD), or even attention deficit disorder (ADD or ADHD), you may wish to eliminate all sources of cow's milk and gluten from your child's diet and give the GFCF protocol a try.

To help predict how successful this might be, I recommend that parents consult with their pediatrician, and with one of the labs listed in the Resources section at the back of this book, in order to have a blood and urine analysis performed. Since the opiate compounds are larger than normal proteins, they often stimulate an immune response and the production of antibodies, which can be measured in the blood. The bulk of these opiate peptides are also excreted into the urine, and can be detected there through urinalysis. Both of these tests are a worthwhile expense, as they will provide some quick feedback on how your child's body is currently responding to specific foods.

Before changing your child's diet, you should be aware of several things. First, even with the assistance of a pediatrician, some people find this change requires great dedication and vigilance. It means more than directly eliminating all dairy, wheat, oats, barley, and rye (all of which contain gluten) from the diet. Because many commercially prepared foods include casein in some form, and because gluten is an ingredient in many prepared foods, you should seek help from a dietician who can help you identify and eliminate all foods that may be offensive.

Second, the gluten- and casein-free diet (GFCF) protocol is not something one can do half-heartedly. Some parents hope they can only make certain dietary modifications and still produce dramatic results, but the evidence indicates this is simply not the case. You need comprehensive exclusion of the potentially offending proteins to see a recovery or improvement.

Third, parents should be aware that removing casein and gluten from their child's diet can result in symptoms of withdrawal. Speaking from Dr. Robert Cade's office, Malcolm Privette cautioned that some children will exhibit "classic" withdrawal symptoms, including sweating and dilated pupils. They may even express rage after being deprived of the food source of the opiates. These compounds have been giving the child an exaggerated sense of pleasure. Parents need to be prepared for such reactions — which can be good indications that you are going to see behavioral improvements.

While some children take longer to show signs of improvement, and others show no improvement, a significant proportion of those studied by Dr. Cade and his associates did recover and enter into mainstream schools as are a growing number of children today whose parents are employing the GFCF diet. Yet patience is essential. Depending on the individual, it may take some time for the peptides to be expelled from the brain and for the full effects to be seen.

Early intervention also appears critical. There seems to be a limited window in which the GFCF diet may result in improvement. After a certain time, chronic exposure to the opiate compounds may result in irreversible damage.

There is substantial support available. If your own pediatrician is not supportive, be sure to consult the ANDI website (see the Resources section at the back of this book) for a listing of physicians who do support dietary intervention in the treatment of autism and other conditions. The Resources section also contains books, support organizations, and materials to help assure your success with this protocol.

Be sure you read all labels on food packages and look for any reference to casein in its various processed forms, as well as references to whey. Just because a product is labeled "Dairy Free" does not guarantee it is free of dairy proteins. For example, some of Solgar brand's probiotics are labeled "Dairy Free" but contain casein.

You will not only need to eliminate the obvious products — including milk, cream, butter, sour cream, buttermilk, and yogurt — but will also need to be aware of other casein-based ingredients, including ammonium caseinate, calcium caseinate, potassium caseinate, and sodium caseinate. For a comprehensive list of ingredients derived from milk proteins, see Chapter 9. Gluten is found in wheat, rye, barley, and oats and is often used in commercial gravies, hard candies, and lipstick.

Ear Infections

Most parents are quite familiar with the fact that the most common health ailment diagnosed in infants and young children is ear infection.[72] Seventy-five percent of children in the United States suffer from at least one ear infection by their third birthday,[73] and nearly half will suffer from three or more episodes before their fourth birthday. One third of all medical office visits for children are for ear infections. The cost of these visits, excluding prescriptions given and surgical procedures performed, exceeds $2.5 billion annually.

Some people, including well-intentioned pediatricians, maintain that these ear infections are a normal part of growing up. But we are wrong to equate "common" with "normal." It is common for American men to develop heart disease; indeed, one out of two will develop the disease during their lifetimes. However, it is not normal. We know this because hundreds of millions of men in other parts of the world do not succumb to heart disease. Likewise, we know that in certain parts of the world, ear infections in infants and children — referred to in the medical world as *otitis media* — occur far less frequently.

Most pediatricians advise placing the child on a course of antibiotics, usually amoxicillin, to treat ear infections. Some medical practitioners even suggest placing children with recurrent ear infections on antibiotics for the winter months, as a preventative measure.[74] Yet research has shown that children given antibiotics recover more slowly from their condition, and are more likely to experience recurrent infections, compared to children not treated with antibiotics.

Reports have shown that antibiotics perform no better than placebos when given to children with ear infections.[75] Contrary to conventional wisdom, it has been shown that up to 80 percent of all ear infections resolve themselves without drugs, if given sufficient time.[76] Moreover, antibiotic therapy presents a host of other problems nobody would wish upon a child.

As with any illness, if we wish to prevent the occurrence of ear infection, we must know its cause. Conventional wisdom offers that a child is more susceptible to ear infection because of the shorter length, and more horizontal position, of the Eustachian tubes in their ears. Eustachian tubes allow fluid that normally collects in the middle ear to drain to the back of the throat. In adults they are more vertical, and hence drain more effectively.

However, when children develop a cold or sore throat, the tubes can become congested, allowing fluid to accumulate in the middle-ear area. The warm, stagnant fluid becomes an ideal breeding ground for bacteria and viruses. As more bacteria grow, more fluid is retained.

Studies have shown that nearly half of all cases of ear infection have been preceded by either nasal or bronchial congestion or by another respiratory condition.[77] The common wisdom is to assume that such symptoms were initially caused by a bacterial infection. But a blockage of the tube can also be instigated by food allergy,[78] and one of the most frequent allergens in infants and young children is cow's milk.

It should be telling that we see far fewer ear infections in children who are breastfed.[79] The longer children are breastfed, the greater their protection.

"The most frequently missed cause of recurrent ear fluid in infants and young children," writes Doris J. Rapp, M.D., "is an undetected sensitivity to milk."[80] Dr. Rapp is the founder of the Practical Allergy Foundation, a clinical professor at the State University of New York at Buffalo, and a bestselling author. Some parents are starting to make the connection. "It's amazing," observed one mother about her son, "when he gets any sort of milk product, he gets an ear infection within three days."[81]

Allergic reactions to foods often activate defense chemicals in the body, as the body tries to rid itself of what it perceives as a foreign invader. Reactions may include the production of mucus, the production and release of fluids, and the swelling of the throat, nasal passages, and Eustachian tubes in the ear.[82] When the Eustachian tubes swell, the pressure can impinge on the eardrum, causing it to become painful. Fluid can also become trapped, creating the opportunity for bacteria to grow. However, if we simply attack the bacteria with an antibiotic, we have failed to address the underlying cause. Therefore, as is often the case, the risk of the infection recurring is very high.

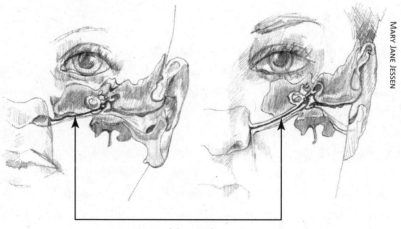

Infant   Adult

MARY JANE JESSEN

Eustachian Tube

Taking the time to identify food allergens may pay off very well for parents and their children. In one study of 104 children with ear infections, all allergenic foods were removed from their diet for sixteen weeks. In 86 percent of the children, the ear infection was resolved completely. In the final stage of the study, the instigating foods were reintroduced to the diet. In 94 percent of the children, fluid began accumulating in their ears. Of the various foods identified as allergenic in the children, the most common was cow's milk![83]

One of the most effective preventative steps a mother can take is to breastfeed her child, and do so as long as possible. Dr. Ruth Lawrence, professor of pediatrics and obstetrics at the University of Rochester School of Medicine in New York and spokeswoman for the American Academy of Pediatrics, has noted that children who are breastfed not only have fewer ear infections, but are also at reduced risk for diarrhea, rashes (eczema), and allergies than formula-fed children.

Studies have shown that exclusively breastfeeding an infant during the first four to six months slashes the risk of ear infections by 50 percent.[84] The longer a mother exclusively breastfeeds her child (and does not drink cow's milk and related foods herself), the greater the protection her child will receive against ear infections.[85]

A study of children with ear infections showed that those who were breastfed exclusively for the first four months of life had only half the risk of recurrent infection as those fed formula. For those infants breastfed exclusively for six months or more, infections returned only one-tenth as often as for the formula and mixed-diet group.[86]

In another study of breastfed versus formula-fed infants, researchers found prolonged ear infections (lasting up to ten days) were five times more common in formula-fed infants during the first year of a child's life. In the second year of life, the formula-fed children were still adversely affected, with ear infections occurring 3.6 times more than in the breastfed infants.[87]

While cow's milk is not the only potential allergen, it is the most common. Other foods that may cause allergic reactions include wheat, corn, citrus fruits (oranges, lemons, limes, and grapefruit), egg whites, soy, and peanuts.

At the time of this writing, a major pharmaceutical firm is promoting a vaccine developed with the hope of ending the scourge of childhood ear infections.[88] This demonstrates a well-intentioned effort to address the symptom while failing to address the cause. As a parent, if you can save your child from ever having to experience the discomfort and trauma of a serious ear infection simply by making appropriate dietary adjustments, why would you not make this your first line of defense?

Ear Tubes

As I stated earlier, antibiotics rarely eliminate ear infections; in many cases, they not only fail to improve the condition, but worsen it considerably. Antibiotics address a symptom, such as the bacteria that may breed in the middle ear, but they do nothing to address the cause. Therefore, the problem is left to repeat itself. Chronic and difficult-to-resolve ear infections often lead doctors to order one of the most common surgeries performed on children today. The procedure is called *myringotomy* and involves surgically placing tubes (grommets) in the ears.

The tubes are placed in the ear to help drain the accumulated fluid, which continues to serve as a breeding ground for bacteria. This surgery requires a general anesthetic, which itself poses a health risk. Studies have also shown that the procedure poses the risk of permanent damage to the tympanic membrane, atrophy of the eardrum, and consequential hearing loss. In one study of ninety-eight children who underwent the surgery, there was a 21 percent increase in deafness in the ears in which the tubes were placed. According to the American Academy of Otolaryngology–Head and Neck Surgery, about 700,000 children undergo this risky operation annually, generating some $1.4 billion in revenue![89] Disturbingly, a study that looked at 6,600 such surgeries found that 60 percent were unnecessary.[90]

Today, most medical experts consider drugs and surgery to be the best tools available for addressing ear infections in children. However, this is a perspective based upon a medical paradigm devoted to the treatment of disease and the mitigation of symptoms *once they exist*. A different approach is to ask why our children are so vulnerable to these infections in the first place? How might we *prevent* the infections from occurring, and thereby avoid having to consider drugs and surgery? While removing potential food allergens from a child's diet is not a panacea, it involves no major costs, poses no harm, and can have a powerfully healing effect in many cases.

Eczema (Skin Rash)

Eczema is one of the most frequent symptoms of allergy to cow's milk in infants.[91] Some children are exquisitely sensitive to cow's milk, and develop a severe rash just from having skin contact with it.[92] Surprisingly, however, some pediatricians are unaware of this fact and continue to encourage milk consumption when children are suffering from this highly irritating condition. As a child I suffered from extensive eczema on the inside of my arms and on the backs of my legs. But my pediatrician refused to consider the role milk was playing. Eventually my mother made the decision to eliminate milk and my relief was rapid and complete.

The benefits of breastfeeding apply here as well. Again, by totally eliminating cow's milk from the diet, you can easily determine whether or not it is playing a role in a case of eczema. If it is not, you may wish to consider eliminating other common food allergens — such as soy, citrus, wheat, nuts, and fish — to see if this remedies the condition.

Gastrointestinal Problems

Cow's milk can be linked to surprisingly severe digestive problems in children. As we'll see in this section, breastfeeding and dietary changes can help significantly.

Colic

Colic is a condition in which infants experience severe abdominal pain, produce a chronic, high-pitched scream, and exhibit a tendency toward excessive spitting up. The condition makes for both a miserable child and miserable parents, and can result in malnutrition.

While some people dismiss colic as the behavior of a "difficult child," substantial evidence suggests that it may be a symptom of allergy to cow's milk,[93] and simply removing cow's milk and associated products from both the child's and parents' diets can produce the docile infant parents hoped for.[94] Infants may be exposed to the offending bovine proteins through cow's milk-based formula or through breast milk containing cow's-milk proteins originating in the mother's diet.

Researchers at Washington University School of Medicine showed that when a mother consumes even small amounts of cow's milk, bovine proteins still manage to get absorbed by her intestine and enter her breast milk, where they will be passed to her breastfeeding infant. For example, mothers of colicky children have significantly higher concentrations of cow's-milk protein in their breast milk when sampled.[95] So even if the child is not fed a cow's-milk formula, if the infant's mother continues to drink cow's milk and eat dairy products herself and breastfeeds her infant, the colic induced by the cow's milk will not be remedied.[96]

In Anne Lamott's bestselling book *Operating Instructions,* she described how her newborn was severely colicky, and how this drove her to the brink of insanity. Eventually a friend advised her to stop eating ice cream and other dairy products. She did so, and shortly thereafter, her baby returned to a more docile state. Some days later, the author forgot and resumed her regular diet containing cow's milk, only for her son Sam to resume his fitful and screaming state.[97]

In a study reported in the *European Journal of Pediatrics,* children with recurrent vomiting — a frequent symptom in colic — were not responding to conventional therapy. The researchers found that "a striking improvement occurred" within 24 hours of adopting a diet free of cow's milk."[98]

In a study of nineteen breastfed infants not directly consuming cow's milk, yet still colicky, 68 percent were cured once cow's milk was eliminated from the mother's diet.[99] In another study reported in *Lancet,* colic disappeared from thirteen of eighteen breastfeeding children once their mothers were taken off cow's milk.[100]

In a study of sixty-six breastfeeding infants with colic, cow's milk was removed from the mother's and infant's diet, and in more than half of the group the colic disappeared entirely.[101] Another study tested twenty-seven infants with severe colic, some crying up to five-and-a-half hours a day.[102] When the infants were given a formula free of cow's milk, symptoms disappeared in twenty-four of the infants.

While cow's milk has been established as a common cause of colic in infants, it is important to note that it is not the only potential culprit. Some infants are extremely sensitive and will react to other food elements that end up in mother's milk, including garlic, legumes (beans), broccoli, and even soy. In cases where colic is not cured by the elimination of cow's milk, these and other foods in the mother's diet should be considered.

Intestinal Bleeding

Though rarely mentioned to parents, occult (hidden) gastrointestinal blood loss caused by consumption of cow's milk is quite common in infants.[103] It has been documented in medical journals dating back to 1954.[104] The loss of blood is quite serious, and can lead to iron-deficiency.[105] Such blood loss appears to be instigated by a protein in cow's milk called *bovine serum albumin* (BSA).

Frank Oski, M.D., former director of pediatrics at Johns Hopkins University School of Medicine, has cautioned that, although the bleeding is steady and quite significant (as much as 5 milliliters a day), it occurs slowly, in amounts too small to be detected by the parent's naked eye[106] (this is why the condition is called *occult*). So without the required chemical test, such blood loss often goes unnoticed.

Conservative estimates are that 15 to 20 percent of children under two years of age suffer from iron-deficiency anemia, and much of it may be caused by such blood loss caused by ingesting cow's milk.[107] In one study, a breastfed infant developed iron deficiency just four weeks after switching to cow's-milk feeding.[108] Another study found that the incidence of iron deficiency can be as high as 62 percent among infants who have been fed cow's milk before the age of six months;[109] by comparison, the incidence of iron deficiency among infants fed cow's milk after ten months was only 6 percent. It also seems that the blood loss increases or decreases as intake of cow's milk increases or decreases, respectively.[110]

Gastrointestinal bleeding not only poses the threat of iron-deficiency anemia, but even more disconcertingly, it seems to affect brain development. Iron loss brought about by intestinal bleeding is sufficient to interfere with brain development at its most critical period, meaning it can ultimately affect future intelligence. This impaired development may result in the child's brain's never reaching its full potential for growth.

An important study of three hundred children reported in the *Lancet* showed that, on average, children who had been breastfed had an intelligence quotient (I.Q.) that was 10 percent higher than their counterparts who were fed on cow's milk, when tested at eight years of age.[111]

Why is consumption of cow's milk associated with this iron deficiency, which can restrain brain development? Cow's milk contains very little iron (about 0.5 mg per liter). Dr. Oski states that "milk is so deficient in iron that an infant would have to drink an impossible 31 quarts a day to get the government's recommended daily allowance (RDA) of 15 mg."[112] Additionally, only 5 to 10 percent of this iron is absorbed by the infant. To compound the problem, cow's milk's excessive protein and calcium interfere with the absorption of iron from other foods. Coupled with the fact that cow's milk can cause direct iron loss through intestinal bleeding, this would seem to stack the odds against an infant's immediate or long-term full health potential.

Although some parents hope to make up for potential iron deficiencies by feeding iron-fortified foods to their infants, this may not be an effective remedy. Even when infants are fed such foods, they may still suffer from iron-deficiency anemia if they are fed cow's milk. This suggests the blood loss from intestinal bleeding is so severe that it offsets supplemental iron.

Breast milk, on the other hand, has more iron than cow's milk, and is better absorbed by the infant, because nature formulated it to be so. It also does not cause the severe irritation to the gastrointestinal tissue (or the resulting blood loss and iron deficiencies) seen in children who are given cow's milk.

Constipation

Constipation is a well-known condition in which there is difficulty in eliminating hard waste from the body. Some parents describe their children not defecating for up to fifteen days. A number of studies show a relationship between consumption of cow's milk and constipation, and a marked improvement when the offending milk is removed.[113]

In a case reported in the *Journal of Allergy and Clinical Immunology*, a five-year-old boy was admitted to the hospital with constipation and anal fistula and fissures. The boy had already been admitted to the hospital when two months old for acute enteritis, and at six months for diarrhea. From ages six to 12 months, he was hospitalized on six occasions because of wheezing and bronchiospasms. At the age of two years and six months, he was admitted again, this time with anal fistula and fissures. At four years old, he entered the hospital yet again to have surgery performed on his fissures, which reappeared thirty days later. Finally, after all of these interventions, cow's milk was considered a suspect, and eliminated from his diet. Within two weeks, the boy's constipation corrected itself, and after two months, the anal fissures and fistula were healed completely.[114]

In another case reported in the *New England Journal of Medicine*, a double-blind, crossover study was performed with sixty-five children aged eleven to seventy-two months suffering from constipation. The children had failed to defecate for anywhere from three to fifteen days; forty-nine of them had anal fissures. All had been treated by gastroenterologists and given laxatives, but none had benefited from the treatment. The children were given either cow's milk or soy milk for two weeks, then no milk at all for one week. Then the feedings were reversed, so that those who had received soy milk were now fed cow's milk. While fed soy milk, 68 percent of the group (44 children) responded positively to the therapy, producing eight or more bowel movements during the second phase of the study. Further, in those who responded positively, anal fissures and pain with defecation were alleviated.[115]

Intestinal Obstruction

Another problem linked to consumption of cow's milk by infants is intestinal obstruction.[116] While constipation can occur even for extended time periods without pain, obstruction typically results in severe, focused pain.

Infants only absorb 60 to 70 percent of the butterfat in milk. The remaining 30 to 40 percent of fat turns into calcium soaps, and finally thick curds, which are believed to sometimes create a blockage. Symptoms of this blockage include abdominal distention, extreme weight loss, and vomiting. In some cases, the blockage is so significant it can be palpated (felt) in the lower abdomen area.

Colitis

Colitis, also known as inflammatory bowel disease, can result in bloody diarrhea, abdominal cramps, fever, and colic in infants. In the most extreme cases, known as *necrotizing enterocolitis,* the condition can result in death.[117] Although a number of potential causes have been identified, including the use of antibiotics, food allergy can instigate the condition.

In a study published in *Archives of Disease in Childhood,* researchers found an allergic reaction to foods was the cause of colitis in infants under the age of two. Cow's milk, the authors wrote, was the most common culprit. After it was excluded from the diet, the infants recovered completely.[118]

Remember that breastfeeding is best for the child, but it can pose a serious risk if the mother is still drinking milk, because allergenic bovine proteins consumed by a mother can pass into her breast milk.[119] In a case reported in *Clinical Pediatrics,* an exclusively breastfed four-day-old infant was admitted to the hospital with profuse rectal bleeding.[120] After performing a battery of tests, medical personnel determined that the infant's *hematocrit level** had fallen from just 38 percent to 30 percent in the previous eight hours.

Eventually, they learned that the mother had been consuming four to five glasses of milk a day. They determined that the offending proteins from the cow's milk eventually made their way into the mother's breast milk and affected the infant, who was severely allergic. The protein led to iron loss through intestinal bleeding.

Bovine Growth Hormone, IGF-1, and Children

In Chapter Five, we looked at some very serious risks that may be associated with consuming milk from cows treated with the bioengineered hormone

---

* Hematocrit level represents the volume of erythrocytes (mature red blood cells) in a given volume of blood after being packed by centrifuge. Normal hematocrit levels for a newborn range from 49 percent to 54 percent.

rBGH. These included heightened risk of breast cancer in women and of prostate cancer in men.

Milk produced by rBGH-treated cows may pose a special threat to children. According to cancer authority Dr. Samuel Epstein, milk from these cows may lead to "dangerous premature growth in infants." Dr. Epstein's note of caution is based upon the way rBGH appears to boost IGF-1 levels in cow's milk. Researchers already know that acromegaliacs — people who suffer from exaggerated growth of their hands, head and feet — are victims of excessive levels of IGF-1.[121]

Exposure to elevated levels of IGF-1 may also increase a child's susceptibility to developing cancer because fetuses and infants' breast cells are known to be highly sensitive to hormonal influences. There is concern that the cells may get "imprinted" by exposure to elevated IGF-1 levels; this "imprinting" may make the tissue highly sensitized to mammography, and to exposure to endocrine-disrupting industrial chemicals later in life. Ultimately, this may boost future risk of developing breast cancer.

Diabetes, Type I

Diabetes can severely compromise quality of life and result in premature death. Diabetes is the leading cause of blindness, and substantially increases the risk of heart disease, kidney damage, and, in extreme cases, amputation of limbs compromised by reduced circulation. There are two types of diabetes: Type I, or juvenile diabetes, and Type II, formerly called adult-onset diabetes. Since more and more younger people are now developing this second, more common version of the disease, it is now more appropriately referred to just as Type II.

Type I diabetes is primarily an autoimmune disease. It occurs when the body attacks itself. It is characterized by a damaged pancreas's inability to produce the hormone insulin. Insulin is responsible for metabolizing glucose (the body's source of fuel) out of the bloodstream and into cells. This is necessary after carbohydrate consumption, when blood glucose levels begin to rise. In Type I diabetes, the body fails to produce insulin, and the blood level of glucose (also known as blood sugar) begins to rise to dangerous levels.

In the case of Type II diabetes, the pancreas can still produce insulin. But the body does not respond to its presence as it should — a situation referred to as *insulin resistance*. Type II diabetes accounts for approximately 90 percent of all cases of the disease, and although its incidence is growing at an alarming rate, it can often be managed well by making healthful lifestyle choices. Essential to that lifestyle are a low-fat diet and a regular exercise program.

Type I diabetes presents a grimmer situation because, regardless of efforts made to modify their lifestyles, sufferers are relegated to a lifetime of multiple daily injections of insulin, insulin pump therapy, and constant glucose monitoring.

At the 59th Annual Scientific Sessions of the American Diabetes Association, scientists presented studies showing evidence that cow's milk presents a serious risk for an autoimmune reaction that may lead to the development of Type I diabetes in susceptible children.[122] The medical literature supporting this hypothesis is quite substantial;[123] there are now nearly a hundred studies on the subject, and the American Academy of Pediatrics has formally acknowledged the validity of the problem.[124]

The theory supporting this correlation takes us back to the discussion of beta-casomorphin-7 (BCM7) in the section on autism. In the case of type I diabetes, BCM7 happens to have a sequence of four amino acids identical to a sequence in GLUT2, the glucose-transporting molecule that resides in the insulin-producing (islet) cells of the pancreas. This sequence is believed to instigate an immune response to BCM7. However, since GLUT2 also has this same sequence, it too is suspect, and thus the insulin-producing cells it resides within are also attacked. In this response, the body's immune cells, called *T cells*, attack the islet cells of the pancreas over time. This damages the pancreas to the point where it can no longer produce enough insulin, and Type I diabetes results.[125]

One international study found that as milk consumption in a country rose, so did the incidence of Type I diabetes.[126] And, when we scan world populations, it becomes clear that the more cow's milk is consumed, particularly by children, the higher the incidence of juvenile diabetes.[127] For example, Finland has one of the highest intakes of dairy products in the world. Interestingly, the country also has the world's highest rate of insulin-dependent diabetes, with the disease afflicting forty out of every thousand children. And in Puerto Rico, where a surprising 95 percent of mothers feed their children cow's milk-based formulas instead of breast-feeding, the incidence of diabetes is almost ten times that of countries such as Cuba, where breastfeeding is almost ubiquitous.[128]

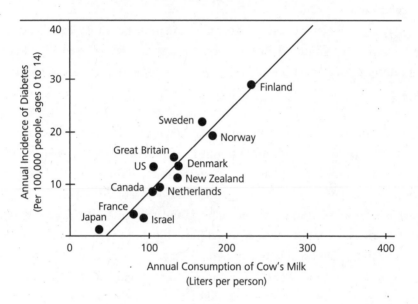

In one case researchers found that 51 percent of Type I diabetes suffer-ers had antibodies to beta-casein, compared to only 2.7 percent of controls subjects who were diabetes free.[129]

Finnish researchers looked at the risk of diabetes in 173 newborn chil-dren who each had a relative suffering with diabetes. In a double-blind study, half of the children were given, in addition to their mother's milk, a supplement based on cow's milk, while the other half were given a predi-gested formula. Neither the parents nor the researchers knew which child was receiving the standard cow's-milk supplement. In the eighty-four children consuming the predigested formula, three children developed antibodies seen in children who develop diabetes. However, in the group who received the standard cow's-milk formula, ten of the children had developed these antibodies.

A study of 142 diabetic children published in the *New England Journal of Medicine* found that all these children had substantial blood levels of antibodies to this same protein.[130] Researchers have shown that children with more types of autoimmune antibodies are more likely to eventually develop diabetes. In the Finnish study, three of the children had a single type of antibody, while the remainder had developed two or more different antibodies. Suvi M. Virtanen, a nutritional epidemiologist and coauthor of the Finnish study, says the presence of a single type of antibody in susceptible children places them at a 40 percent risk of developing Type I diabetes within a decade. If they have three types of antibodies, their risk of developing Type I diabetes climbs to between 80 and 90 percent.[131]

In another study, 725 children were first genetically tested to determine their susceptibility to diabetes. Then they were monitored for eleven years. The children who drank more than three glasses of milk a day had five times the risk of developing diabetes than children who drank less than three glasses.[132]

Apparently, the earlier a child is exposed to the protein, the greater the risk of an autoimmune response. An Australian study showed children given cow's-milk formula in the first three months of their lives were 52 percent more likely to develop diabetes than those not fed cow's milk. When asked what he thought of the hypothesized link between cow's milk and diabetes, Dr. Neville Howard, an Australian pediatric endocrinologist, replied, "There is a relationship to early weaning. Our epidemiology did show a significance of cow's-milk feeding as a factor in the development of Australian kids with diabetes."[133] Dr. Howard is leading researchers in the largest international study of its kind, including twenty countries, to see if conclusive evidence can be found.

So substantial is the evidence supporting the theory that proteins in cow's milk elicit diabetes that in 1994, the American Academy of Pediatrics issued this statement: "Early exposure of infants to cow's-milk protein may be an important factor in the initiation of the B-cell destructive process in some individuals .... The avoidance of cow's-milk protein for the first several months of life may reduce the later development of IDDM or delay its onset in susceptible people"[134]

Obviously, not all children exposed to cow's milk develop diabetes. So far, no one knows how to detect, in advance, which child will be susceptible to developing diabetes after exposure to cow's milk. Yet should parents knowingly take such a risk — possibly condemning their children to lives of exogenous insulin dependency, sharply reduced quality of life, and the further risk of many other health complications associated with diabetes?

Behavioral and Learning Problems

As we saw in the section on pesticide contamination of cow's milk in Chapter Six, American children are experiencing an epidemic of learning disabilities. It is estimated that twelve million Americans under the age of eighteen are suffering from one or more learning, developmental, or behavioral disabilities today.[135] The number of children diagnosed with ADHD alone rose from ninety thousand in 1990 to nearly six million in 1998.[136] It is difficult not to notice the reports of how contentious, angry, and downright violent a sizeable portion of the youth of America have become. Worse, newspapers and magazines are filled with stories of children committing heinous crimes, and generally disregarding authority figures in their lives.

A study from the *American Journal of Public Health* found that in two cities, 18 to 20 percent of fifth-graders were taking prescription drugs for behavioral problems.[137] Another study of a Michigan state Medicaid program found 223 children under age three who were already taking psychiatric medications, with 45 percent of the group receiving multiple drugs.[138]

From 1975 to 2000, US prescriptions for Ritalin climbed from 150,000 to over six million. By 2000, 85 percent of worldwide prescriptions for the drug were given to Americans, with about one in eight children receiving a prescription.[139] At least 2.5 million children are currently taking psychostimulant drugs such as Ritalin, Adderall-XR, and Concerta for their symptoms.[140] In 2005, an estimated $2 billion worth of medications for inattention alone were prescribed in the United States.[141] There are now at least twelve drugs approved for children by the FDA, including stimulants, antidepressants, mood stabilizers, antipsychotics, and antianxiety drugs.[142]

Ultimately, these drugs follow the traditional American medical model and treat symptoms — making children more compliant, calm, and focused — without addressing root causes. Many parents, and children, stand firmly by their use of prescription drugs as a critical aid providing improvements in various conditions. For some, there may be no more effective treatment. However, we should ask how many of these children (and adults) might benefit from an initial, thorough examination of the types and qualities of foods they consume, to identify deficiencies or excesses, allergic reactions, and exposures to contaminants, which may — individually or collectively —be causing disturbances in brain function.

All medications present the risk of side effects, and some of the psycho-stimulants, in particular, have been reported to increase the risk of sudden death[143] from heart failure, as well as depression, stunting of growth,[144] unintended weight loss,[145] emotional blunting,[146] and the development of tics similar to those seen in children with Tourette's syndrome.[147] One popular prescription has been shown to cause tumor growth in animals.[148]

Prescription medication has been the mainstay, and continues to be the first-line approach, in treating all sorts of psychological, behavioral, and learning disorders in children. Though there is still a great deal of reluctance to embrace the idea, it is now well documented that the foods we eat can have a profound impact on our moods and mental performance, our abilities to learn, and our behaviors.[149]

Foods have an effect on the physical nature and function of brain cells, on the balance of neurotransmitters, and even on the proper flow of blood and oxygen to the brain. In the same way the human heart can be choked by excesses of saturated fat and cholesterol, placing us at risk of heart disease, an unhealthful diet (or one containing undetected allergens) can expose us to irritating and possibly disabling immune reactions. Such a diet can also lead to deficits in nutrients critical to proper brain function, mood, and our general sense of well-being.[150]

Moreover, many foods today are laced with pesticide residues that may also interfere with proper nervous system function. An important example that is often overlooked is the fact that many children and adults are chronically exposed to low levels of *organophosphate* and *carbamate* pesticide chemicals through the foods they eat. By design, many of these chemicals interfere with the proper functioning of the nervous system. They do this by blocking the action of the enzyme *cholinesterase*, which is required to break down the neurotransmitter *acetylcholine*.[151] This neurotransmitter blockage disturbs nerve conduction. In cases of accidental poisoning by such chemicals, observed symptoms include muscle twitching, vision problems, hypertension, and mood swings. Might a child with a genetic predisposition, who is chronically exposed to such chemicals, display these symptoms in the classroom setting and be mistakenly diagnosed with a behavioral or learning disorder?

Obviously, many factors are contributing to the behavioral problems currently being seen in American children. These may include hyper-stimulation from technology, and even stress caused by the inappropriate, unachievable expectations many parents place on their children. The American Academy of Pediatrics has acknowledged that watching TV is not only inappropriate for young children, but actually changes the way in which their brains grow, resulting in attention problems later in life.[152]

To some, to suggest that food can affect mood and behavior, let alone scholastic performance, sounds too simple to be true. And other lifestyle modifications, such as limiting exposure to media, may be in order. But evidence suggests we may be able to make inexpensive yet powerful dietary modifications in both children and adults, to improve their performance and psychological wellness.

Can Foods Influence Behavior and Learning Ability?

Fifty years ago, physicians such as Dr. Frederic Speer and Dr. Albert Rowe documented in the medical literature the way foods can affect mood and behavior. But this idea was brought to the wider attention of parents and health-care practitioners in 1973. The messenger was a Californian allergist, Benjamin Feingold, M.D., who presented his information to the American Medical Association before publishing his related book, *Why Your Child Is Hyperactive*. Dr. Feingold's work focused primarily on the abundance of food additives, such as artificial coloring, sweeteners, and preservatives.

Thirty-seven years ago, a leading expert was already alarmed at the incidence of hyperactive and attention-deficient children![153] Dr. Feingold's work, focused on the powerful role foods and additives could play in a child's (or adult's) behavior, would be followed by that of other prominent physicians, including Drs. Doris J. Rapp, William Crook, Robert Mendelsohn, and Keith Conners.

Dr. Paul Buisseret, of Guy's, King's and St Thomas' School of Medicine in London, England, is another expert who shed light on the food-behavior relationship. While treating a group of seventy-nine children for abdominal pain, diarrhea, or constipation, he made an unexpected discovery. All of the children's conditions were relieved after cow's milk was removed from their diets. While he had fully expected to see improvements in the GI problems, Dr. Buisseret noted something else. Approximately one-third of these children happened to be suffering from psychological disturbances, which also improved significantly when the milk was removed from their diets.[154]

In another study, researchers studying chronic juvenile delinquents found that they consumed more than twice as much milk as their control-group counterparts.[155] Still another researcher, Alexander Schauss of Tacoma, Washington, author of the book *Diet, Crime, and Delinquency,* documents a relationship between dietary factors and violent and criminal youth. In some of his research, he compared delinquent children to children of a similar background who were not problematic, and noted the delinquent adolescents consumed ten times as much milk.[156] Exorbitant consumption of any food is often a flag for possible food allergy. One of the best-known pediatricians in the United States, a man who has had extraordinary results treating thousands of children, is Dr. William G. Crook. He reports the food most frequently causing allergies is cow's milk, followed by corn and sugar.[157]

Darrell Klute of Olean, New York, whose son, Jamal, had been diagnosed with severe allergy to cow's milk (among other foods), understands the food-behavior link well. Despite his diligent efforts to be sure his son's diet is free of all allergens, occasionally something slips by. He says within minutes of his son's ingesting an allergen, he becomes "uncontrollable."

The literature on the subject of child behavior is replete with such anecdotal accounts of children affected in powerful ways by the foods they eat. It seems that both children and adults can be affected — on a chronic low-grade level — by certain foods, which lead them to behave in undesirable ways. They can become irritable, fidgety, unruly, depressed, hyperactive, angry, or drowsy.

As the authors of a study in *Annals of Allergy* stated: "Through a simple elimination diet, symptoms can be controlled. Elimination of the causes of ADHD is preferable to the pharmacological therapy of this condition."[158] Some have suggested that as many as 75 percent of the children currently taking Ritalin may actually not need the drug, and could instead be treated simply, safely, and effectively through diet.[159]

If we use drugs to treat the symptoms of children's behavioral problems but fail to address the true causes, what long-term good are we doing them? Further, if the cause of a particular case is indeed dietary, and doctors fail to present dietary intervention as a treatment option, on what ethical grounds are they standing?

As we have seen earlier, despite the fact few parents are aware of the powerful role of food in their child's behavior, and few doctors suggest dietary changes as a treatment option, the medical literature is replete with well-conducted studies substantiating the fact that diet is a potentially critical player in behavioral disorders.

Doris J. Rapp, M.D., is a known expert in working with hyperactive children who has provided relief for thousands of children and their parents. She is the author of many bestselling books, including *Is This Your Child?* In the *Journal of Learning Disabilities* she described using double-blind studies to determine whether children are affected by food allergies. Her results are nothing less than fantastic. By addressing diet — particularly dairy products — she has helped children regain their focus and state of calm without resorting to medications.[160]

The March 1985 issue of the journal *Lancet* reported that sixty-two of seventy-six hyperactive children improved significantly when their diet was changed to remove cow's milk, among other foods. The January 1989 issue of *Journal of Pediatrics* reported that, in some cases, headaches and hyperactivity were related to diet. In the same month, the journal *Pediatrics* reported a ten-week study of twenty-four hyperactive children who were given a prudent diet free of likely antigens. More than half improved with the dietary changes.

Another study, published in the *Journal of Orthomolecular Psychiatry*, showed as many as 80 percent of a group of juvenile delinquents were found to have allergies to cow's milk; in some cases, the tendency for the youths to act out or become problematic could be predicted by the amount of cow's milk they were drinking.[161] Pediatrician William Crook was so convinced by the studies he was reading in the medical literature that he set up his own five-year clinical study of how dietary changes affected hyperactive children in his practice. An amazing 74 percent of the children exhibited a "clear-cut improvement" after common food allergens were removed from their diets. In Dr. Crook's study, cow's milk was an instigator in nearly 40 percent of cases.[162]

It's not just allergies that may take a toll on our children's nervous system and interfere with their ability to conduct themselves socially and academically. Additives such as coloring agents, preservatives, sweeteners (natural and artificial), and flavor enhancers may also be playing a role.

Research has shown that nutritional deficiencies early in life can increase the risk that a child will turn aggressive and violent. After tracking the nutritional, cognitive, and behavioral development of one thousand children for fourteen years, University of Southern California researchers reported those children who had experienced prior nutritional deficiencies were 41 percent more likely to show aggressive behavior than their well-fed counterparts. By age seventeen, they were 51 percent more likely to demonstrate violent and antisocial behaviors.[163] The researchers focused specifically on the childrens' and adolescents' tendencies to lie, cheat, get into fights, bully others, vandalize property, and use obscene language. The greater the number of indicators of malnutrition, the greater the antisocial behavior.

There are hopeful models in which children have been transformed by dietary changes. These stories offer a window into the potential that awaits us if we are simply willing to pay attention to what is going into our children's bodies.

One of the most exciting stories in recent years came from Appleton Central Alternative High School in Appleton, Wisconsin. ABC News reported it, but clearly not enough people heard the story. In its past, Appleton Central was a hotbed of violence. Children brought weapons to school, there were high rates of dropouts, expulsions, and drug use, and the principal's office was overrun with disciplinary concerns.

All this changed when a private company, Natural Ovens, was charged with overhauling the food program. They discarded pizza, French fries, sugar-laden sodas, and all entrees that contained chemical additives such as colorings and preservatives. In place of these foods, they provided purified water, real fruit juice, whole-grain breads, and bountiful offerings of fresh fruits and vegetables, among other things. They even went so far as to replace rectangular tables with round tables that allowed the children to interact more.

By all accounts, the dividends were enormous. School principal LuAnn Coenen reported, "I can say without hesitation that it's changed my job as a principal. Since we've started this program, I have had zero weapons on campus, zero expulsions from the school, zero premature deaths or suicides, zero drugs or alcohol on campus. Those are major statistics."[164] "Since the introduction of the food program," says teacher Mary Bruyette, "I have noticed an enormous difference in the behavior of my students in the classroom. They're on task, they are attentive. They can concentrate for longer periods of time. I don't have disruptions in class or the difficulties with student behavior I experienced before we started the food program."

When asked how the new foods were affecting them, one student, named Taylor, reported that she was "able to concentrate better" and was "not as tired" and had "more energy." Another student reported, "Now that I can concentrate, I think it's easier to get along with people."

Please understand that while cow's milk is consistently implicated as a leading cause of food allergy, and while allergy can manifest itself in a variety of symptoms — including behavioral problems and learning difficulties — milk is not the only food allergen that parents or doctors should consider. Besides the additives discussed earlier, potential food allergens include wheat, soy, citrus, and chocolate.

Discussion of these potential allergens goes beyond the scope of this book. However, I urge any concerned parent to look more deeply into this topic. Any adverse condition is worth addressing through dietary intervention before beginning prescription medications. For support, see the Resources section at the end of this book.

Overweight and Obese

As mentioned already, the American population is seriously overweight, and our children are no exception. Today 1 in 3 children and teens is overweight or obese.[165] With extra weight comes risk, not only for numerous health problems, but for social problems as well. Children can be brutal to overweight peers, and few things are as painful during childhood as being excluded from athletic games, parties, and other activities because of the restricted mobility a weight problem brings.

Such exclusion, and a general sense of not fitting in with others, may be why the Centers for Disease Control and Prevention found that children who perceived themselves as overweight are more than twice as likely to commit suicide as children of a healthy body weight.[166] Overweight children are also prone to grow up to become overweight adults, and to thereby live with elevated risks of cancer, heart disease, and other chronic conditions compromising the quality and length of their lives.

The additional protein and fat in cow's milk does no help at all to children struggling with their weight. The largest study of its kind, published in *Archives of Pediatrics & Adolescent Medicine,* reviewed more than twelve thousand children aged nine to fourteen from every state in the nation. It found that the more milk the children drank, the fatter they became — even if they followed the current federal recommendation of three daily servings. Children who drank low-fat milk were also at higher risk for weight gain, which suggests that the hormones in milk may be playing a bigger role than the fat itself.

Since there is no nutritional requirement for milk and since the risk for a host of health problems — including some cancers associated with milk consumption in adolescence[167] — rises with its consumption, why introduce a child to cow's milk in the first place?

In this chapter, we have reviewed the leading health problems in infants and children possibly associated with the consumption of cow's milk. While some of these problems, such as colic, gastrointestinal obstructions, and the like, can produce uncomfortable and irritating symptoms, a number of others, such as Type I diabetes and autism, have profound, lifelong implications for the sufferers and their families.

It would be a deeply unfortunate outcome for any child to have to suffer one of these conditions simply because their caregivers were unaware of the risks associated with cow's-milk consumption, or were under the impression that the risks were justified because of the fallacious belief that children require cow's milk to be healthy.

In the next chapter, we'll explore the real causes of osteoporosis, and look closely at the critical lifestyle factors the milk commercials and print ads, and even many well-intending doctors, never bring up.

Seven

The Real Causes of Osteoporosis

Dairy has been considered a health food, and that's an unfortunate myth.[1]
— T. Colin Campbell, Ph.D. Author, *The China Study*

In 1997, a study of calcium intake and bone health made national headlines. The study warned of an American epidemic of osteoporosis. The cause of this epidemic, the study suggested, was that Americans were "passing by the dairy case."[2] The study, and its conclusion, seemed to be a thinly disguised promotional campaign for the dairy industry. Yet when it was released to the press, numerous newspapers gave unquestioning endorsements. *The Oakland Tribune* titled its front-page article "Every Body *Still* Needs Milk,"[3] a modified version of the California Milk Advisory Board's famous marketing slogan.

The events mentioned above reveal a classic case whereby the results of a single study are released to the media, which in turn does little or no independent follow-up before relaying the data to the public, thereby confirming it. Had any of the newspaper editors chosen to do rudimentary research, they would have found a plethora of evidence refuting the study's claim. The headline-making story should be the fact that nearly 70 percent of the studies investigating whether cow's milk and calcium supplements truly make a substantial difference in the risk for bone fracture indicate they do *not*.

Is it shocking no major newspaper challenged the claim America's problem with osteoporosis is a consequence of not consuming the milk of another species? Yes. It is shocking that numerous credentialed, respected, well-meaning health-care professionals continue to believe and promote this idea with no scientific basis in fact, an idea that any serious investigative research would expose as fallacy. Unfortunately, it reflects the status quo of culture conditioned for decades by aggressive dairy industry advertising propaganda and special interest influence. In this matter of milk and human health, our collective common sense has been put out to pasture. Take a moment and ask yourself a simple question: *Does it really make sense that humans must "nurse" from cows for their entire lives to fulfill their calcium needs?* The idea is clearly preposterous. It is also scientifically refutable, as this book will show.

Since many people drink cow's milk believing it will protect them from osteoporosis, it is essential to understand this disease and its causes.

What Is Osteoporosis?

The term *osteoporosis* is familiar to millions of people. Many believe it is caused by a dietary calcium deficiency, and can be effectively treated by increased dairy and calcium intake. This prevailing theory is a new wives' tale propagated by the dairy industry and promoted by a poorly informed health-care system.

Osteoporosis — *osteo* meaning bone, and *porosis* meaning porosity — is the name for the progressive narrowing and increasing frailty of bones. It significantly increases the risk of bone fractures. As osteoporosis advances, the marrow cavity at the center of the bone becomes larger and the porosity of the bone increases, reducing its density and strength. (It should be noted that a certain amount of bone loss is a normal phenomenon in both men and women that occurs in the healthiest of humans as they age.)

Our skeletons are made up of two types of bone: *trabecular* (about 20 percent of bone) and *cortical* (about 80 percent). Trabecular bone comprises the "spongy" interior of the bone, forming a mesh-like inner structure. Cortical bone forms the denser, compact outer shell.

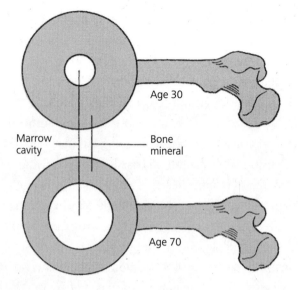

Fractures due to this thinning of the bones occur most frequently in the *distal forearm* (*Colles' fractures*) until about age seventy-five. From this age onward, the hip becomes the predominant site of fracture.[4] Other bones prone to fracture because of osteoporosis include the pelvis, rib, wrist, and vertebrae. One in three women and one in five men over the age of fifty can expect to sustain an osteoporotic fracture in their lifetime.[5]

In advanced cases, a mere sneeze can cause a rib to fracture, or lifting a heavy bag of groceries can fracture a wrist. When osteoporosis affects the spine, an individual vertebra can fail in what is called a compression fracture. Several compression fractures can result in a spinal slump, forming the hump in the upper back most often seen in elderly women, and therefore referred to as a "dowager's hump." According to the National Osteoporosis Foundation, twelve million Americans over the age of fifty are affected by osteoporosis today. Another forty million have osteopenia, or mild thinning of the bones, and most don't know it.

The Centers for Disease Control and Prevention report that 340,000 Americans a year — 80 percent of them women — are hospitalized, for an average of three weeks, due to a hip fracture. Only a quarter to a half of these people will regain their prior level of mobility;[6] one in five will be institutionalized due of their fracture.[7] Twenty percent of those who undergo surgery after a hip fracture die within twelve months of the procedure, a far greater percentage than their counterparts of the same age who have not suffered a fracture.[8] Another 700,000 will suffer a vertebral fracture, 250,000 a wrist fracture, and 300,000 will fracture another bone.

Globally, the World Health Organization estimates 30 percent of women over the age of fifty have osteoporosis.[9] Some authorities question the diagnostic criteria on which this shocking estimate is based. For example, osteoporosis is widely diagnosed based on criteria using "young white women" as a standard of bone health. Therefore, older women, postmenopausal women, and women of color cannot be certain that their diagnosis, and potential treatments such as prescription drugs, are justified.[10]

This statistical quibble doesn't negate the fact that osteoporosis is a major problem. But certain current admonishments to women should be carefully considered. These include recommendations to get a bone mineral density (BMD) test the day they reach menopause, if not sooner, and to begin taking prescription drugs to treat their "diseased" bones if test results do not reflect the density of a woman in her youth.

Surgery and one year of rehabilitation after a hip fracture cost an estimated $23,000, with the average lifetime cost of a hip fracture at $81,300.[11] Total health-care costs associated with treating osteoporosis in the United States now exceed $18 billion annually. To be sure, osteoporosis has also become big business for drugmakers. The world's seven major pharmaceutical markets now ante up some $9 billion for drugs aimed at combating osteoporosis.[12]

Even more disconcerting, osteoporosis rates are climbing in the United States and many other industrialized nations, with the disease striking an increasingly younger population.[13] In some areas, the rate has doubled in only a decade! If we remain on this trajectory, estimates are that the worldwide incidence of hip fracture will increase 240 percent in women and 310 percent in men by 2050.[14]

Osteoporosis isn't something one suddenly develops at a particular age. The disease develops over many years until it becomes noticeable. An osteoporotic fracture is an advanced symptom of an existing disease that has been quietly brewing in the bones for decades.

Hip Fracture Incidence by Region and Sex

Country	Women	Men
United States	101.6	50.5
New Zealand	96.8	35.2
Sweden	87.2	38.2
Jerusalem	69.9	42.8
United Kingdom	63.1	29.3
Holland	51.1	28.5
Finland	49.9	27.4
Yugoslavia	39.2	37.9
Hong Kong	31.3	27.2
Singapore	15.3	26.5
South Africa Bantu	5.3	5.6

* Per 100,000 population.

Our bones are living tissue. They are continually regenerated through-out our lifetime in a process called *remodeling*. This involves two kinds of special cells: *osteoclasts,* which break down and remove old bone material, and *osteoblasts,* whose purpose is to repair small-scale damage and build bone back up by secreting collagen, the foundation from which bone is formed once calcium has then been integrated. By age fifty, the structure of our bones will have been completely rebuilt about five times through this remodeling process. In osteoporosis, old bone is reabsorbed faster than new bone is formed.

Conventionally accepted risk factors for osteoporosis include a fam-ily history of the disease, being female, being Caucasian, being thin, early menopause, sedentary living, smoking, coffee, soft-drink and alcohol consumption, and hyperthyroidism. Yet, conventional wisdom also holds osteoporosis is largely a consequence of calcium deficiency, and the solu-tion, as the ads keep telling us, is to "bone up" with a sufficient quantity of milk each day. This erroneous concept has taken hold in the minds of health professionals and consumers alike.

The reality is that Americans consume plenty of calcium, rank among the top consumers of dairy products in the world, and also suffer one of the highest rates of osteoporosis in the world. Clearly, we are missing very important pieces of the puzzle. These pieces relate to the synergy or interplay of varied factors which combine to set the stage for osteoporosis.

Dr. Meir Stampfer,* professor of nutrition and bone health research at Harvard University's School of Public Health, says: "High milk intake and better bones is not well-established."[15] Dr. Walter Willett, principal investigator of the Harvard Nurses' Study, author of more than a thousand scientific articles, says, "Consuming plenty of dairy products is being portrayed as a key way to prevent osteoporosis and broken bones. But not only does this fail to fit the bill as a proven prevention strategy, it doesn't even come close." Dr. Willett leaves no question about what the enormous amount of research has taught him, saying, "Dairy products shouldn't occupy a prominent place in our diet, nor should they be the centerpiece of the national strategy to prevent osteoporosis."[16] Dr. Julian Whitaker, director of the Whitaker Wellness Institute, observes: "In only two generations, the rate of hip fractures in the United States has quadrupled, and it is currently one of the highest rates in the world. Americans are also near the top of the chart for dairy consumption." In his wellness letter, Dr. Whitaker asks, "Would someone please tell me why we keep telling our children that dairy foods strengthen their bones?"[17] The concern expressed by these medical authorities is echoed in the findings from numerous studies. Although there have certainly been studies that reach a conclusion supporting the message we keep hearing about consuming more dairy and more calcium, the clear majority simply do not support this conventional wisdom.

A case-control study of elderly Americans published in the *American Journal of Epidemiology* showed that supplementing the diet with cow's milk did not reduce the incidence of bone fracture at all.[18] The Harvard Nurses Study, which included more than seventy-seven thousand women, found women who drank three or more glasses of milk a day had no reduced risk of hip or arm fractures during a twelve-year follow-up period, when compared with women who drank little or no milk. The Health Professionals

---

* Dr. Stampfer was designated the most frequently cited scientist in the field of clinical medicine during the decade 1995–2005.

Follow-Up Study, also from Harvard researchers, reviewed forty-three thousand men, and found no relationship between calcium intake and bone fracture. A meta-analysis of six prospective studies involving a total of 39,563 men and women examined milk consumption and risk of bone fracture. The authors concluded that people who consumed less than one glass of milk a day were at no greater risk of bone fracture.[19] No significant benefit was shown even after adjustments were made for weight, menopausal status, smoking, and alcohol consumption. In fact, once again, the women who drank the most milk had a higher incidence of fractures than the women who drank no milk at all.[20]

An Australian study of elderly men and women reported in the *American Journal of Epidemiology* found no benefit to bone health in people who consumed more dairy products, while those with the highest levels of dairy consumption showed almost double the risk of bone fracture![21] Another Australian study found increased dairy consumption increased the risk of bone fractures in men and women. Those who consumed the most dairy products had double the rate of hip fracture of those who ate the least dairy products. A further Swedish study of sixty thousand women published in the journal *Bone* indicated no association between calcium intake and risk of bone fracture.[22]

One of the most telling discoveries about bone health came from Dr. T. Colin Campbell. Campbell is perhaps best known for heading the Study on Diet, Nutrition, and Disease in the People's Republic of China, considered the "Grand Prix" of such studies. His collected data have taught us a great deal about the relationship between lifestyle and risk of diseases, including osteoporosis. His research team's findings, detailed in an extraordinary book called *The China Study*, indicate that, "Ironically, osteoporosis tends to occur in countries where calcium intake is highest and most of it comes from protein-rich dairy products." (These countries include the United States, Canada, Sweden, the Netherlands, Australia, New Zealand, and northwestern Europe).[23]

In the US, where some reports have indicated the average daily calcium intake is 1,143 mg, osteoporosis is near-epidemic; in China, where intake is a modest 544 mg, the disease is quite rare. The Chinese data, Campbell said, "indicate that people need less calcium than we think and can get adequate amounts from vegetables."[24]

Bring on the Calcium, Right?

Calcium intake has become a national obsession in the United States, with a record 119 new calcium-fortified food products introduced in 1999 alone. Even over-the-counter drugs, including a famous brand of aspirin, are marketed as "great sources of calcium." Calcium is now added to candy bars, orange juice, breakfast cereal, margarine, and many other products. Many people take an excess of calcium, simply because it has been added to so many common foods.[25]

"The more calcium, the better" is the prevailing wisdom around bone health. But there is no compelling evidence to vindicate this obsession with a single nutrient. Blaming weak bones on low calcium intake is misleading to the public. If simply consuming more calcium were the answer to bone loss, then countries like America, where a relatively large amount of calcium is consumed, should have a correspondingly low incidence of bone fracture. But this is not the case, a fact many credible health writers, doctors, and nutritionists fail to notice.

Americans are routinely told they need to consume 800 to 1,200 mg of calcium a day. Yet women in the high-risk category for bone fracture who routinely consume more than 1,000 mg of calcium a day are actually found to be at increased risk of bone fracture.[26] The World Health Organization, in its own calcium recommendations, notes that countries with the highest calcium intake frequently have the highest hip-fracture rates. While calcium is important to bone health, drowning the body in calcium has proven to be a counterproductive strategy.

A number of studies over the last several decades on the relationship between calcium intake and bone health illuminate this conundrum. One of particular interest, which looked at Bantu women in Africa, was conducted by Dr. R. A. Walker and published in the journal *Clinical Science* in 1972. Walker reported that only 5 percent of Bantu women consumed more than 500 mg of calcium a day, with the majority consuming from 175 to 475 mg — a calcium deficiency by US standards. We would expect these calcium-deprived Bantu to show corresponding poor bone health. Instead, Dr. Walker found that the Bantu women were in excellent overall health, with very strong bones and teeth and a rare incidence of fractures. Even more confounding is the fact that Bantu women give birth to, and breastfeed, an average of six children in their lifetime — both processes which place great calcium demands on the mother.

A more recent survey found the average daily calcium intake of the general population of native South Africans to be a mere 196 mg, less than a fifth the intake of African Americans, who consume an average of 1,000 mg a day. Does the extra 804 mg give African Americans added protection against bone fracture? Apparently not — their bone fracture rate is nine times higher than their South African counterparts![27] These findings illustrate the fundamental fact regarding calcium and bone health — it's not the quantity of calcium we consume that makes bones healthy, but the quantity of calcium the body *retains*.

South African Bantus exemplify the fact that bone health can be maintained on a fraction of the US–prescribed calcium intake. And the women of Papua New Guinea show the Bantus are not an anomaly in this respect. American women consume thirty-two times more dairy than their sisters in Papua, and suffer forty-seven times the rate of broken hips.[28] On the other end of the scale, the Inuit population of northern Canada consumes an average of 2,000 mg of calcium per day, derived primarily from the many edible fish bones in their diet. That's 800 mg more than the inflated US recommended daily dosage. It may be no coincidence that the Inuit have one of the highest rates of osteoporosis in the world.[29] But despite their huge intake of calcium, most is washed away in their urine.

Is there something special about Bantu and Papuan women? Perhaps one secret of their bone health is that — like the women of Singapore, Spain, Yugoslavia, and other nations who share their low calcium intake and high bone health — they don't consume enormous quantities of dairy products.

Another well-known study on calcium intake and bone health was led by Dr. B. Lawrence Riggs at the famous Mayo Clinic. Dr. Riggs studied more than a hundred women between the ages of twenty-three and eighty-eight, whose calcium intake ranged from 269 to 2,000 mg a day. The women's bone density was measured regularly over a period of up to six years. Even when taking into account age, menopause status, and estrogen levels, Dr. Riggs reported: "We found no correlation between calcium intake levels and bone loss, not even a trend." When comparing women consuming 500 mg to those consuming 1,400 mg of calcium a day, the rate of bone loss was nearly identical![30]

More recently, the journal *Pediatrics* published the results of a large study of girls, aged twelve to eighteen, who were tracked for six years. Since the average female adolescent gains between 40 and 60 percent of her peak skeletal mass during this period, the intention of the study was to determine whether higher intake of calcium at this time of life would lead to greater bone density later in life — and presumably, a lowered risk of hip fracture. Calcium intake in the girls ranged 500 to 1,500 mg a day. "We were surprised to find our hypothesis refuted," reported the researchers. "Calcium intake was not associated with hip Bone Mineral Density at 18 years, or with total body bone mineral gain."[31]

	Average Calcuim Intake	Source of Calcuim	Incidence of Osteooporosis
USA	1,143 mg (milligrams)	Primarily Dairy Products	Epidemic
China	544 mg	Primarily Vegetables	Rare

Data derived from the Study on Diet, Nutrition, and Disease in the People's Republic of China.

What About Calcium Supplements?

If consuming lots of milk and dairy products isn't the bone health panacea we have been told it is, what about taking calcium pills? Selling calcium tablets is big business. Today, manufacturers move close to $200 million worth of them annually, and the demand continues to grow. Some twenty million American households are consuming calcium supplements.[32] Many people believe they will benefit by adding calcium to their diet in supplement form. A minority of studies show some benefit. Yet the majority of the research does not support supplementation as a means for preventing bone fracture. One reason may be the fact that calcium fortification, whether through calcium-rich foods or calcium pills, fails to address what appears to be the root cause of bone loss.

For example, in one study of calcium supplementation, women given 500 milligram of calcium supplements a day suffered bone loss at the same rate as their counterparts who took no supplements.[33] A Women's Health Initiative (WHI) study reported in the *British Medical Journal* found no difference in the risk of bone fracture between women receiving 1,000 mg of calcium in pill form and 800 I.U. (International Units) of vitamin D, and women who did not receive these supplements. The 3,300 women participants underwent a seven-year randomized follow-up study. Researchers found "no evidence that calcium and vitamin D supplementation reduces the risk of clinical fractures in women with one or more risk factors for hip fracture."[34] Another double-blind study of post-menopausal women given either 2,000 mg of calcium supplementation or a placebo (a "dummy pill") showed the same rate of bone loss for both groups.[35]

Can Excess Calcium Be a Problem?

It appears our excessive calcium consumption, whether by way of foods or supplements, isn't helping our bones stay strong and healthy. So we must consider the potential problems and effects of calcium mega-dosing. Mark Hegsted, former Harvard University professor of nutrition, emeritus, cautioned: "It will be embarrassing enough if the current calcium hype is simply useless; it will be immeasurably worse if the recommendations are actually detrimental to health."[36] How could excess calcium be detrimental?

We've seen studies showing societies consuming large amounts of calcium frequently show corresponding higher rates of hip fracture — in some cases, the highest rates. Besides not reliably eliminating the risk of fractures, studies have shown that calcium supplements may contribute other problems, such as iron deficiency. Researchers at Tufts University found iron retention decreased by 45 percent in post-menopausal subjects who were given 500 mg of supplemental calcium with meals. Other research has shown that calcium supplements in doses of between 300 and 600 mg, taken with meals, can reduce iron absorption by up to 62 percent.[37] A large number of American women are already nearly iron-deficient, and don't need this additional factor working against them.

Studies have also confirmed that most calcium supplements are contaminated with lead — extraordinary amounts, in some cases. Some calcium supplements have as much as 20 micrograms of lead per daily dose of calcium![38] Lead accumulates in the bones and is toxic to humans, particularly children. Since an estimated 50 percent of pregnant women take calcium supplements, this presents a potentially serious problem to mothers and their unborn children. Lead can damage the developing nervous system of a fetus or a growing baby.

Some researchers believe the body's ability to absorb calcium, and form new bone, may actually be degraded by habitual excess consumption through diet and supplements. Over time, this calcium onslaught may prematurely exhaust the reproductive capacity of the osteoblasts, our bone-building cells, thus diminishing new bone-matrix formation and resulting in porous, fracture-prone bones. Studies show that excessive calcium supplementation can also interfere with parathyroid hormone, further disrupting bone integrity.[39]

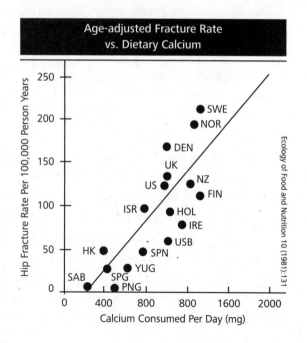

Excessive calcium consumption may also disturb the body chemistry in ways that interfere with the absorption and utilization of other important elements essential to bone health and integrity, such as magnesium. When magnesium is in short supply, calcium is more likely to end up being deposited in soft tissues, contributing to the risk of kidney stones, arthritis, and atherosclerosis. Calcium excess may also compromise the immune system, our first line of defense against disease. Magnesium plays an important role in the development and proper functioning of immune cells. Yet excess calcium displaces magnesium ions, and in doing so, may impair the function of key immune factors such as *leukocytes* (white blood cells). [40]

The True Causes of Osteoporosis

As with most degenerative diseases, osteoporosis is a multi-factorial disease, meaning many factors contribute to the overall risk. These may include genetics, race, and sex, as well as lifestyle factors such as exercise, diet, smoking, alcohol consumption, and others. Let's examine these risk factors to see how they may be taking a toll on our bones. Research indicates that one of the most important risk factors is an excessive intake of dietary protein in general, and, perhaps more importantly, of total protein derived from animal products.[41]

Too Much Protein

We covet protein in America. Not only do we eat protein-rich meals three or more times a day, but many of us also consume protein supplements in the form of powders, pills, and "energy bars." Moreover, over the past decade, there has been an unfortunate resurgence of fad diet books touting the alleged virtues of a high-protein diet, and judging from book sales, Americans are eating up this nutritional lore. Today, the average American's total protein intake can be excessive, up to four times the body's actual needs. And now the dairy industry has unveiled a new milk, directed at children, containing four additional grams of protein per serving.[42] "Protein is a nutrient that is so highly regarded by everyone, including investigators themselves," says Dr. T. Colin Campbell, "that there is a tremendous bias against considering its ability to control disease."

While protein is an essential nutrient, and it's important to bone health, the human body needs a relatively small amount to perform its tasks. When that amount is exceeded, as is common in the United States, the likelihood of disease rises. Researchers have found that excess protein, particularly when derived from animal sources, leads to a condition known as *metabolic acidosis*. When this condition is prolonged, it ultimately results in *acid-induced bone dissolution*.[43] Simple biochemistry will explain why.

For the myriad chemical reactions that occur in the body, a slightly alkaline state is required, with a pH (potential hydrogen) level slightly above 7.0. The pH is simply a reference to the acid-base balance of bodily fluids, including blood, urine, saliva, and extra- and intracellular fluids. Using the kidneys, lungs, and other systems, the body works to maintain an acid-base balance as a matter of course.

All foods vary in their potential to promote an acid or alkaline ash.* Generally speaking, fruits and vegetables are alkalinizing, whereas meats, poultry, seafood, grains, some legumes and highly processed foods are acidifying. To buffer acidity, the body draws upon *alkalinizing* calcium, potassium, and magnesium, which are eventually excreted in the urine.[44] The storehouse for 99 percent of our calcium is the skeletal system — the bones. In an effort to restore an alkaline state, the body will mobilize calcium by calling upon the osteoclast cells to break down bone and free the calcium. If this happens occasionally, it is not of great concern. The problem is that many of us are consuming a highly acid-producing diet on a regular basis, so our bodies are literally hemorrhaging calcium around the clock. Due to this compensatory response, over a prolonged period, the mineral content in bone, and bone mass, will begin to drop.[45] With age, our body's ability to excrete acid declines due to a decrease in kidney function.[46]

Numerous studies dating back as far as seventy years document how, as dietary animal protein intake increases, more calcium is excreted in the urine.[47] The following graph, which appeared in the journal *Calcified*

---

* The acid-producing potential of a food is calculated using the Potential Renal Acid Load (PRAL) formula which determines its acid or alkaline load. Negative numbers mean the food is alkaline-forming; positive numbers mean the food is acid-forming.

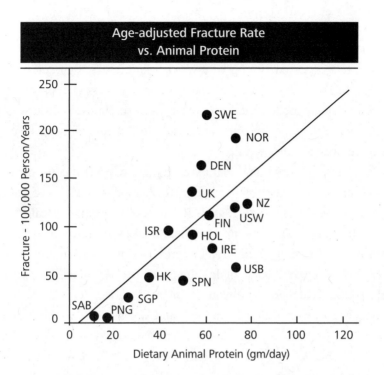

Age-adjusted Fracture Rate vs. Animal Protein

Tissue International in 1992, relates protein consumption to incidence of hip fracture.

To examine the influence of protein on calcium balance, researchers placed individuals on a high-protein diet containing a progressively larger calcium intake. Surprisingly, even when the subjects were consuming 1,451 mg of calcium a day, they were still in negative calcium balance![48]

In response to their findings, the researchers stated: "Our data indicate that high-protein diets cause a negative calcium balance to occur even in the presence of more than adequate dietary calcium. Osteoporosis would seem to be an inevitable outcome of continued consumption of a high-protein diet".

This conclusion was stated another way in the _American Journal of Clinical Nutrition:_ "The consumption of high-calcium diets is unlikely to prevent the negative calcium balance and probable bone loss induced by the consumption of high-protein diets."[49] If you take nothing else away from this book, remember these two quotes. Together with sedentary living, substantial evidence indicates this to be the core factor in why Americans are at such high risk for bone fracture.

In a related statement, noted physician and best-selling author Dean Ornish, M.D., writes: "The real cause of osteoporosis in this country is not insufficient calcium intake, it's excessive excretion of calcium in the urine. Even calcium supplementation is often not enough to make up for the increased calcium excretion."[50]

Some research has found that for each gram of protein consumed, calcium excretion increases by 1 to 2 mg;[51] the National Academy of Sciences maintains the figure is 1 to 1.5 mg. Regardless of how much calcium we add, either through diet or supplementation, we will continue to lose calcium unless we reduce our protein consumption sufficiently.[52] With all other factors remaining equal, doubling your protein intake may increase the amount of calcium lost in your urine by 50 percent.[53]

Suggested protein intakes for men and women are 56 grams and 44 grams a day, respectively. Yet most American men and women exceed this, consuming between 70 and 100 grams of protein.[54] Those recurrently popular high-protein diets recommend a protein intake of between 71 and 162 grams a day.[55]

The sample menu below illustrates how easy it is to exceed the suggested protein intake by following a typical Western diet.

BREAKFAST
3-egg cheddar cheese omelet, 25 grams protein
2 slices Canadian bacon, 12 grams protein
1 cup hash brown potatoes, 2 grams protein
1 cup orange juice, 1.4 grams protein

LUNCH
Cheesecake Factory's Santa Fe Grilled Chicken Salad, 86 grams protein
Chocolate Peanut Butter Cookie Dough Cheesecake, 17 grams protein
Iced tea, 0 grams protein

DINNER
6-ounce steak, 42 grams protein
Medium baked potato with 1 oz sour cream, I tablespoon butter,

7.3 grams protein

1 cup broccoli, 1 pat butter, 6 grams protein

1 8-ounce glass whole milk, 8 grams protein

DESSERT

2 scoops Cold Stone Creamery Amaretto ice cream, 10 grams protein

Suggested daily protein intake for a man/woman: 56/44 grams

Total protein intake from the sample menu: 216.7 grams

A study in the *Journal of Nutrition* further illustrates this phenomenon. Women participating in this study first consumed 46 grams of protein daily for sixty days. Then their diet was adjusted to 123 grams of protein daily for another sixty days. During both phases of the diet, their intakes of calcium, phosphorus, and magnesium were kept constant (at 500, 900, and 350 mg a day, respectively). Researchers discovered that when the subjects increased their protein intake to 123 grams a day, the amount of calcium they excreted in their urine went from 113 to 212 mg daily.[56] In another study, researchers examined women who were typically consuming one and a half times the recommended protein intake of 0.8 grams per kilogram of body weight. Their protein intake was adjusted to meet the RDI. Calcium excretion levels were measured before and after the dietary change. The researchers found that after the reduction in protein, calcium excretion dropped by 32 percent and bone loss by 17 percent.[57]

Animal Protein

It's easy to exceed your protein needs and potentially boost your risk of osteoporosis if you consume the average American meat- and dairy-centered diet. Many Americans eat meat or dairy products in some form at least three times a day. Some studies have shown that vegetarians have a greater bone density than omnivores even when their calcium intake is equivalent.[58]

While excess protein in general causes calcium losses due to the acid production, animal protein, with its higher content of sulfur-containing amino acids that are metabolized to sulfuric acid,[59] appears to worsen the leaching process by creating an increasingly acidic environment.[60] Conversely, plant foods contain a good supply of minerals that are effective at neutralizing the acid formed by animal protein. As stated in *Calcified Tissue International*: "Omnivore diets can induce a more negative calcium balance than less-acidogenic vegetarian diets matched for total protein."[61] The World Health Organization has formally recognized this relationship, stating, "the accumulated data indicate that the adverse effect of protein, in particular animal (but not vegetable) protein, might outweigh the positive effect of calcium intake on calcium balance."[62]

Over time, this calcium loss leads to a decline in both the mineral content and mass of the bone. As animal consumption goes up, so does the rate of fracture. Yet as vegetable-derived protein goes up, fracture rate drops. Researchers from the University of California, San Francisco conducted a study of hip fracture rates in elderly women worldwide. In the thirty-three countries they surveyed, they found that the highest rates of hip fracture occurred in those countries where animal protein consumption was the highest. In the countries where hip fracture incidence was the lowest, vegetable protein exceeded animal protein intake. "Over decades," stated the authors, "the magnitude of daily positive acid balance (blood acidity) may be sufficient to induce osteoporosis. Moderation of animal food consumption and an increased ratio of vegetable/animal food consumption may confer a protective effect."[63]

By age sixty-five, women who have followed a meat-centered diet have lost, on average, 35 percent of their bone mass, while women who have followed a plant-centered diet have only lost about half of that amount: 18 percent. Registered dietician Bob LeRoy says: "Epidemiologists have found more evidence linking osteoporosis risk with animal protein consumption than with any other food factor, plausibly explaining the irony that most abundantly calcium consuming nations endure the most broken hips."[64] Dr. Campbell adds, "The correlation between animal protein [intake] and fracture rates in different societies is as strong as that between lung cancer and smoking."[65]

In a National Institutes of Health study published in the *American Journal of Clinical Nutrition*, researchers found that women who derived the most dietary protein from animal sources had three times the rate of bone loss, and 3.7 times the rate of hip fractures, compared to women who obtained most of their protein from vegetable sources.[66]

Research consistently shows that those populations deriving the greatest amount of their protein from animals have the highest incidence of hip fractures.[67] Furthermore, people who derive the greatest amount of protein from meat may lose bone mass nearly four times as fast as those who consume the least meat.[68]

In parts of the world where protein is consumed in moderation — particularly areas where it is derived from plant sources — osteoporosis is not nearly the problem it is in the United States.[69] Even when protein is eaten beyond basic needs, if it comes from plant sources, the leaching process is minimized.[70]

Rates of hip fracture in Chinese women are a fraction of those for American women of comparable age.[71] Osteoporosis rates for women in Yugoslavia, Singapore, and Chile are also significantly less than rates for women in the United States.[72] Rates are lowest in Africa[73] where, as in China, dairy is not a staple food for most people. The average animal-based protein intake in Africa is also a fraction of what it is in America.[74] Other factors, such as the level of physical exercise, also play an integral role in these statistics, but this does not diminish the significance of dietary choices.

By modifying our protein intake, both its source and its quantity, we can significantly reduce a major risk factor for osteoporosis and other diseases. Studies show that these simple dietary modifications minimize our loss of calcium and improve overall bone health. One study reported in the *American Journal of Clinical Nutrition* found that eliminating animal protein from the diet cut calcium loss by more than 50 percent.[75]

The state of acidosis caused by excess consumption of protein, in particular animal protein, has two other deleterious effects. First, it promotes osteoclastic action and suppresses osteoblastic action;[76] you will recall that osteoclasts are responsible for breaking down and removing old bone material, while osteoblasts do the opposite, repairing tiny structural damage and rebuilding new bone. Second, in experimental models researchers have noted that acidosis can lead to skeletal muscle catabolism, that is, the atrophy of skeletal muscles, which decreases muscle mass.[77] It has been theorized that the body does this to use glutamine from muscle to produce the ammonia needed to excrete the acid. So while bone is being depleted to counter the acidosis, so may be muscle. This may be an overlooked factor in elderly people's susceptibility to falling, since often it is the fall that precipitates the fracture and not the other way around.

Acid Diet
↓
Systemic Acidity
↓
Increased osteoclast activity (bone break down)
↓
Increased urinary calcium excretion (loss of calcium)
↓
Decreased osteoblast activity (bone formation)
↓
Reduced bone mineral content and bone mass
↓
Muscle catabolism (breakdown)
↓
Decreased stability
↓
Increased risk of fall
↓
Increased risk of bone fracture

The ideal is to be sure that your diet is rich with alkalinizing foods that can offset the effect of acidifying foods. This means eating a diet that is rich in fruits and vegetables and avoiding the foods that contain excessive levels of animal protein, sodium, and sugar, and a dearth of agents that promote an alkaline state. More specifically, it means cutting back dramatically on meats, seafood, dairy products and processed foods.

Fruits and vegetables come in a great package. Along with their health-supporting fiber and their protective phytochemicals, they are rich in the vitamins and minerals essential to bone health and that promote an alkaline state. In Chapter Nine you'll find a comprehensive list that identifies which foods are most acidifying and which are most alkalinizing.

Sodium

It is common knowledge that a high-sodium diet is unhealthy, the primary concern being sodium's propensity to increase blood pressure. Yet we now know that excess sodium also plays a negative role in bone health.[78] High sodium diets seem to encourage calcium loss. And a high sodium/ high protein diet, which is quite common in the US, packs a double whammy.[79]

Studies show that for each gram of sodium one consumes, approximately 15 mg of calcium will be excreted from the body.[80] For each gram of sodium consumed beyond actual needs, an adult women could lose an additional 1 percent of her bone mass per year.[81] Although we need no more than 1,000 mg of sodium daily, the average American consumes 3–4,000 mg, and some as much as 8,000 mg![82] Some fast-food burgers and other heavily salted dishes contain over 1,200 mg just by themselves. We don't know exactly why sodium accelerates calcium loss. But we know that it does. We also know that when excess sodium is present, the kidneys' blood filtration rate increases considerably, while their capacity to capture calcium and return it to the bloodstream is diminished. The table below shows how easy it is to overload on sodium.

Sodium Content of Some Common Foods

Food Item (and Serving Size)	Sodium Content (Typical)
Soy sauce, 1 Tbs	1,200 mg (milligrams)
Canned tomato juice, 6 oz.	659 mg
Bacon, 2 slices	274 mg
Canned chicken noodle soup, 1 cup	1,107 mg
Corn chips, 3 oz.	693 mg

A study published in the *New England Journal of Medicine* in 2010 reported that reducing the amount of sodium in our diet by just a half-teaspoon of sodium a day could prevent almost a hundred thousand heart attacks a year.[83] Not a bad dividend for improving bone health.

Alcohol

The majority of studies show that alcohol harms bone health, but not all show an increase in risk of bone fracture.[84] Alcohol negatively affects the bones in a number of ways. First, it interferes with the function of osteoblasts, which are essential to new bone formation.[85] Alcohol also undermines bone health by inhibiting the absorption, and accelerating the excretion, of several nutrients essential to bone health, including vitamin C, zinc, copper, calcium, and magnesium. In excess, alcohol can also damage the liver, which plays a key role in metabolizing vitamin D, another element essential to bone health. People who consume large amounts of alcohol tend to have poor diets, and are therefore already likely to be deficient in nutrients important to bone health. Finally, alcohol consumption can compromise our sense of balance and coordination, and thereby increase our risk of falling.

Smoking

Smoking significantly contributes to poor bone health. Nicotine reduces the sensitivity of receptors for certain calcium-regulating hormones. And many toxic chemical additives in cigarettes, such as cadmium and lead, also undermine bone health.

A study of smoking/nonsmoking identical twins showed a 44-percent increased risk of bone fracture in the twin who smoked long-term.[86] It is estimated a woman who smokes a pack of cigarettes a day in her adulthood will lose up to 10 percent additional bone mass by menopause.

The best evidence for the role of smoking in bone deterioration comes from a meta-analysis of twenty-nine existing studies, which found one in eight hip fractures could be attributed to smoking.[87] Regardless of age, the risk of bone fracture is greater for smokers. But between the ages of sixty and eighty, the elevation in risk goes from 17 percent to 71 percent.[88] Smoking and alcohol consumption significantly increase the risk of osteoporosis in men. Dr. Charles W. Slemenda and colleagues, of the Indiana

University School of Medicine, have shown these detrimental practices outweigh heredity as male risk factors.[89]

Refined Sugar

As we saw above, the average American consumes 390 soft drinks per year. Now consider that the average carbonated soft drink contains about ten teaspoons of sugar! In addition to the many health problems sugar is known to cause, sugar interferes with calcium absorption, thereby increasing the risk of osteoporosis.[90] Sugar is acidic, so its consumption makes the body increasingly acidic. As mentioned, the body prefers an alkaline state, and to achieve this, buffers acidity, ultimately drawing on calcium. The more sugar we eat, the more imbalanced our body chemistry becomes, and the less our body is able to utilize minerals found in healthy foods.

Caffeine

Caffeine delivers more than a "rush" to the user. In addition to raising cholesterol and taxing the adrenal glands, this widely used stimulant causes the body to excrete calcium in the urine.[91] A number of studies show that the more caffeine a person consumes, the more difficult it is to retain calcium.[92] Some studies have shown that caffeine consumption lowers bone mineral density, potentially increasing the risk for fracture.[93] Others have specifically linked caffeine consumption to a greater risk of bone fracture.[94] However, several other studies have not shown either association.

It's estimated that a hundred million Americans consume three to four cups of coffee a day, which adds up to forty-three gallons a year.[95] At 90 to 150 mg of caffeine per cup, this is an enormous amount of caffeine, even before factoring in the caffeine in sodas, teas, chocolate, many common medications, and even some bottled waters. Moreover, a cup of coffee used to mean a five-ounce serving; these days it's not unusual to see people nursing a thirty-ounce cup. One study showed that two cups of coffee a day could result in the loss of an additional 15 mg of calcium. Another study found that women who consume four cups of coffee a day triple their risk of hip fracture, compared to women who drink little or no coffee.[96] There will be more studies evaluating this relationship and hopefully a more definitive finding will become evident. For now, given that osteo-porosis is a multifactorial disease involving a number of lifestyle factors, it would seem prudent to take into consideration the potential role of caf-feine and decrease your caffeine intake.

Dieting

It is estimated that nearly half of American women consume less than 1,500 calories a day in an effort to achieve and maintain a slim figure. Some con-sume far fewer. This fixation with dieting poses two threats to bone health. First, extremely low-calorie diets often cause the menstrual period to cease, which encourages bone loss. Second, ultra-low-calorie diets virtually assure an inadequate supply of all of the nutrients essential to bone health.

Over the last decade a storm of best-selling books have touted high-protein diets as the solution to body-weight problems. As you now know, a high-protein diet virtually guarantees a negative calcium balance. These medically inappropriate fad diets do more harm than good, and their calcium and bone-depleting effects can have lifelong, even crippling consequences.

Anorexia

Most women with anorexia nervosa — the intentional, severely restricted intake of food — also suffer from detrimental bone loss. The condition reduces levels of circulating estrogen to as much as one third of the normal level, which adversely affects calcium balance. Anorexic women tend to absorb less and excrete more calcium.[97] This extremely serious disorder requires intervention by experienced specialists.

Hyperthyroidism

Hyperthyroidism is a condition in which the body secretes excessive levels of thyroid hormone. This condition causes more bone to be degenerated than is rebuilt.

Hysterectomies

The United States has more hysterectomy operations than any other nation; by age sixty, more than half of American women have had their uterus removed. Even if the ovaries are left intact, bone loss often accelerates soon after this procedure. This is because after as many as half of all hysterectomies, the ovaries stop functioning prematurely, which in turn prematurely accelerates bone loss.[98]

Heavy Metals

Aluminum is hazardous to humans in many ways, not the least being its possible influence on brain degeneration. But aluminum also promotes calcium loss, reduces calcium absorption, and interferes with the mineralization process and the ability of bones to self-repair.[99] Most aluminum exposure comes from contaminated foods, aluminum foil, aluminum-containing antacids,[100] aluminum cookware, conventional antiperspirants, unfiltered drinking water,[101] and conventional baking powder. It is possible, with some effort, to avoid all these sources.

Cadmium also alters calcium metabolism, and may cause damage to the kidneys. Cadmium reaches us through cigarette smoke, pesticides, fertilizers, gasoline, paint, and the incineration of waste.

Lead inhibits calcium absorption and suppresses vitamin D function. It also accumulates in the bone, displacing calcium. Lead is one of the most pervasive contaminants of our environment. Enormous amounts of this heavy metal were deposited in our air and soils from the leaded fuels used prior to the 1980s. Today, lead is found in older household paints, leaded crystal (glassware and vases), unfiltered drinking water, pottery glazes, pesticides, hair-coloring agents, and food cans.

Medications

Some medications are known to increase the risk of bone fracture, either by accelerating bone loss or by interfering with proper calcium metabolism. These include anti-seizure and anti-anxiety medications, corticosteroids,[102] anti-coagulants, thyroid hormone,[103] aluminum-containing antacids,[104] and possibly thiazide diuretics. In the first year of taking a corticosteroid prescription, we may lose up to 14 percent of bone mineral content. Recent findings have also shown a link between a popular cardiac medication and a 25-percent increased risk of bone fracture in men.[105] If you are taking any of these medications, you may wish to ask your physician if there are alternatives that are not detrimental to bone health.

Lack of Exercise

Exercise is a major factor in keeping bones strong. Unfortunately, too many public health organizations and health practitioners choose to promote milk and yogurt rather than spread the word about how truly powerful exercise can be in lowering the risk of bone fracture. It may be the ever-larger TVs and the endless array of channels keeping us anchored to the couch, or our computers and video games, or the increasing periods of time many of us spend sitting in a car, bus or train during our daily commutes, but Americans are getting less exercise than ever. According to the Centers for Disease Control and Prevention, 55 percent of Americans don't get the minimum weekly exercise for disease prevention and 26 percent get no exercise at all.

Have you ever broken an arm or a leg, and had that limb in a cast for a few weeks or months? Remember how the muscle looked when your doctor finally removed the cast? Chances are it had atrophied and was noticeably smaller than the other limb you had been using. Like muscles atrophied in a cast, bones become frail and even smaller with disuse. To remain strong, they must have weight bear down on them through some form of exercise. There is a direct relationship between moderate bone stress and bone strength, because weight-bearing exercise stimulates the tissue's electrical potentials and facilitates production of new and stronger bone.[106] Without this moderate stress, bones will de-mineralize.

Active individuals who exercise regularly generally have up to 40 percent greater bone mass than their peers who don't exercise.[107] That's an enormous protective advantage! The most physically active adolescents will have greater bone density at age eighteen than their sedentary counterparts,[108] and will carry this bone-health advantage into adulthood. Numerous long-term studies of tens of thousands of people from all over the world have shown the benefits of frequent exercise. Consistently, we see a 40- to 60-percent reduction in risk of fracture. And the benefit carries over from youth to late in life, as those who exercised and were most physically active in their youth see a large reduction in risk later on. One case-control study found that by age forty-five, women who managed to exercise at least four times per week as teenagers had one-fourth the bone-fracture risk of those who exercised only once a week.[109] Other studies have shown that people with the greatest level of physical activity in their youth reduced their risk of bone fracture by as much as 60 percent, compared to those least active. In addition to increasing bone mass and strength, regular exercise helps one keep muscles strong and retain balance and coordination. More often than not, bone fractures are precipitated by a fall. So if we can keep our muscular strength, coordination, and sense of balance, we can reduce the risk of falling in the first place.

We have learned about inactivity and bone health from the space shuttle missions. On Earth, gravity ensures that all we need to do is move our bodies — by walking, jogging or running, or climbing steps. But NASA space physiologists have determined that in space, the lack of gravity leads to bone under-stimulation, which causes astronauts to lose bone mass through mineral depletion at a rate of 1 to 1.5 percent a month, mostly in the hip and lower spine. In 1996, astronaut Norman Thagard lost 11.7 percent of his bone minerals during an extended, 115-day stint in space. Researchers at Johnson Space Center have developed and use an array of space exercise equipment, including a special bicycle built for two, to help astronauts maintain their bone health while in orbit.

Even if you bypassed exercise as a teen, you can still significantly increase your bone mass today through weight-bearing exercises. When it comes to strengthening bones, a little exercise can go a long way. In one study, a program of weight-bearing exercise increased participants' bone mass by 5 percent in as little as nine months.[110] Another study showed women who exercised three times weekly for twenty-two months increased their bone mass by more than 6 percent, while a counterpart group of sedentary women lost bone mass in the same period.[111] Another study, conducted at the University of Toronto, showed a 7.5 percent increase in bone mass in just twelve months among post-menopausal women between the ages of fifty and sixty-two who exercised regularly.[112] In a study at a Toronto hospital, an 8-percent increase in bone mass was found over the same period.

Even eighty-year-old women have increased their bone mass with as little as thirty minutes of exercise, three times a week.[113] Most studies have shown that people can increase their bone density from 1 to 7 percent with an exercise regime lasting six months to a year.

Women who are more active not only build stronger bones, but suffer fewer fractures.[114] Athletes are even better off, with bone mass as much as fifty percent greater than that of non-athletes. It has been estimated for each 1 percent bone mass is increased, the risk of bone fracture decreases by 6 percent![115] So a 5-percent increase is theoretically good for a 30-percent reduction!

A study published in *Pediatrics,* the official journal of the American Academy of Pediatrics, highlighted the bone-building benefits of incorporating exercise early in life.[116] The study tracked a group of girls for six years, from ages twelve to eighteen — again, the critical period in which young girls acquire between 40 and 60 percent of their lifetime skeletal mass. Those who exercised regularly had greater bone density by age eighteen than their sedentary counterparts. The researchers discovered that the dietary intake of calcium had no impact on bone density. Instead, the girls' involvement with sports and exercise was the decisive factor and primary predictor of bone growth in adulthood.[117]

Evidence clearly shows that it is never too late to benefit from the bone-building effects of exercise. Since her diagnosis of breast cancer in 1982, Ruth Heidrich, author of *A Race for Life,* has won nearly a thousand trophies and medals for marathon and triathlon competitions. Even more impressive, despite a family history of osteoporosis, she has consistently increased her bone mass since her forties. At age sixty-three, she retained a bone mass greater than that of the average thirty-year-old American woman. Her secret, she says, is regular exercise, combined with a vegetarian diet.[118]

Fluoride

According to the Centers for Disease Control and Prevention, approximately 145 million Americans[119] are drinking artificially fluoridated water, and approximately two-thirds of the US drinking water is fluoridated. The fluoridation of drinking water was introduced with the stated intention of reducing tooth decay in the population. The government-recommended dose is between 0.7 and 1.2 mg per liter of water.

It seems that fluoride — when consumed in fluoridated drinking water and in all of the numerous beverages and canned foods made with it (juice, beer, vegetables, fruits, etc.) — can cause bone to grow in a deformed manner. It also seems that this chemical ion can weaken bone structure, making bones more brittle and ultimately elevating the risk of fracture.[120]

The effects of fluoride exposure also seem to be cumulative. We may only see symptoms over an extended time, rather than immediately after exposure. Like plaque building up in arteries and setting the stage for heart disease, fluoride may build up in the body and its deleterious effects may grow, proportionate to the duration and level of exposure.

If we look closely, the relationship between fluoridation of community water and elevation of risk for hip fracture is quite compelling. This is evidenced in at least eight respectable studies, four of which have been published in the *Journal of the American Medical Association (JAMA)* since 1990. All show that hip fracture rates are higher in communities where fluoridation is used in the municipal water system, as summarized:[121]

- In 1986, M.R. Sowers and colleagues, in a retrospective study, found an increased fracture rate in both pre- and post-menopausal women proportional to their water-fluoride exposure.[122]

- In 1991, M.R. Sowers and colleagues completed a prospective study, again showing fluoridated water exposure was correlated with more than double the fracture rates compared to areas without fluoridation.[123]

- In 1991, Jacobsen and colleagues showed a strong positive correlation of hip fracture to fluoridation.[124]

- In 1991, C. Cooper and colleagues showed a statistically significant increase of hip fracture incidence in England, proportional to fluoride content of drinking water.[125]

- In 1991, C. Keller compared hip fracture rates in 216 US counties with natural fluoride concentrations in drinking water, and found significantly higher fracture rates in counties with fluoride levels higher than 1.2 ppm (parts per million).[126]

- D.S. May and M.G. Wilson reported finding that, as the percentage of people exposed to fluoride in water increased, the hip fracture-rate generally increased.[127]

- In 1992, C. Danielson and colleagues reported the risk of hip fracture was approximately 30 percent higher for women and 40 percent higher for men in fluoridated communities. Among seventy-five-year-old women, the risk was about twice as high in fluoridated communities.[128]

- In 1995, H. Jaqmin-Gedda and colleagues, scientists from the University of Bordeaux, France, studied hip fracture rates in seventy-five civil parishes in southwestern France. They found hip fracture was 86 percent more likely in parishes with water fluoride levels higher than 0.11 ppm.[129]

There are other studies worth noting. For example, in one study published in the *American Journal of Epidemiology,* researchers who had examined the impact of water fluoridation on bone health reported: "Residence in the higher-fluoride community was associated with a significantly lower radial bone mass in premenopausal and post-menopausal women, an increased rate of radial bone mass loss ... and significantly more fractures."[130] Studies have shown the same thing in other countries. For example, a study of water fluoridation in France reported "a deleterious effect of fluoride in drinking water on the risk of hip fractures."[131]

It is worth noting that the National Federation of Federal Employees, a union comprised of scientists, engineers, lawyers, and other professionals at the headquarters of the Environmental Protection Agency (EPA) charged with assessing the safety of drinking water, sponsored the California state initiative to prohibit fluoridation of drinking water. In a formal statement, Dr. J. William Hirzy, vice president of the federation, said, "We conclude that the health and welfare of the public is not served by the addition of this substance [fluoride] ... a hazardous waste of the fertilizer industry ... to the public water supply."[132] At least fourteen countries have already come to the same conclusion and have outlawed fluoridation of drinking water.

Water fluoridation appears to be one more overlooked factor that may be contributing to osteoporosis and other health problems, in the United States and elsewhere. Tens of millions of Americans are exposed to it, whether they like it or not.

As an additive, fluoride has no place in drinking water, and poses many other threats in addition to its apparent negative impact on bone health. Because it is also found in many toothpastes, mouthwashes, dental treatments, and all the products made from fluoridated water, most of us are unwittingly consuming far more than the dubious "safe level" added to drinking water. Scientists at Indiana University decided to investigate fluoride exposure through foods and, in October 2002, reported their findings in *Community Dentistry and Oral Epidemiology*. Specifically, they looked at children aged three to five, and determined that they were significantly overexposed to fluoride from cumulative sources including French fries, potato chips, white bread, ketchup, and soft drinks.*

A Recipe For Osteoporosis

The causes of osteoporosis are not so mysterious; the American lifestyle is a recipe almost guaranteed to produce bone disease. The average American eats a highly acidic, high-protein diet centered upon meat, fish and dairy products, the very foods that cause bones to be robbed of their minerals. The diet is sorely deficient in fruits and vegetables, the alkaline foods that are rich in essential bone building materials and that help to buffer the acidity of all the meat, fish and dairy consumed. This same diet is loaded with excessive sodium, sugar, and caffeine and highly processed and nutritionally deficient convenience foods. The average American also consumes an average four hundred acidic soft drinks a year, plus as many as one

---

* If you are concerned about excessive fluoride ingestion, you may wish to consider installing a water filtration system in your home. The very best is a reverse-osmosis multifiltration system, which will remove up to 99 percent of the fluoride as well as most of the other contaminants commonly found in tap water. Another step you can take is to avoid the use of fluoride-containing toothpaste. Still another is to check the label before drinking bottled water, as many distributors now add fluoride to their water before bottling it.

thousand cups of coffee. Add to this the chronic drip feed of artificial fluoridation from canned foods, condiments, beer and wine, fast foods, and tap water and widespread vitamin D deficiency. Compounding this is the fact that more than half of America fails to get the minimum amount of exercise that is essential to supporting bone health. No wonder America is facing an osteoporosis epidemic.

Women and men can dramatically alter their risk of osteoporosis. Each of us can counteract, minimize and even negate all of the risk factors addressed in this chapter without resorting to unnecessary prescription medications. We can do this by making simple, healthy lifestyle changes. If we don't, no amount of hormones or prescription drugs will give us healthy bones or bodies.

Eight

The Hidden Costs of Dairy Products

Cow's milk in the past has always been oversold as the perfect food, but we are now seeing that it isn't the perfect food at all and the government really shouldn't be behind any efforts to promote it as such.

— Dr. Benjamin Spock[1]

Today, it is estimated there are roughly ten million cows producing milk for human consumption in the United States, each yielding an average of approximately 18,204 pounds of milk, with a collective output of roughly 182 billion pounds of milk annually.[2] Few of us could begin to imagine how this phenomenal output is achieved, nor at what cost.

As Americans continue to concentrate around large cities and their suburbs, we become increasingly disconnected from the Earth, from agriculture, and from farming communities. The foods sold in our stores are delivered in brightly colored and immaculate packaging and displayed in pristine refrigerated cases, devoid of any evidence of the industry practices employed to produce them.

As our world population swells toward seven billion people, we face the undeniable realities of global warming, toxic waterways, the destruction of coral-reef systems, unprecedented smog in our airways, and the dramatic shrinking of our forests. Many people are asking what they can do to reduce their impact on the Earth and her resources. Likewise, there is a growing consciousness about the welfare and needs of the animals residing on this planet, with television channels devoted entirely to the subject.

Yet even with this consciousness, certain critical questions are still not being considered, such as: How is the food I consume produced, and how was it delivered to the stores? What are the labors involved? What resources are consumed? What unseen costs may be burdening the animals involved in food production? Finally, what impact does conventional food production have on our environment? In this chapter, we'll look closely at the many impacts caused by our overconsumption of dairy products — impacts affecting not only our personal health and the health of millions of animals, but the health of our planet.

Since the milk of a cow is not essential to human health, does not protect us from bone fracture, and, in the end, poses certain risks to our health, consideration of the impacts discussed in this chapter becomes all the more important.

A Cow's Life

Most of us have a rather romantic mental picture of how cow's milk is produced. That picture may include a small dairy farm in the country, where a single farmer clad in overalls rises with the sun, fetches his milking pail, and heads to the pasture to bring old Bessie in to be milked. That image of yesteryear has been replaced by something few readers could conjure in their minds. As Peter Martin of the London *Sunday Times* put it, "The modern high-yield dairy cow is a pitiful, ramshackle embodiment of market-driven exploitation."[3] Although there are still many small dairies left that do fit the image we hold in our minds, most modern dairies are not the soft, rolling hills and lush, green pastures portrayed in some milk commercials on television.

In the past few decades, some important books have been written about what really happens at the average factory farm. Elaborating on the conditions of modern industrial dairy farms, and their treatment of the ten million cows now employed for milking, is beyond the scope of this book. In his classic *Diet for a New America*, Pulitzer Prize–nominated author John Robbins wrote a succinct summary:

> The trouble seems to stem from the modern cow's insistence
> in asserting her fundamental nature. She still wants to do what

cows have always done: devotedly care for her young, quietly forage and ruminate, and patiently live with the rhythms of the Earth.

Such outdated ideas, of course, put her at cross purposes with an industry that looks upon her as a four-legged milk pump, a machine whose purpose is to provide milk for profit. She is bred, fed, medicated, inseminated, and manipulated to a single purpose — maximum milk production at minimum cost.

The industry points today with considerable pride to the fact that the average commercial cow now gives three or more times as much milk in a year as her bucolic ancestors. They don't mention that her udder is so large that her calves would have a hard time suckling from it, and might easily damage it if they were allowed to try. Nor do they mention that under natural conditions, Old Bessie would live 20 to 25 years. In the unbelievably stressful world of today's dairy factories, however, she is so severely exploited that she will be lucky if she sees her fourth birthday.[4]

For a cow to produce milk, she must become pregnant, which is handled through artificial insemination. The first insemination occurs at age fifteen months; she will be inseminated again a mere sixty days later.[5] It astounds people to learn that while fifty years ago, a cow may have produced some two thousand pounds of milk annually, today's cows produce upward of fifty thousand pounds a year. At least one celebrated dairy cow, who bears the unsentimental name "0-500" on a Chatfield, Minnesota, dairy farm, has produced an astounding 70,300 pounds of milk in one year — enough to fill a milk tanker truck one-and-a-half times![6] And agribusiness keeps devising new food additives designed to make cows produce still more milk per pound of feed.[7]

The milk is extracted from Bessie three times a day by electronic milking machines. Stray voltage from the machines occasionally shocks the cow in the process, causing fear, panic, and sometimes even death. It has been reported that a dairy farm can lose several hundred cows a year just to stray electrical voltage.[8]

The four years of Bessie's life are likely spent confined in a concrete stall. Administering the genetically engineered growth hormone rBGH may cause her already painfully large udder to grow to an even more obscene size, ultimately making it drag on the ground. This will, in turn, boost the chances of infection, necessitating the administration of antibiotics.

Peter Martin, who wrote an exposé of dairy myths, took a tour of a local dairy producer to see for himself what life was like for a modern bovine. He recalled the experience of seeing one of these poor cows, a "shed-housed fermentation vat on legs, teats dragging on the ground, it's a sight to frighten children — a giant, 650-kilo, emaciated ectomorph resembling Frankenstein's goat."[9]

Since she is regularly being impregnated so that she will keep producing milk, a dairy cow is constantly producing offspring. But her relationship with her newborn is ever-so-brief. Most calves are removed from their mothers immediately at birth; the remainder within twenty-four hours.[10] If she gives birth to a female, her offspring will likely join the unfortunate ranks of her mother and other dairy cattle. If the calf is male, it is often shipped off to a veal farm. There, the calf will spend fourteen to seventeen weeks confined in a crate that prohibits him from moving, and will deliberately be fed a diet nearly devoid of iron. If the calf were to move, his muscles would develop normally, making his flesh unacceptably tough to those who eat veal; if he were fed the iron he needs, his flesh would turn a natural red, another undesirable outcome.

Until September of 2009 one might not have been able to imagine the kinds of deplorable conditions and shocking treatment of animals that can occur at a dairy farm. On this date things changed when the animal welfare advocacy group People for the Ethical Treatment of Animals (PETA) released an investigative video in which dairy cows are lying in accumulated feces and urine, others are milked from feces-smeared udders, and yet others cows are brutally kicked and electrocuted by farm workers. Several of the cows are clearly ill and too weak to stand. The footage, which was shot over a period of months, was given to PETA by a former employee of the dairy farm. After multiple attempts to convince his employer to provide better care and conditions for the animals failed, the worker decided to take his concerns to the local authorities, and ultimately to the public, filing fifteen counts of animal abuse and neglect with the Pennsylvania court. When one sees these kinds of images it is a normal response to reassure oneself that such unconscionable treatment of animals must be a rare exception and that most dairy farms must be run, by people who seek to assure the welfare of cows they keep.

Yet on January 26, 2010, the ability to reject the possibility that the whistleblower's video might represent a broader problem, if not a culture, within the industry became much more difficult. On that day Mercy for Animals, an animal welfare advocacy group, released a chilling investigative video that was aired by major television networks, including ABC World News. The footage revealed filthy conditions, acts of violence, grisly routine procedures such as tail docking and the burning of horn buds, as well as depriving sick and wounded cows of veterinary care.[11] Calling it "mind-blowing" and "horrifying," CNN's Emmy Award-winning journalist Jane Velez-Mitchell warned viewers that there are scenes in the video "so horrible we cannot show them to you on camera."[12] In one scene a worker hits a curious cow in the face with a metal wrench: he later brags about this to a fellow worker. In another scene a cow with a prolapsed uterus (protruding outside her body) is reportedly left for days without medical attention. Other footage reveals multiple open wounds on the cows, some literally dripping pus. In the milking parlor cows are crowded together with feces caked to their hindquarters, as inches away, milk is extracted from their udders. Cows stand on floors hoof-deep in feces and urine and newborn calves are dragged away from their mothers by one leg.

This footage elicited a strong outcry from many who viewed it. Some posted their reactions on news websites. However, industry spokespersons interviewed about the video insisted that the footage, though deplorable, was an anomaly in the industry, some using the refrain of "one bad apple" in reference to the 7,000 cow dairy farm where the abuse was reported to take place. Yet, four months later, a new video from an Ohio dairy farm investigation surfaced. By now, any hope that the "one bad apple" in an industry claim had credence was dashed. In this new video workers are shown beating cows with their fists and with crowbars, stabbing them in their sides and overfull udders with pitchforks, kicking them in the udders and in the head, and a calf is thrown to the ground and its head is repeatedly stomped on. In another scene a cow's nostrils are wired to a gate before a worker begins smashing its head with a steel bar.[13] After viewing the footage veterinarian Dr. Debra Teachout observed, "The fact that there are several different people captured in the acts of malicious attacks on the calves and cows suggests an exceedingly permissive and even supportive atmosphere for animal cruelty to become the norm at this facility ... There is obviously no respect for the animals or for their welfare at all ... The lives of the calves and cows at this farm are full of terror and pain." Dr. Temple Grandin, an associate professor of livestock behavior at Colorado State University and advisor to the US Department of Agriculture said, "The handling of both the calves and cows was atrocious animal abuse ... These people were deliberately torturing animals and their behavior was totally sickening."

Because I've met a few, I'm certain there are many dairy farmers who are truly concerned for the welfare of the animals from which they profit and seek to provide adequate and timely veterinary care to their cows and to create an environment that is as clean as such environments can be. They, too, would be as horrified as the rest of us to see the kinds of abuse revealed in these investigations. Yet clearly, if this kind of abuse and neglect can occur over a period of months in three different states at large dairy facilities, the USDA's oversight is frightfully deficient and a culture of neglect and abuse has been allowed to spread.

Although not all of the common practices of dairy farming were depicted in these videos, let's take a closer look at a few of them.

Tail Docking

Dairy cows also undergo the cruel abuse of tail docking, the amputation of half or more of the tail. Docking, which originated on Australian dairy farms, involves placing a very tight rubber ring around a portion of the tail to cut off the blood and oxygen supply to the area beyond the ring. In some cases, the tail is allowed to simply fall off of its own accord after the tissue has died. However, it is also common for farmers to simply cut the tail off, without anaesthetics, using a pair of pruning shears. Super-hot scissors may also be used to simultaneously cauterize the cut.[14]

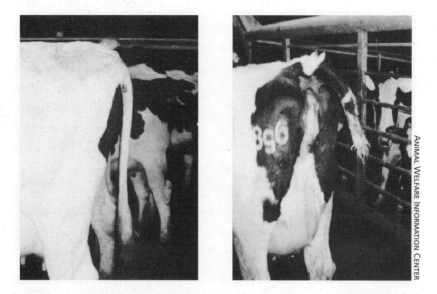

Intact tail (left) and tail that has been partially removed (right)

Some dairy farmers dock cows' tails because they believe that a full-length tail may become soiled in excrement and urine when the animal lies down on its filthy stall floor and could infect the cow's udder, possibly leading to mastitis.[15] It would seem, however, that a more direct possibility for infection is the contact of the udder with the floor when a cow lies down in its stall.

A dairy-farmer survey found that the prevailing justifications for docking a dairy cow's tail were related to farm worker comfort and convenience, and offered no benefit to the cow. The number-one reason was to spare workers the annoyance of having a tail in their face while they hook up milking machines. The second-ranking reason was ease of access to the udder from the rear, and the third was a reduction in milking time.[16]

Such are the risks when an animal designed to roam pastures is forced to remain in a tiny stall where its feces and urine gather around its feet. Humane farmers have suggested simple alternatives to mutilating dairy cattle's tails, such as providing fresh straw bedding each day, slatted floor boards (rather than concrete) that allow waste to drain away, and regular sanitization of the stalls. Allowing cows to graze at pasture could also do wonders. Cows have tails for a good reason —to swat irritating flies away from their bodies. As of January 2010, the practice of tail docking became illegal in California. Perhaps other states will follow its lead.

Another questionable procedure to which dairy cows are subjected is the removal of "extra" or *supernumerary* teats (nipples) from their udders. According to the third edition of the textbook *Practical Techniques for Dairy Farmers,* the appearance of supernumerary teats is quite common. Moreover, the text cautions that if these teats are not removed, they may become functional — that is, they may produce milk just as the other teats do. This begs the question: Why are these teats considered "undesirable" to a dairy farmer? The answer, according to the text, is that milking machines are designed with an ideal udder structure in mind. Should nature deviate from this mechanical ideal by providing more teats, it could make placement of the "teatcup" challenging for the farmer.

Surprisingly, the text also says, "At any rate, extra teats detract from an udder's general appearance." It is surprising to learn that a farmer could be concerned in the slightest with the "general appearance" of a cow's udder. After all, these cows are not paraded before judges at an animal fair, but are routinely confined to cement floor stalls with little or no room to move. The only people who see their teats are the workers who place the milking machines onto the udder.

Aesthetically pleasing or not, extra teats are routinely removed from cows by a simple and merciless procedure involving no anesthetic. In short, the cow is placed on its side, its back legs are spread, and the teat is sliced off the udder with a pair of scissors, the preferred tool of use. The text advises that dull scissors are even better, as they "tend to crush the blood vessels as they cut," which minimizes bleeding.[17]

Dehorning

Not surprisingly, a cow's horns can cause injury to other cows when the animals are kept in cramped quarters. An injured cow is a less-productive cow — growth and milk production are reduced — and therefore, horns are routinely removed, again, without anesthetic.

In calves under ten weeks of age, the procedure is referred to as "disbudding," and involves using a hot iron (hot-iron cautery) to destroy the horn's "bud" (root) tissue. In older cows, farmers use a saw, shears, or wire.

As with having a nipple crimped off with scissors, we can only imagine the pain the animals feel during and after this inhumane procedure. All of the procedures have been shown to result in elevated serum levels of the stress hormone cortisol.[18] Studies have also shown that use of local anesthetic, sedative, and anti-inflammatory medications sharply reduces the pain response and distress that cows experience.[19] However, presumably because the administration of such agents is both costly and time-consuming, US farms commonly forgo them.[20].

Few of us even think of the unfortunate existence of these creatures when we reach for a gallon of milk from the dairy case at our supermarket. Yet each time we do so, we unwittingly vote with our dollars and endorse such cruelty. In light of all these disclosures, to say a dairy cow's life is stressful would seem to be an understatement. Veterinary scientist Neil Forsberg of Oregon State University says, "In situations where producers manage their dairy herds to get as much milk production as possible, cows may suffer physical and metabolic stress, which weakens their immune systems, making them more susceptible to disease."

Forsberg suspects this may be the cause of Hemorrhagic Bowel Syndrome (HBS) or "bloody gut," a condition that causes blood clots in the small intestine, which in turn obstruct and enlarge the bowel. Considered a significant and growing problem in dairy herds, it causes the animals to suffer severe distress, and not infrequently, sudden death.[21]

Milking the Taxpayer!

Born of the New Deal-era, our government began subsidizing and regulating the milk industry with the Federal Milk Marketing Order in 1937, followed by a price support program in 1949. In 2002, an income support program was added. Each month, the marketing order program, under which two-thirds of all dairy products are produced, specifies a minimum price that will be paid for these times. The balance is produced under a California state regulatory system. The rate that processors pay for the milk is dependent upon how they will use it. The price support program guarantees that the government will step in and buy, at a set price, whatever amount of butter, cheese, and nonfat dry milk is produced, even if the demand for the product is absent and it must go into cold storage. Since 1950, American dairies have produced far more milk than consumers demand.[22] This policy keeps the price of dairy products high as it insulates the industry from the price influence of actual demand. In 2002, the Milk Income Loss Contract policy was established. The purpose of this program is to provide cash payouts to dairy producers in the event that market prices dip below a specified threshold. What product is not sent to storage is dumped into public schools, where children are required to consume the stuff, contributing to the health problems reviewed in Chapter Six. The remaining surpluses end up in refrigerated storage centers. Between the years 1980 and 1985, it was reported that the government spent, on average, $2.1 billion of our tax dollars each year buying up the overproduction of cow's milk.[23]

In 1986–1987, hoping to reduce the burden of this milk price-support program, Congress hatched an idea that entailed dairy farmers simply killing off portions of their milk-producing herds. Ultimately, the fourteen thousand farmers who participated would send 1.5 million cows to their graves.[24] Yet this drastic mass slaughter hardly addressed the long-term problem. According to *Consumer Reports,* in 1991, the government still spent $757 million buying up surplus milk.

In December 2001, Senate leaders introduced their legislative plan to award milk producers an additional $2 billion in subsidies, on top of their already staggering handouts. This was intended to support the farmers through the year 2006.[25] In 2009, Congress added another $350 million to the over $1 billion that had been paid that year through the Income Support and Price Support Programs.[26]

Since it was invented for the purpose of boosting milk yields, and given the regular surpluses from milk producers, one wonders where the logic was found in introducing rBGH to the dairy industry. Consumers Union estimates the boost in milk yields caused by the use of rBGH alone may account for $200 million annually to buy up the additional surpluses.

In the end, the cost to taxpayers of these dairy policies can be as high as $2.5 billion a year.[27] It's not hard to imagine the benefits of the many social, environmental, and humanitarian programs those wasted billions could have been spent on. David Stockman, budget director for the Reagan administration, may have assessed the multi-billion-dollar subsidies paid to the dairy industry most accurately when he called them "probably the single most worthless, lacking-in-merit program in the entire federal budget." Transcending the politics of subsidies may pose a formidable challenge, however, since nearly half of our congressional leaders receive campaign contributions from the National Dairy Council.

The Environmental Connection

In the United States, dairy farming is concentrated in two areas: California, the leading dairy-producing state, and Wisconsin. In California today over one million cows are part of the dairy business that generates $47 billion a year. There are nearly ten million dairy cows at work to meet America's demand for milk.

These massive armies of dairy cows require a great deal of food to produce so much milk. Consequently, enormous tracts of land in the United States and elsewhere are not available to grow food for human beings, because they are used to grow food for cows.

In addition to all the milk they produce, cows produce a lot of something else — something that isn't discussed at school or pictured on the milk cartons we bring home from the supermarket. It's a product the dairy industry would prefer not to have to deal with, but it is a natural consequence of all those cows: urine and manure.

The average dairy cow produces 120 pounds of manure every day![28] That's about the same quantity produced by twenty-four people. According to a Senate Committee on Agriculture, Nutrition and Forestry study, the quantity of urine and manure that California's dairy herds produce annually is equivalent to the waste produced by a city of twenty-one million people! The same report indicated that even a small dairy farm of two hundred cows can produce as much waste as a city of ten thousand people.[29] Of course, this cow waste is not processed through plumbing and treatment plants the way human waste is. Too often it makes its way into our groundwater, streams, and rivers, poisoning them. An EPA study estimated that in total, US dairy cows produce 54 billion pounds of manure annually. That's over two and a half times the amount produced by humans.[30]

Years ago, when the number of dairy cattle was far more manageable, the intent was to collect the urine and manure and store it in leakproof lagoons, and then use it to fertilize crops.

Today, however, there are so many cows producing so much waste that the holding lagoons can't accommodate it, and there aren't enough crops to be fertilized by this tonnage. Moreover, when heavy rains come, much of the waste can make its way into local rivers and, ultimately, into the aquifers that supply drinking water to large communities.[31] In the summer months, these manure lagoons sometimes catch fire and require fire crews to intervene.[32]

Over the years, dozens of dairy-farm workers have actually drowned in what has been described as a "stew of liquefied manure." This happens when the overflowing slurry from the lagoons is pumped into concrete holding structures. The deadly gases produced by the liquefied waste have overcome workers who enter the structure for routine maintenance. After passing out, they fall into the soup of waste, where they drown.[33]

Some of the holding lagoons are collapsing, overflowing into roadside ditches and creeks that feed rivers — and worse, leaching into groundwater, including the aquifers that provide drinking water to millions of people. Today, 60 percent of America's rivers have been designated "impaired" by the Environmental Protection Agency (EPA), with animal waste one of the major pollutants.[34] Furthermore, the waste produced by dairy cows (and by cows raised for beef) is much more concentrated than municipal sewage — by one set of measurements, 160 times more concentrated overall, yielding 200 times the concentration of ammonia.[35]

So what's wrong with this waste getting into creeks, rivers, and drinking water? In a word, nitrates. Nitrates choke rivers by causing radical growth and decay of algae, which in turn depletes the water of oxygen — ultimately rendering it uninhabitable for fish. Nitrates entering drinking water are also dangerous to humans, and can even cause death in infants. Animal waste is also riddled with parasites, bacteria, and viruses, and is the primary suspect in the increasing occurrence of blooms of toxic microbes in water. Between 1984 and 1996, nitrate levels measured in public water systems in California's Central Valley increased by 400 percent!

Reports have indicated that some dairies intentionally discharge their waste into surrounding soils and streams. The *Chicago Tribune* reported a classic case of a farmer illegally discharging animal waste into a local river in 1998. "It's the worst I have ever seen. This has killed off everything in 4.1 miles," said Steve Pescatelli, regional stream biologist for the Department of Natural Resources.[36] The biologist was referring to Little Indian Creek in Kendall County, Illinois. The discharge of animal waste had so contaminated this body of water that an estimated hundred thousand fish were killed, including minnows, quillback, redhorse, carp, stone cats, rock bass, and small-mouth bass. In another case at a large dairy in Elmwood, Illinois, in February 2001, millions of gallons of manure spilled from a holding lagoon into the nearby Kickapoo Creek.[37]

In yet another case, a Nevada dairy farm with five thousand dairy cattle was charged with intentionally dumping 1.7 million gallons of liquefied waste into the local environment.[38] The waste made its way into California's Amargosa River, a full eight miles away, causing massive contamination. In this case, the company that operates the farm was fined $500,000 for its transgression! However, this sizeable fine will do nothing to reverse the environmental damage.

In Milwaukee, Wisconsin, in 1993, some 400,000 people were sickened and at least a hundred died after they were exposed, through their drinking water, to the deadly pathogen *Cryptosporidium*. This parasite was ultimately traced to dairy-cattle manure.[39]

In a United States Senate hearing it was revealed that dairy operations in Waco, Texas, upstream of Lake Waco, were producing 5.7 million pounds of manure daily that land applications could not absorb. The runoff found its way into the lake, a source of drinking water for 150,000 people. Researchers estimated that 44 percent of the phosphorus found in the lake was brought there in dairy waste. The city has spent millions of dollars addressing such water pollution.[40]

Gary Conover, representing the Western United Dairymen — California's biggest dairy lobby — has said: "We know there are illegal discharges of dairy wastes when they can't control their overflows." He added, "We agree those dairymen need to follow the regulations."[41] Yet if the holding lagoons are already overflowing, and if existing crops cannot accommodate all of the waste as fertilizer, and if the number of dairy cows continues to swell by some 38,000 a year, how does a dairy farmer comply with waste-handling regulations?

Research has shown that the advent of synthetic rBGH has only worsened the problem of contending with increasing animal waste. The hormone increases a dairy cow's appetite and the quantity of milk she produces. As milk production increases, so does the total amount of waste the cow produces.[42]

Scientists have discovered a new problem accompanying all of this waste entering our waterways: pharmaceutical pollution. As we saw in Chapter Five, cows are routinely treated with hormones. They are also commonly given antibiotics, both to accelerate growth and to treat illness. Other drugs may be administered for various conditions. Unfortunately, this stew of drugs is eventually excreted in animal waste, and pharmaceutical residue is now showing up in waterways downstream of factory farms.[43] Preliminary tests indicate that drug-laden waste is having an undesirable effect on aquatic life. The question remains: What effect are these waste-borne drugs having on humans who depend on such water?

Our ecosystems have limited capacity to accommodate this concentrated and contaminated waste. Regardless of the regulations for handling such waste, more cows necessarily mean more waste — and consequently, excess toxins, which the planet is running out of ways to absorb. Rather than establishing more regulations on how to handle the waste, a more proactive stance would be to not produce it in the first place.

If Americans were as well educated about the health risks associated with dairy consumption as they are about which celebrities have milk mustaches, perhaps there would no longer be a need for these "megadairies" and the environmental degradation they bring.

Cows and Methane Gas

Many people will be surprised to learn methane gas is twenty-three times more powerful than carbon dioxide as a greenhouse gas. Methane is the gas released by the flatulence and belches of beef and dairy cattle. According to Michael Abberton of the British Department for the Environment, Food and Rural Affairs, an average dairy cow will release between one and two hundred liters of methane a day.[44]

Cows in the United States produce an estimated hundred million tons of methane gas annually, which represents about 20 percent of the country's total annual emissions of the gas. The more cows we raise for milk and beef, the more flatulence, and therefore the more methane gas emitted into the atmosphere.

Lost Resources

Despite the fact that humans have no need for the milk of a cow, and would be far healthier if we were to eliminate cow's milk from our diets completely, huge quantities of resources are consumed to enable cows to produce the milk demanded by Americans.

The average dairy cow today must consume approximately eighty pounds of food a day to keep producing so much milk. This includes grass, sorghum, hay, grain, corn, and more. To grow the sheer tonnage to meet the needs of these cows requires huge expanses of agricultural land — land that could be growing truly healthful food for the world's population.

All this food for cows soaks up water, to the tune of 45 gallons a day per cow.[45] Very few places on Earth brag of having too much water; many places are imperiled by having precious little. The estimated one million dairy cows in California alone, a state that often faces serious droughts, use up 45 million gallons of water every single day of the year. The California Farm Bureau Federation reported that when all dairy farming and milk processing water needs are taken into consideration, 48.3 gallons of water are used to produce one eight-ounce glass of milk.[46]

The Drug-Resistance Connection

We have all heard about drug-resistant bacteria. In Chapter Five, we reviewed how the antibiotic drugs used to help humans fight illness are now often impotent against microbial invaders. Experts are pointing the finger at the widespread abuse of antibiotics in factory farms. Many are calling for an immediate ban on farm use of such mainstays of human treatment as penicillin, tetracycline, and erythromycin.[47]

Drug resistance develops because not all bacteria are susceptible to a given drug. A certain percentage of bacteria may survive the drug, due to their genetic makeup. Once the weaker bacteria are killed, these stronger bacteria flourish. When the same drug is used against these resistant bacteria, they shrug it off and continue to multiply.

Some bacteria are particularly troublesome when they develop resistance to a second or third drug. *The New England Journal of Medicine* has reported that there is now a strain of salmonella bacteria that resists the effects of five different antibiotics.[48] The number of cases of human infection by this strain of bacteria has multiplied by thirty in the last decade and a half. Within a span of six years, drug resistance in the *Campylobacter* bacterium rose to 13 percent from no previous resistance at all.

Antibiotics were originally used to treat sick animals in the same way they were used with humans. These antibiotics have been incorporated into animal feed as a matter of routine, whether animals are sick or not. Much of the misuse of antibiotics on factory farms is due to the peculiar fact that they make the animals grow faster and put on more weight — which offers great financial advantage to farmers.[49]

According to Dr. Tamar Barlam, director of the Antibiotic Resistance Project at the Center for Science in the Public Interest, there is strong evidence that wholesale administration of important antibiotics to farm animals is increasing bacterial resistance. He has stated the "bacteria can then infect people, and jump to other organisms that are in humans."[50]

Such cases are reported with increasing frequency. An example occurred at a Vermont dairy farm, where nine members of the farming family developed an illness caused by salmonella bacteria that were resistant to five leading antibiotics. Eventually, thirteen dairy cows died from the infection.[51]

The sordid conditions of most factory farms contribute to the spread of bacteria. In the interest of larger profits, factory farms often confine large numbers of animals into very tight spaces. For example, there are 19,000 concentrated animal feeding operations (CAFOs) in the US, where up to 100,000 hens, 700 dairy cattle and 2,500 pigs may be sequestered.[52] Because of their close proximity to one another, the animals spread the bacteria easily. Contact with those animals, or exposure to unpasteurized milk, can spread the disease to a human. It is now estimated that the United States is facing an annual cost of $30 billion just to contend with the problem of drug resistance.

There is no human requirement for the milk of a cow, or of any other nonhuman species. It should therefore be apparent that we could avoid many of the destructive environmental consequences of large-scale dairy farms, as well as much of the misery imposed upon the cows inhabiting them. It takes only our imagination to see how we could lighten the burden on our overtaxed planet simply by reducing and eliminating dependence upon cow's milk.

In the next chapter we'll look at the simple steps you can take to make the transition from dairy, the types and quantities of nutrients needed to support bone health, and how best to get those nutrients.

Nine

Calcium Without Cow's Milk:
Making the Transition

Dairy products shouldn't occupy a prominent place in our diet, nor should they be the centerpiece of the national strategy to prevent osteoporosis.

— Walter Willett, M.D., M.P.H., Dr. P.H.

By now you understand that cow's milk was never intended for human consumption. It is neither essential for human health nor does its consumption assure bone integrity in humans. According to the USDA's latest Pesticide Data Program findings, cow's milk is a product that is consistently contaminated with dangerous chemical residues including known carcinogens, neurotoxins, and developmental and reproductive toxicants.[1] Cow's milk also contains nearly 60 different hormones and growth factors that may pose risks to our health. Reliance upon cow's milk is associated with risk for numerous serious illnesses, including forms of cancer and heart disease, and cow's milk is one of the most allergenic foods contributing to a host of symptoms in those predisposed. With this in mind, it's time to turn our attention toward healthful foods and lifestyle choices that provide the nutrients essential for and are protective of bone health.

One of the most important strategies is to adopt a diet that promotes alkalinity over acidity.

Where Will I Get the Calcium I Need?

One of the first questions many people ask when they consider eliminating dairy from their diet is: "Where will I ever get the calcium I need?" Imagine if you didn't need to obsess any longer about calcium intake. What if you didn't need to examine every label and count every milligram of calcium to be sure you were getting enough? Wouldn't life be easier?

It's not only unnecessary to get our calcium from cow's milk; it's counterproductive. Indeed, evidence suggests our early ancestors derived their dietary calcium from roots, tubers, nuts, and leafy greens. By eating in this way, they were able to adequately meet their calcium needs.[2]

While we surely need calcium in our diet, we need much less than we've been led to believe. And we can certainly obtain the calcium we need from foods other than milk. Just a little study of the nutrient composition of foods shows that there is a plethora of calcium sources other than cow's milk. After all, to repeat my question from an earlier chapter, where do cows get *their* calcium? Certainly not from suckling milk from horses or pigs! As nature intended, they get it from eating greens, which in turn get the calcium from the soil in which they grow. Likewise, powerful animals such as gorillas and elephants, both with substantial bones, as well as all of the other species in the animal kingdom, do not seek out the milk of another species. They derive their calcium from the plants they eat.

Calcium occurs in many foods. If you begin to make leafy greens, vegetables and fruits the centerpiece of your diet, you will not only be able to obtain the calcium you need, your calcium needs will be less. This is because you will retain more of the calcium you ingest than if you were following a diet centered upon meat, cheese and processed foods. As you will see in the table provided in the next section there is a plethora of foods from which to get not only the calcium but all of the other nutrients essential to bone health.

How Much Calcium Do We Need?

The Food and Nutrition Board (FNB) at the Institute of Medicine of the National Academies suggests the calcium intakes found on the following page. Remember, however, that these blanket recommendations, inflated as they are, have not succeeded in assuring the bone health of Americans. The academy's analysis of what are called "balance studies" indicated that

Recommended Daily Dietary Intake for Calcium

Age	Male	Female	Pregnant	Lactating
Birth to 6 months	210 mg	210 mg		
7–12 months	270 mg	270 mg		
1–3 years	500 mg	500 mg		
4–8 years	800 mg	800 mg		
9–13 years	1,300 mg	1,300 mg		
14–18 years	1,300 mg	1,300 mg	1,300 mg	1,300 mg
19–50 years	1,000 mg	1,000 mg	1,000 mg	1,000 mg
50+ years	1,200 mg	1,200 mg		

humans need about 550 mg of calcium a day. For "good measure," they roughly doubled that figure, assuming this would help ensure that 95 percent of Americans met their calcium quota.[3] The National Health Service in England recommends a calcium intake of 700 mg per day.[4]

According to the World Health Organization (WHO), an intake of between 400 and 500 mg of calcium a day "is required to prevent osteoporosis."[5] Some studies have shown there is little benefit to exceeding this amount.[6] However, many health organizations stand by the US Food and Nutrition Board's DRI of 1,000 mg for adults age 19–50 and 1,200 mg from age 50 onward. As you have read, there are many people the world over who consume as little as 300 mg of calcium a day — including people in Japan, Peru, South Africa, and India — and they maintain good health and strong bones, and have a relatively low incidence of osteoporosis.[7]

The WHO, which acknowledges the paradox of worldwide hip fracture rates being highest in countries with higher calcium intakes, suggests calcium intake recommendations are best made according to diet and lifestyle. From looking at varying lifestyles around the world, there is a well-developed picture of the lifestyle choices of those with the lowest risk of bone fracture. We know that a sedentary lifestyle in which a person gets little exercise and consumes a diet centered upon meat and dairy products, and that's high in sodium, caffeine, and sugar, is very unlikely to support bone health, nor health in general. So if you follow a typical diet like the sample menu on page 174, your calcium needs are going to be greater because of your heightened loss of calcium; and, as researchers have cautioned, consuming enormous amounts of calcium may not be enough to offset this destructive dietary choice.

So we have the option of making the same deleterious choices we have been making for decades, and getting the same results, or we can adopt change in favor of a different outcome, one in which we substantially lower our risk.

A diet that regularly includes adequate calories from the foods listed in the table below can't help but provide adequate calcium and other nutrients essential to bone health. Many fortified foods, such as orange juice and certain breakfast cereals, as well as a host of fortified beverages (see table below), also provide an abundance of calcium. For example, three-quarters of a cup of Total Plus breakfast cereal provides about 1,000 mg of calcium per serving, 300 mg of which is absorbed. Basic Four cereal provides 306 mg of calcium per cup of cereal, 93 mg of which is absorbed.

Remember, however, while adequate calcium intake is important, it is the retention of that calcium that really counts. As we will see later in this

Calcium in Fortified Nondairy Beverages (per 8-oz serving)	
DairiFree	275 mg
Edensoy Extra	200 mg
Pacific Almond, Low-Fat	250 mg
Pacific Rice, Fat-Free	150 mg
Pacific Hazelnut	250 mg
Pacific Hemp Milk	500 mg
Rice Dream, Enriched	300 mg
Soy Dream, Enriched	300 mg
Vitasoy, Enriched	300 mg
Westsoy Plus	300 mg
Westbrae Natural Rice Drink	250 mg
Westbrae Oat Plus	300 mg
White Wave	300 mg

Sources of Calcium			
Milligrams of calcium per 3.5-oz serving			
Agar seaweed	567 mg	Lima beans	55 mg
Almond butter (1 tbsp)	43 mg	Maple syrup (1/4 cup)	53 mg
Almonds (1 cup)	377 mg	Mustard greens	104 mg
Amaranth (1 cup)	298 mg	Navel orange	56 mg
Arugula	309 mg	Navy beans	128 mg
Barley	57 mg	Okra	176 mg
Bibb lettuce	35 mg	Onion	57 mg
Black beans	47 mg	Orange juice (fortified)	350 mg
Blackstrap molasses (2 tbsp)	344 mg	Peanuts	74 mg
Boston lettuce	35 mg	Peas	95 mg
Brazil nuts	186 mg	Pinto beans	82 mg
Broccoli (1 cup)	83 mg	Pistachios	131 mg
Brussels sprouts (8)	56 mg	Quinoa (1 cup)	102 mg
Butternut squash	80 mg	Raisins	53 mg
Chicory (curly endive)	100 mg	Rhubarb	115 mg
Chickpeas	80 mg	Romaine lettuce	68 mg
Collard greens	148 mg	Sesame seeds (1 oz)	280 mg
Corn bread (one 2-oz. dairy-free piece)	133 mg	Soybeans	175 mg
Dandelion greens	147 mg	Soy milk (fortified)	200-300 mg
Dulse seaweed	296 mg	Soy yogurt (6 oz)	250 mg
Escarole (endive)	52 mg	Sunflower seeds	126 mg
Figs, dried (1 cup)	286 mg	Sweet potato	70 mg
Great northern beans	121 mg	Swiss chard	102 mg
Green beans	58 mg	Tahini (2 tbsp)	128 mg
Hazelnuts	209 mg	Tempeh	154 mg
Hiziki seaweed	1,400 mg	Turnip greens	197 mg
Kale	94 mg	Wakame seaweed	1,300 mg
Kelp seaweed	1,093 mg	Walnuts	83 mg
Kombu seaweed	800 mg	Watercress	120 mg
Lentils	37 mg	White beans	161 mg

chapter, when alkaline foods such as fresh fruit are added to the breakfast cereal and mixed vegetables and tomato sauce are added to the pasta, these healthful additions provide the base needed to buffer the acid potential of these foods and make them more supportive of bone health.

Water as a Source of Calcium

People often forget that drinking water is a source of calcium and other minerals. Depending on where you live and the brand of bottled water

Calcium Concentration in US and Canadian Tap Waters (mg/L)

Region	City	Calcium Average	Calcium Range
Northeast	New York	18.8	5.4–83.3
	Philadelphia	67.3	33.6–103.6
	Nassau	12.9	0.1–24.8
	Delaware	61	22–100
	Cleveland, OH	33	N/A
	Columbus	47.6	39.6–50.8
	Pittsburgh	53.2	27.2–79.2
	Average	42.0	
Midwest	Indianapolis	89.8	53–110
	Chicago	30.8	30.2–21.3
	Omaha	57.6	39–90
	Wichita	24.4	N/A
	St. Paul	25	20–30
	Detroit	25	24–29
	Average	42.1	
Southwest	San Antonio	72	63–86
	Las Vegas	74	N/A
	Dallas	47.2	28.4–89.2
	Houston	38	37.1–38.8
	Oklahoma City	57	24–90
	Phoenix	131	82–180
	Average	81.1	

you have access to, water consumption alone could contribute 13 (tap) to 54 percent (mineral) of the suggested daily calcium intake. For example, if you live in Montgomery, Alabama, at 8.3 mg per liter, your tap water won't add a substantial amount of calcium to your diet. However, if you live in Phoenix, Arizona, your tap water yields about 131 mg per liter (about four eight-ounce servings). The calcium content of bottled water varies almost as much as tap water. If you drink Acquafina or Sparklettes bottled water, the calcium is negligible. Yet if San Pellegrino is your brand, you'll be

Calcium Concentration in US and Canadian Tap Waters (mg/L) cont.

Region	City	Calcium Average	Calcium Range
West Coast	Los Angeles	35	21–96
	San Francisco	16	4.0–31
	San Diego	125.2	101.2–150
	San Jose	97.5	58–192
	Portland	34.4	N/A
	Seattle	22	18–26
	Tacoma	74	N/A
	Average	57.7	
South	Jacksonville	120	60–168
	Washington, DC	43.5	43–45
	Durham	11.3	N/A
	Nashville, TN	30.4	N/A
	Memphis	19.2	N/A
	Montgomery	8.2	2.54–12.4
	Miami	68	24–112
	Average	42.9	
Ontario	Toronto	34	31.8–35.9
	Kitchener	135.5	75.2–180
	Waterloo	125.9	92.5–220
British Columbia	Vancouver	1.4	0.93–2.59
Quebec	Montreal	32	30–34
Nova Scotia	Halifax	6.8	N/A

getting 208 mg of calcium per liter. If you have access to Prince Noir water from France, you'll get 528 mg of calcium per liter.[8]

Where Will I Get the Vitamin D I Need?

Vitamin D is actually a hormone synthesized by the body when the skin is exposed to sunlight. It is essential for the absorption of calcium and the mineralization of bone. Although it can be obtained from some fish and fortified foods, most of us acquire it from the sun. Normally, just thirty minutes in the sun a day, twice weekly, between 10 a.m. and 3 p.m., will supply our vitamin D reserves. However, recent surveys show that many Americans, especially the elderly, are not getting enough vitamin D. There are several reasons for this. While the elderly have always spent more time indoors, with our increasingly sedentary lifestyles, people of all ages are spending more time before televisions, gaming consoles, and computers. If we don't get outside, we don't get the sun required to make vitamin D. Secondly, when we do get outside, the widespread adoption of sunscreen could be interfering with our exposure to the ultraviolet light that stimulates the skin to produce vitamin D.[9]

Regular alcohol consumption, which by itself reduces calcium absorption, is often overlooked when it comes to the body's use of vitamin D. Alcohol interferes with enzymes that help convert vitamin D to its active form. If you live north of San Francisco and Philadelphia (draw an imaginary line across the US) or in another climate with little sun exposure, you will need to take a vitamin D supplement from November through February. Also overlooked may be the role of the increasing incidence of obesity in the US. As body fat mass increases, the bioavailability of vitamin D decreases, as it is increasingly stored in fat and its release into the circulation may be hampered.[10] If you are African-American, you may only produce about half the vitamin D that a lighter pigmented individual will. Generally, after age fifty, the ability of the body to convert vitamin D to its active form diminishes.

A flurry of studies on vitamin D have been released in the last few years, a number of which suggest the vitamin has a much broader role in health than previously thought, including the prevention of cancer, hypertension,

IBS, and Type-1 diabetes. A number of experts have called upon the government to substantially raise the RDI for vitamin D. Given that surveys show that between 75 and 95 percent of hip fracture patients are deficient in vitamin D and that a large percent of the general population tested has sub-optimal levels, it would be sensible to have your own vitamin D levels tested.

The recommended intake of vitamin D is 200 IU (International Units), or 5 micrograms, daily for individuals aged 19–50. From ages 51–70 the suggested intake rises to 400 IU. After age 70, 600 IU is suggested.

Vitamin K

Until relatively recently, the importance of vitamin K outside of its role in blood clotting was not well recognized. It is now acknowledged that this vitamin plays a role in supporting bone density and maintaining calcium balance. Vitamin K is required for the production of osteocalcin, a noncollagenous protein found in the bone matrix that regulates the mineralization of bone. Some surveys have shown a greater tendency toward bone fracture in women who have lower levels of vitamin K. Apparently not all of us are getting adequate levels of vitamin K, and this may be due to how few leafy green vegetables grace the plates of the average American. Foods rich in vitamin K also happen to be those which promote an alkaline state. The currently recommended intake for vitamin K is 90 micrograms a day for women and 120 micrograms a day for men.

Food sources of vitamin K

Kale	Turnip greens	Broccoli
Swiss chard	Brussel sprouts	Spinach
Collards	Endive lettuce	
Parsley	Romaine lettuce	

Making The Transition

One of the first things you may wish to do is identify a nondairy beverage that you enjoy with cold cereal, in baking, or simply to drink by the glass. As the serious health risks associated with cow's milk and milk products have become increasingly apparent, and the failure of cow's milk to deliver on the promise of strong bones has become clearer, there has been a surge of interest in healthful alternative beverages.

Again, it is important to remember that these alternatives don't exist because cow's milk *needs* to be replaced by anything. In other words, although superior health can be achieved without dairy products, some of us have grown accustomed to having cold and hot breakfast cereals with milk, or smoothies and shakes made from milk, not to mention ice cream. Healthful and tasty versions of these and other dishes can be prepared using any number of available soy, rice, hazelnut, almond, or oat beverages, many of which work quite well in recipes normally requiring cow's milk or cream. See the table on page 212 for nutrient information on leading brands of non-dairy beverages. A variety of nondairy beverages are fortified with calcium for those who are accustomed to relying upon a liquid for their calcium intake. These great-tasting replacements can be used just like cow's milk on cold or hot cereals and in your favorite recipes requiring milk. Soy, nut, and other nondairy beverages are sold in eight-ounce aseptic containers that need not be refrigerated until they are opened. They are available in flavors such as chocolate, mocha, and vanilla, but most taste just fine without flavoring.

You can use mashed tofu as a substitute in recipes that call for ricotta or cottage cheese. There is now a plethora of ice creams and other frozen desserts made from soybeans, rice, coconut, and fruit. Or you can make your own ice cream at home. Check out books like *The Vegan Scoop: 150 Recipes for Dairy-Free Ice Cream that Tastes Better Than the "Real" Thing* by Wheeler Del Torro.

Although soy- and rice-based cheeses are often recommended to cheese lovers, be aware that these alternative products may contain casein, a cow's-milk protein, which is added to soy cheese to give it a "stretchy" consistency as it melts. A new cheese product from Daiya Foods has set the bar high for nondairy cheeses. Unlike other cheese-like products, this one is not made from soy and does not contain casein. It stretches, melts, and tastes like the cheese you know, but is much lower in fat and contains no cholesterol or dairy proteins. Some markets and a variety of pizzerias and other restaurants are now offering this option to their customers; for a directory of these establishments, visit: daiyafoods.com/where/index.aspx

We owe it to ourselves and our children to take an intelligent stance and refuse to buy into the age-old mythology that humans need cow's milk. Our health and that of our children will be sharply improved as soon as we give our bodies a complete break from all cow's milk and related foods. You will be giving your children a tremendous gift by never starting them on cow's milk, ensuring they will not be faced with all of the health threats discussed in this book, and challenged years later to eliminate cow's milk from their diets.

If you suffer from milk protein allergy or a condition for which you want to be sure you are not consuming cow's milk proteins, you will want to be sure to be aware of certain ingredients indicating the presence of cow's milk protein. This chart shows you what to look for.

Ingredients Indicating the Presence of a Milk Product or Protein

Ammonium caseinate	Demineralized whey	Natural flavoring
Artificial butter flavor	Dry milk solids	Opta (fat replacer)
Butter fat	Half & half	Potassium caseinate
Buttermilk	Hydrolized casein	Rennet casein
Butter solids	Lactose	Simplesse (fat replacer)
Calcium caseinate	Lactoferrin	Sodium caseinate
Caramel color	Lactalbumin	Sour cream
Casein	Lactalbumin phosphate	Sour cream solids
Caseinate	Magnesium caseinate	Sour milk solids
Cream	Milk derivative	Yogurt
Curds	Milk protein	Whey
Delactosed whey	Milk solids	Whey protein concentrate

Choose Bone-Supporting Foods

Recall that in Chapter Seven we looked at how important it is to immune function, metabolism, enzyme production, and countless other processes, that our body maintains an alkaline state. This is the ideal climate within which the myriad of chemical reactions and processes in our body occurs.

A healthful diet composed of adequate alkaline-producing foods will support proper pH. But we now know that the typical American diet, with its focus on beef, chicken, fish, cheese, and canned and highly processed foods, promotes an acid environment.

When our body becomes more acidic it takes a number of compensatory measures to restore the proper pH: the kidneys excrete fixed acid and the lungs expel volatile acid. But the body can become overwhelmed in the absence of adequate alkaline-forming foods and due to the decline of kidney function with age. We've noted that one response is to draw calcium and other minerals from the bones in an effort to buffer the acidity. While the bones are capable of enduring this process occasionally without harm, a chronic draw of calcium from the bones will result in a loss of bone mass and subsequent weakening of the bones. In a state of acidosis, the bone-building cells, osteoblasts, are inhibited while the activity of bone dismantling cells, osteoclasts, is increased.[11]

The ideal diet to support bone health is one that is centered upon foods that are alkaline and rich in bone-supporting nutrients. This is not to say that one should never eat acid-forming foods; our bodies need some of the foods that are minimally acid-forming. If the majority of the foods you eat daily are alkaline-forming and rich in nutrients that support bone health, you'll be on the right path. An important step is simply becoming familiar with which foods are acid-forming and which are alkaline-forming. One of the most acid-producing diets one can follow is the low-carb diet, which is nearly devoid of fruits and vegetables and rich in meat, fish, dairy and eggs. By design, it is deficient in the very foods that are most important to bone health and centered upon those most damaging.

Calculations have been made to determine a food's potential renal acid load (PRAL). The calculation is based upon the values for the five nutrients (calcium, magnesium, phosphorus, potassium, and protein) in foods that are most determinant of whether an acid or alkaline state is promoted.[12] The PRAL values are represented in a positive range (acid forming) and a negative range (alkaline forming). The higher the positive number, the greater the acid potential. The higher the negative number the greater the alkaline potential. When we provide adequate alkalinizing foods the body is better able to neutralize acidity without placing great demands upon the bones. The result is improved calcium balance, reduced bone resorption, and an accelerated rate of bone formation. Coupled with a minimal intake of caffeine, salt, alcohol, and refined sugar, and the addition of a regular bone building exercise routine, you have a recipe for lasting bone integrity! The formula is quite simple. Make fresh fruits and vegetables the foundation of your diet. These foods, unlike meats and dairy products, are rich in the nutrients your body needs to support bone integrity, including boron, calcium, copper, iron, magnesium, manganese, potassium, phosphorus, silica, zinc, essential fatty acids (EFA), and vitamins A, B_6, C, D, K, and folic acid. Vitamin B_{12} is also a player in bone health. Since it is not reliably found in foods of plant origin, if you are consuming no foods derived from animals, vitamin B_{12} needs to be obtained from a vitamin supplement. Protein is also essential to bone health, but excessive protein is detrimental to bone health. The same foods that are richest in nutrients that support bone health are also moderate in protein content, so you are less likely to consume excessive amounts.

For years the evidence has mounted that a diet centered upon fruits and vegetables lowers risk of cancer, heart disease, stroke, hypertension, type-II diabetes, obesity, digestive disorders, even Alzheimer's and Parkinson's disease. It lowers cholesterol levels and blood pressure and is rich in the fiber, carotenoids, flavonoids, and other phytochemicals that have been shown to protect against cancer. These are all the other wonderful benefits, in addition to promoting bone health, that you gain as you include more fruits and vegetables in your diet.

As a simple guiding principle, be sure you are getting a couple of servings of fruits and vegetables with every meal. Your goal should be to eat at least six to eight servings of fruits and vegetables a day. Make fresh fruit and vegetables your snack foods. Some of the alkaline superstars vegetables are broccoli, collard greens, dandelion greens, endive, mustard greens, kale. Try to squeeze them into one meal a day. Alkaline fruits include cantaloupe, dates, nectarines, raspberries, and watermelon. Blend up whole fruit into smoothies. Add fruit to your hot or cold breakfast cereal. Put fruit in or on your pancakes, waffles, and baked muffins. If you haven't

Potential Renal Acid Load (PRAL) values for selected foods, per 100 grams (3.5 oz)

Food	PRAL Values	Food	PRAL Values	Food	PRAL Values
Fruits/Juice		Leeks	-1.8	Salami	11.6
Apples	-2.2	Lettuce, green	-3.14	Shrimp	10.45
Apple juice	-2.2	Lettuce, iceberg	-1.6	Salmon	11.11
Apricots	-4.8	Mushrooms, white	-1.4	Turkey	9.9
Apricots, dehydrated	-33.0	Onions	-1.5	Trout	10.8
		Spinach	-14.0	Tuna, blue fin	18.14
Avocado	-8.61	Sweet potato, baked with skin	-8.18	Veal	9.0
Bananas	-5.51			**Grains**	
Black currents	-6.50	Tomatoes	-4.07	Bread, rye	4.1
Blackberries	-5.06	Zucchini	-4.76	Bread, wholegrain	1.8
Cherries	-3.82	**Dairy Products / Eggs**		Bread, white	3.7
Dates, Medjoo	-13.67	Buttermilk	0.5	Corn, yellow	2.96
Figs, dried	-14.05	Butter	0.43	Cornflakes	6.0
Grape juice	-1.0	Cheese, blue	11.96	Oats	13.31
Lemon juice	-2.5	Cheese, Camembert	14.6	Pasta, egg	6.4
Nectarine	-3.05			Quinoa	-0.19
Orange juice	-2.9	Cheese, cheddar	18.98	Rice, brown	12.5
Oranges	-2.7	Cheese, cottage	8.33	Rice, white, precooked	4.6
Peaches	-3.11	Cheese, goat	16.50		
Pineapple	-2.7	Cheese, Mozzarella	15.28	**Beans/Legumes**	
Raisins	-21.0	Cheese, Parmesan	27.78	Adzuki	-2.98
Raspberries	-2.40	Cream, sour	1.2	Baked, canned	-0.8
Strawberries	-2.2	Egg, whole	8.2	Chickpeas	2.6
Watermelon	-1.9	Egg, white	1.1	Green	-3.1
Vegetables		Egg, yolk	23.4	Lentils, green or brown	3.5
Artichoke	-4.69	Milk, whole	0.7		
Asparagus	-0.4	Milk, non-fat	0.03	Lima	-4.07
Broccoli	-3.57	Yogurt, plain	1.5	Pinto	-1.20
Beet greens	-19.56	**Meat/Fish**		Tofu, firm	-0.60
Beets	-4.98	Bacon	25.00	Peas	1.2
Cabbage, red	-4.29	Beef, lean	7.8	**Nuts/Seeds**	
Carrots	-4.9	Chicken	8.7	Cashews	6.4
Cauliflower	-4.0	Corned beef, canned	13.2	Hazelnuts	-2.8
Celery	-5.2			Macadamia	-0.45
Cucumber	-0.8	Ham	10.45	Peanuts	8.3
Eggplant	-3.4	Herring	7.0	Pistachio	-2.0
Kale	-4.22	Hot dog	6.7	Pumpkin seeds	-14.33

Source: Remer, Thomas and Friedrich Manz, "Potential renal acid load of foods and its influence on urine pH," *Journal of the American Dietetic Association* 95 (1995):791-97.

been fond of vegetables in the past or you feel uninspired about preparing them, check out the Resources section at the end of this book for a list of cookbooks that will give you an entirely different (and delicious) experience of what it's like to enjoy meals that are rich in health promoting foods.

Fruit and Vegetable Serving Size Examples

1-piece of fruit	6-ounces fruit juice
½-cup of grapes	1-cup lettuce, spinach, kale or chard
½-cup cut fruit, dried fruit or berries	½-cup baby carrots
	½-large sweet potato

Minimize Alcohol Consumption

Recall from Chapter Seven that alcohol consumption has been shown to be damaging to bone. It not only interferes with the absorption of and promotes the excretion of nutrients essential to healthy bone, but it can lead to liver damage that will interfere with vitamin D metabolism. Alcohol can interfere with the action of osteoblast cells that are essential to new bone formation. Alcohol also compromises our sense of balance and coordination and thereby increases our risk of falling. For these reasons you may want to reduce consumption of or entirely eliminate alcohol from your lifestyle.

Minimize Caffeine Intake

We know caffeine contributes to calcium losses so be sure to reduce caffeine intake. Remember that caffeine occurs in coffee, tea, soft drinks, chocolate, and some sports drinks. Collectively, you may be consuming far more caffeine than you imagine.

Minimize Sodium Intake

Reducing sodium intake requires more than ignoring the salt shaker. This is because many canned, cured, and processed foods contain substantial amounts of sodium. Simply by avoiding processed foods you will make great strides in reducing sodium. Many of us are unaware of how much sodium is in our diet. So pay attention to food labels as well as how often you apply salt to your meals. Beware that foods like cured fish, fast food hamburgers, and canned soups can contain thousands of mg of sodium. If you are accustomed to adding salt to your food, consider experimenting with herbs and spices as a seasoning alternative.

Seasoning Combinations for Legumes and Vegetables

Beans, dried	Basil, oregano, dill, savory, sage, cumin, garlic, parsley, bay leaf
Beans, green	Basil, dill, marjoram, rosemary, oregano, savory
Beans, lima	Basil, chives, marjoram, savory
Beets	Tarragon, dill, basil, thyme, cardamom seed
Broccoli	Tarragon, marjoram, oregano, basil, garlic
Brussel sprouts	Basil, dill, caraway, thyme
Cabbage	Caraway, celery seed, savory, dill, garlic
Carrots	Basil, dill, coriander, parsley
Cauliflower	Basil, rosemary, tarragon
Eggplant	Basil, oregano, rosemary, sage, onion, garlic
Onions	Oregano, thyme, basil
Peas	Basil, mint, savory, dill
Potatoes	Dill, chives, marjoram, parsley
Spinach	Rosemary, garlic, tarragon, thyme,
Squash	Basil, dill, oregano
Tomatoes	Basil, bay leaf, oregano, dill, garlic, savory, parsley

Get Exercised

For optimal bone health, regular exercise is not an option, it's a require-ment. Over the past decades, it has become increasingly clear that regular exercise doesn't just make us feel good, it offers tremendous benefits in terms of disease prevention and longevity. Getting plenty of exercise, not drinking cow's milk like the celebrities featured in the milk-mustache ads, is a truly effective way to help prevent, and even reverse, the bone loss associated with osteoporosis. A substantial amount of research has been done to assess the value of exercise in reducing the risk of bone fracture. Tens of thousands of subjects have been monitored, in some cases for as long as twenty years. Consistently, the research has shown a 40- to 60-per-cent reduction in the risk of fracture in those who get the most exercise. Here's why. As with muscle that endures micro-tears and is then rebuilt stronger, when we place stress on bone, we cause tiny micro-fractures. This stimulates the osteoclast cells to remove the weakened bone and the osteoblasts to add new, stronger bone. In the absence of weight-bearing stress, older and weaker bone can prevail, and the risk of fracture can go up.

Research into how we can best develop our peak bone mass found it was not calcium intake but rather exercise that most affected our bone mass potential.[13] To be sure, in many of the countries where we see relatively few bone fractures, we also find a physically active population. It's never too late to benefit from the bone-building potential of regular exercise. It's also important to note that the majority of the bone fractures (about 80 percent) seen in osteoporosis cases are not spontaneous but the result of a fall. An estimated thirty percent of people aged 60 or older fall within a 12-month period.[14] Exercise is essential to developing, maintaining, and regaining the balance and coordination that is key to preventing falls. So regular exercise can build greater bone density and develop the muscle tone, balance, and coordination that will keep you on your feet and reduce your chance of falling. A simple walking program has been shown to reduce the risk of falling by up to 60 percent.

Weight-bearing exercise is the type that best supports bone health. Examples include weightlifting, jogging, running, hiking, stair-climbing, step aerobics, dancing, tennis, and racquetball. Even gardening is helpful. At a minimum, you should aim to get thirty minutes of weight-bearing exercise in each day. If you can't fit thirty minutes into your schedule at once, try two fifteen-minute intervals in the day. In recent years tai chi, a martial art, has become a popular way to develop fitness, strength and coordination. Described by some as a "moving meditation" of slow, gentle, movements, tai chi has been shown to reduce the chance of falling after as little as twelve weeks of practice.[15] Many community centers now offer tai chi classes.

While anyone can adopt a regular walking program, or climb stairs, there are some worthwhile benefits to joining a health club. You will be among many other people who share your interest in preserving health, and you will have access to a vast array of the latest equipment to help keep your exercise effective, varied, and interesting. At almost any health club or gym, you will also be able to find competent, certified trainers who can design an exercise regimen appropriate for your personal interests and, if desired, assist you with your exercise program.

Whether you join a club or walk in your neighborhood or hike in the hills, try to find a partner with whom you can do these activities. It's nice to have a companion, and it's also inspiring. You're less likely to forget your daily exercise if you have a partner relying on you to show up. Before any exercise, take time to warm up and even stretch your muscles (see the Resource section for a suggested stretching book). If you are a walker or hiker, vary your route to keep it interesting. If you use a health club facility, try different exercises and machines that train the same muscle group. Throughout your day, take advantage of every opportunity to put greater resistance on your bones. Walk to work if you can, or park farther away so you can walk part of your commute. Take the stairs instead of the elevator, and walk on the escalator instead of standing idle. Adopt a dog from a shelter. You'll provide a home for an animal in need and that animal will give you another important reason to go for a walk.

Remember that exercise in childhood is a key determinant of the bone mass children will have as an adult. Those who begin life with greater bone mass will have more to lose (a good thing) than those who fail to establish an exercise habit early in life. So if you have children, inspire their interest in exercise from an early age. Your own exercise will be a healthy model for them.

Bone-Saving Lifestyle Strategies

Consume 6-8 servings fruits and vegetables daily
Minimize or eliminate coffee
Minimize or eliminate alcohol
Minimize or eliminate soft drinks
Minimize or eliminate animal protein
Consume 500 mg of calcium daily from plant sources
Have vitamin D levels tested and supplement accordingly
Exercise 30-60 minutes daily
Stop smoking

Conclusion

By now it should be perfectly clear that cow's milk is not only unnatural for humans to consume, its inclusion in the diet presents risk for numerous illnesses. The idea that the milk of another species is required for human bone health is not only a silly notion but one the scientific literature has shown to be false. You can see that the question of how to maintain bone health and prevent fracture is not nearly as simple as we have been told. We have seen how an abundance of calcium in the diet not only fails to guarantee bone integrity, but may present other health problems, as well. Contrary to what commercial interest may wish you to believe, no aspect of human health is achieved and maintained with magic bullets. Most health problems are multi-factorial, and many are brought about by lifestyle choices. As such they require that we consider the larger picture, as we design a strategy to overcome and prevent such problems. You now have the information to implement a new and comprehensive strategy for bone health and general health that is supported by hundreds of studies from the scientific literature. Because I've seen the dramatic life-changing effects in those who have adopted these positive lifestyle choices, it excites me to think about the improvements you may enjoy in your own life.

Remember to visit our online book club at www.newsociety.com
to share your thoughts about *Whitewash* and/or other New Society titles.
See you there!

Resources

Recommended Reading

Books

Autism

Lewis, Lisa. *Special Diets for Special Kids.* Arlington, TX: Future Horizons, 1998.

Seroussi, Karen. *Unraveling the Mystery of Autism and PDD: A Mother's Story of Research and Recovery.* New York: Simon & Schuster, 2000.

Breastfeeding

Baumslag, Naomi, and Dia L. Michels. *Milk, Money and Madness: The Culture and Politics of Breast-feeding.* Westport, CT: Bergin & Garney, 1995.

La Leche League. *The Womanly Art of Breastfeeding.* New York: Plume, 1997.

Cookbooks

Bergeron, Ken. *Professional Vegetarian Cooking.* New York: John Wiley and Sons, 1999.

Berley, Peter. *The Modern Vegetarian Kitchen.* New York: HarperCollins, 2000.

Burke, Abbot George. *Simply Heavenly.* Geneva, NE: St. George Press, 1994.

Bronfman, David and Rachelle Bronfman. *CalciYum! Delicious Calcium-Rich, Dairy-Free Vegetarian Recipes.* Ontario, Canada: Bromedia, 1999. To order directly, call 905-474-9620 or e-mail info@bromedia.com.

Costigan, Fran. *Great Good Desserts Naturally!* New York: Good Cakes Productions, 1999.

Johnson, Deborah Page. *The Feel Good Food Guide: Easy Recipes Free of Sugar, Wheat, Eggs, Yeast, Dairy, and Soy!* Lombard, IL: New Page Productions, 2006.

Klein, Roxanne, and Charlie Trotter. *Raw.* Berkeley, CA: Ten Speed Press, 2003.

Martin, Jeanne Marie. *Vegan Delights: Gourmet Vegetarian Specialties.* Madeira Park, BC: Harbour, 1993.

McDougall, Mary. *The McDougall Plan Recipes,* Vol. 1. La Vergne, TN: Ingram Book Company, 1983.

McKenna, Erin. *Babycakes: Vegan, Gluten-Free, and (Mostly) Sugar-Free Recipes from New York's Most Talked-About Bakery.* New York: Clarkson Potter, 2009.

Melina, V., and J. Forest. *Cooking Vegetarian.* Toronto, ON: Macmillan Canada, 1996.

Newkirk, Ingrid. *The Compassionate Cook.* New York: Warner Books, 1993.

Patrick-Goudreau, Colleen. *The Joy of Vegan Baking: The Compassionate Cooks' Traditional Treats and Sinful Sweets.* Beverly: Four Winds Press, 2007.

Raymond, Jennifer. *The Peaceful Palate.* Summertown, TN: Book Publishing Company, 1996; *Fat-Free and Easy.* Summertown, TN: Book Publishing Company, 1996.

Reinfeld, Mark, and Bo Rinaldi. *Vegan World Fusion Cuisine.* Kapaa, HI: Thousand Petals, 2004.

Robertson, Robin. *Vegan Planet.* Boston: Harvard Common Press, 2003.

Saltzman, Joanne. *Amazing Grains: Creating Vegetarian Main Dishes with Whole Grains.* Tiburon, CA: HJ Kramer, 1990.

Stepaniak, Joanne. *The Uncheese Cookbook.* Summertown, TN: Book Publishing Company, 1996.

Vegan Vittles: Down-Home Cooking for Everyone. Summertown, TN: Book Publishing Company, 1996.

Tucker, Eric, and John Westerdahl. *The Millennium Cookbook.* Berkeley, CA: Ten Speed Press, 1998.

Vegetarian Resource Group. *The Vegetarian Journal's Guide to Natural Foods Restaurants in the US and Canada.* Vonore, TN: Avery, 1993.

Wasserman, Deborah. *Simply Vegan: Quick Vegetarian Meals.* Baltimore, MD: Vegetarian Resource Group, 1999.

Fluoride

Bryson, Christopher. *The Fluoride Deception.* New York: Seven Stories, 2004.

Groves, Barry. *Fluoride: Drinking Ourselves to Death?* Dublin, Ireland: Newleaf, 2001.

Hazards of Cow's Milk

Griffin, Vicki, B. *Moooove Over Milk: The Udder Side of Dairy.* Hot Springs, NC: Let's Eat!, 1997. Ordering Information: 800-453-8732.

Oski, Frank A. *Don't Drink Your Milk: New Frightening Medical Facts About the World's Most Overrated Nutrient.* Brushton, NY: Teach Services, 1992.

Hulse, Virgil. *Mad Cows and Milk Gate.* Phoenix, OR: Marble Mountain, 1996.

Lupus

Harrington, Jill. *The Lupus Recovery Diet: Personal Stories, Scientific Studies, and a Program That Really Works in Overcoming Lupus and Rheumatoid Arthritis.* Mill Valley, CA: Harbor Point, 2004.

Nut and Seed Milk Production

Edwards, Edith. *Milk Recipes from Nuts and Seeds.* New York: Teach Services, 1998.

Stretching

Anderson, Bob. *Stretching.* Bolinas, CA: Shelter Publications, 2000.

Vegan Lifestyle and Children

Pavlina, Erin. *Raising Vegan Children in a Non-Vegan World: A Complete Guide for Parents.* Tarzana, CA: VegFamily Publishing, 2003.

Other Resources

Allergies

Allergy Blood Testing, Alletess Medical Laboratory, 216 Pleasant St., Rockland, MA 02370; 800-225-5404.

The Food Allergy Network, 10400 Eaton Place, Suite 107, Fairfax, VA 22030-2208; foodallergy.org

Autism

Basic Information

Autism Network for Dietary Intervention (ANDI), 609-737-8985; fax, 609-737-8453; autismndi.com

ANDI was established by parent researchers Lisa Lewis and Karyn Seroussi to help families around the world get started on, and maintain, an appropriate diet. The ANDI mission is to help parents understand, implement, and maintain dietary intervention for their autistic children. ANDI publishes a newsletter that contains research updates and recipes for gluten-free and casein-free cooking, as well as articles by physicians and parents of autistic children. ANDI also provides a roster of physicians reported to be supportive of the use of dietary intervention for treating autism.

Autism Research Institute, autism.com/ari

Provides basic information about autism as well as current research and alternative treatments. Produces the annual Defeat Autism Now (DAN) conference.

Blood Analysis Laboratories

AAL Reference Laboratory, Inc., 1715 E. Wilshire, #715, Santa Ana, CA 92705; 800-522-2611

This lab specializes in testing urine for opiate peptides.

Alletess Medical Laboratory, 216 Pleasant St., Rockland, MA 02370; 800-225-5404

This lab specializes in detecting antibodies to gluten and casein in the blood.

Autism Research Unit, Dr. Paul Shattock and Paul Whitely, School of Health Sciences, University of Sunderland, Sunderland SR2 7EE, United Kingdom; 001-44 0191 510 8922; fax, 001-44 0191 567 0420; osiris.sunderland.ac.uk/autism/index.html; aru@sunderland.ac.uk

Gluten Free Mall, glutenfreemall.com

Online mall for gluten-free products.

The Great Plains Lab, 9335 West 75th St., Overland Park, KS 66204; 913-341-8949; fax, 913-341-8949; Dr. William Shaw, Ph.D., Director, gpl4u@aol.com; greatplainslaboratory.com/

Great Smokies Diagnostic Laboratory, Martin Lee, Ph.D., Director, 63 Zillicoa St., Asheville, NC 28801; 800-522-4762

Immunosciences Laboratory, Inc., 8730 Wilshire Blvd., Ste. 305, Beverly Hills, CA 90211; 310-657-1077, 800-950-4686; immunsci@ix.netcom.

Support Sites

autism.com/ari

autismndi.com

autism-resources.com

generationrescue.org

gfcfdiet.com

Treatment Centers

Dr. Buttar Clinic, Rashid A. Buttar, D.O., 20721 Torrence Chapel Rd., #101, Cornelius, NC 28031; 704-895-WELL; drbuttar.com

Dr. Sudhir Gupta, University of California, Irvine, sgupta@uci.edu

International Child Development Resource Center, Jeff Bradstreet, M.D., 1688 W. Hibiscus Blvd., Melbourne, FL 32901; 321-953-0278

Recombinant Bovine Growth Hormone (rBGH)

Samuel S. Epstein, M.D. Cancer Prevention Coalition

c/o University of Illinois at Chicago School of Public Health, MC,

922 2121 West Taylor Street, Chicago, IL 60612

312-996-2297, fax 312-413-9898 (*please include a cover sheet*)

Organic Consumers Association, 6771 South Silver Hill Drive, Finland, MN 55603 218-226-4164, fax 218-353-7652, organicconsumers.org

Dr. David Kronfield, Veterinarian and Researcher, Virginia Polytech Institute; 540-231-6763, ext. 6124

Crohn's Disease, Paratuberculosis, and Cow's Milk

crohns.org

johnes.org

John Hermon-Taylor, M.D., Chairman, Department of Surgery, St. George's Hospital Medical School, London, England SW17 0R

Diabetes and Cow's Milk

Outi Vaarala, University of Helsinki, Department of Medicine, Hallituskatu 8, 00100 Helsinki, Finland

Suvi M. Virtanen, University of Tampere, School of Public Health, PO Box 607 (Medisiinarinkatu 3), FIN-33101 Tampere, Finland

Hans-Michael Dosch, Hospital for Sick Children, Division of Immunology and Cancer Research, 555 University Ave., Toronto, Ontario, Canada M5G1X8

Fluoridation and Disease

For detailed information about the health risks posed by water fluoridation, see the definitive book by Barry Groves, *Fluoride: Drinking Ourselves to Death?* (Dublin, Ireland: New Leaf, 2001).

Another excellent compilation and analysis of the scientific research on fluoridation is the sworn affidavit given by John R. Lee, M.D., for the State of Wisconsin Circuit Court. At the time of this writing, the entire document could be obtained at rvi.net/~fluoride/lee.htm

nofluoride.com

J. William Hirzy, Ph.D., Hirzy.John@EPA.gov

Vice President, National Federation of Federal Employees, a union comprised of scientists, engineers, lawyers, and other professionals at the

headquarters of the Environmental Protection Agency who are opposed
to public water fluoridation.

New York State Coalition Opposed to Fluoridation, Inc., nyscof@aol.com,
orgsites.com/ny/nyscof

Fluoride-Free Toothpastes

Nature's Gate, 9200 Mason Ave., Chatsworth, CA 91311; naturesgate.com
Tom's of Maine, PO Box 710, Kennebunk, ME 04043;
tomsofmaine.com

Gluten-Free Diet

Center for Informed Food Choices (CIFC), informedeating.org
Gluten-free, Casein-free Diet Assistance, gfcfdiet.com

Water Filtration Systems

Advanced Water Filters
    7701 E. Gray Rd. , Suite 110
    Scottsdale, AZ 85260
    1-800-453-4206
    support@advancedwaterfilters.com advancedwaterfilters.com
US Pure Water Headquarters
    20 Galli Drive., Suite E
    Novato, CA 94949
    415-883-9900, 800-776-7654
    mdwater@uspurewater.com
    uspurewater.com

Restaurants

The selection of restaurants that follows are the types of establishment
where you will have no trouble finding menu options that are free of dairy
and rich in the nutrients that support bone health. Generally speaking,
you will find the most health-supporting options in restaurants that have
vegetarian options or that specialize in vegetarian or vegan cuisine.

Café Gratitude, 2400 Harrison Street, San Francisco, CA 94110, 415-824-
    4652, cafegratitude.com; 1730 Shattuck Avenue, Berkeley, CA 94709,

510-725-4418; 2200 Fourth Street, San Rafael, CA, 415-578-4928; 206 Healdsburg Avenue, Healdsburg, CA 95448, 707-723-4461; 230 Bay Place, Oakland, CA 94612, 510-250-7779

Vegan, raw foods, fresh juices, nut milks, and desserts that people go out of their way for.

Candle Café, 1307 Third Avenue (at 75th St.), New York, 212-472-0970; also at 154 East 79th Street, New York, 212-537-7179

Award-winning organic, seasonal vegan menu.

Chicago Diner, Vegan Bakery, Natural Catering, Vegetarian Dining, 3411 N. Halsted, Chicago, IL 60657, veggiediner.com

Called by one guest a "delicious vegan mecca with everything good." Rated in 2006 by AOL Cityguide as a "city's best" restaurant.

Foodswings, 295 Grand St., Brooklyn, NY 11211, foodswings.net

Vegan fast food joint.

Greens, Fort Mason Center, Building A, San Francisco, CA 94123, 415-771-6222.

Renowned gourmet vegetarian cuisine with sweeping views of the Golden Gate Bridge and San Francisco bay.

Herbivore, 531 Divisadero (at Fell), San Francisco, CA 94117, 415-885-7133.

Vegan, gourmet international dishes, using some organic ingredients.

Medicine, 161 Sutter Street (at the Crocker Galleria) San Francisco, CA 94104, 415-677-4406.

Serves Shojin cuisine from Japanese Zen Buddhist temples.

Millennium Restaurant at the Savoy Hotel, 580 Geary St., San Francisco, CA 94102; 415-345-3900.

Upscale but informal vegan restaurant offering a mostly organic and totally GMO-free gourmet dining experience. Reservations recommended.

Real Food Daily, Santa Monica–West Hollywood–Beverly Hills, realfood.com

Los Angeles' premiere vegan restaurant dedicated to serving certified organic produce and products.

Sublime, 1431 N. Federal Highway, Ft. Lauderdale, FL, 954-539-9000, sublimeveg.com.

Award-winning, natural and organic restaurant and bar.

Vegetarian House, 520 E. Santa Clara St., San Jose, CA 408-292-3798; vegetarianhouse.us

Restaurant Guides

These guides will provide you with a vast array of quality restaurants where you will be able to dine on fabulous, dairy-free foods.

happycow.com

Online guide to health food stores and restaurants worldwide.

supervegan.com

Vegan web directory that includes a restaurant guide for the New York City area.

vegdining.com

Online guide to vegetarian restaurants around the world.

vegguide.org

Worldwide guide to vegetarian and vegan restaurants, grocers, and more with thousands of listings.

Health Organizations

Food Studies Institute, 60 Cayuga Street, Trumansburg, NY 14886, 607-387-6884. foodstudies.org

FSI is dedicated to improving the health of children through healthful nutrition and education. Offers the groundbreaking "Food is Elementary" curriculum developed by Dr. Antonia Demas.

Healthy School Lunches

healthyschoollunches.org

The Healthy School Lunch Campaign is sponsored by the Physicians Committee for Responsible Medicine and is committed to improving the quality of school lunches through the education of parents, school officials, food service workers and government officials.

Physicians Committee for Responsible Medicine, 5100 Wisconsin Ave., Ste. 400, Washington, D.C. 20016; 202-686-2210; fax, 202-686-2216; pcrm@pcrm.org; pcrm.org

Notes

In this age of Internet research, links are constantly changing and being updated. For web-based research, the notes list the original URL where the information was found; even if the original link is no longer active, the citation provided should allow you to track down the relevant information.

Introduction

1   "Broccoli can heal many ills," *Eagle Tribune*, Apr. 3, 2002; "A dish best served cold?" The Globe and Mail, July 29, 2004.

2   Gerrior, S., "Nutrient Content of the US Food Supply," *Home Economics Research Report*, No. 53 (Washington, DC: US Department of Agriculture, Center of Nutrition Policy and Promotion; 2001).

3   Frassetto, L.A., et al., "Worldwide incidence of hip fracture in elderly women: relation to consumption of animal and vegetable foods," *Journal of Gerontology: Series A, Biological Sciences and Medical Sciences* 55 (2000):M585–92.

4   Hegsted, Mark, "Fractures, calcium, and the modern diet," *American Journal of Clinical Nutrition* 74 (2001):571–73.

5   Cumming, R.G., et al., "Case-control study of risk factors for hip fractures in the elderly," *American Journal of Epidemiology* 139 (1994):493.; Feskanich, D., et al., "Milk, dietary calcium, and bone fractures in women: A 12-year prospective study," *American Journal of Public Health* 87 (1997):992–997.; Feskanich, D., et al., "Calcium, vitamin D, milk

consumption, and hip fractures: A prospective study among postmenopausal women," *American Journal of Clinical Nutrition* 77 (2003):504–11.
6 Hegsted, Mark, "Fractures, calcium, and the modern diet," *American
Journal of Clinical Nutrition* 74 (2001):571–73; Boyles, Salynn, "Type 1
diabetes may double in young kids: researchers say rate of type 1 diabetes
in children growing faster than earlier predictions," *WebMD Health* News
diabetes.webmd.com/news/20090527/type-1-diabetes-may-double-in-
young-kids; Landrigan, P. J., et al., "Living in a chemical world: framing
the future in light of the past," *Annals of the New York Academy of Sciences*
1076 (2006): 657–659.

7   US Department of Health and Human Services. Public Health Service.
The Surgeon General's Report on Nutrition and Health DHHS(PHS)
publication no. 88–5021; New York Times Syndicate, "Go heavy on the
veggies to prevent cancer," July 21, 1999, intelihealth.com/IH/ihtIH/
EMIHC000/333/333/231274.html.

8   Ibid.

9   Cooksey, K., et al., "Getting nutrition education into medical schools:
a computer-based approach," *American Journal of Clinical Nutrition*
72 (suppl) (2000):868S–76S.; Lo, C., "Integrating nutrition as a theme
throughout the medical school curriculum," *American Journal of Clinical
Nutrition* 72 (suppl) (2000):882S–89S.

10   American Obesity Association, "Childhood obesity: prevalence and
identification," and "AOA fact sheets, obesity in the US," obesity.org/
information.

11   Department of Health and Human Services, Center for Disease Control
and Prevention, "Overweight and Obesity," cdc.gov/nccdphp/dnpa/obesity/
index.htm; "Government launches anti-obesity campaign," *Reuters*, Aug.
25, 2004, msnbc.com/id/5817165/; Tanneeru, Manav, "Obesity: a looming
national threat?", CNN.com, Mar. 24, 2006, cnn.com/2006/HEALTH/diet.
fitness/03/24/hb.obesity.epidemic/index.html. heart.org/HEARTORG/
GettingHealthy/Overweight-in-Children_UCM_304054_Article.jsp

12   Hedley, A.A, et al., "Prevalence of overweight and obesity among US children, adolescents, and adults, 1999–2002," JAMA 291 (2004): 2847–2850.

13   Foryet, J., "Limitations of behavioral treatment of obesity: review and
analysis," *Journal of Behavioral Medicine* 4 (1981):97–106.

14   Jones, V.A. Clinical Nutrition & Obesity, *eSection Medscape General
Medicine* 7 (2005):79. Available at: medscape.com/viewarticle/507628.

15 American Diabetes Association, "1 in 3 Americans born in 2000 will develop diabetes," diabetes.org/for-media/scientific-sessions/06-14- 03-2.jsp.

16 US Department of Health and Human Services, Agency for Healthcare Research and Quality, "Osteoporosis-linked fractures rise dramatically," September 2009; ahrq.gov/research/sep09/0909RA36.htm

17 American Cancer Society: cancer.org/docroot/PRO/content/PRO_1_1_Cancer_Statistics_2009_Presentation.asp

18 The National Osteoporosis Foundation; nof.org/grants/; Riggs, B., et al., "The worldwide problem of osteoporosis: insights afforded by epidemiology," *Bone* 17 (1995):505S–11S.

19 Canadian Consensus Conference on Osteoporosis, 2006 Update, *Journal of Obstetrics and Gynecology Canada* February 2006; sogc.org/ jogc/abstracts/200602_SOGCClinicalPracticeGuidelines_2.pdf

20 El-Desouki, Mahmoud, "Osteoporosis in postmenopausal Saudi women using dual x-ray bone densitometry," *Saudi Medical Journal* 24 (2003): 953–56.

Chapter 1

1 Gerrior, S., "Nutrient Content of the US Food Supply," Home Economics Research Report No. 53. (Washington, DC: United States Department of Agriculture, Center of Nutrition Policy and Promotion; 2001).

2 National Institutes of Health. Consensus Development Panel on Optimal Calcium Intake. "NIH Consensus Conference: optimal calcium intake," *JAMA* 272 (1994):1942–48.; US Department of Agriculture, "The food guide pyramid," Hyattsville, MD: Human Nutrition Information Services; 1996 (Home and Garden Bulletin No. 252).

3 Kursban, M.S., "End food industry influence on US diet," *San Francisco Chronicle,* Jan. 7, 2000, A:23.

4 Zamiska, Nicholas, "How milk got a major boost by food panel," *Wall Street Journal* Aug. 30, 2004, B:1.; Letters to the Editor, *New York Times,* Sept. 7, 2004, A:26.

5 National Osteoporosis Foundation, 1232 22nd St., N.W., Washington, DC 20037, 202–223–2226; nof.org.

6 James, Sallie, "Milking the customers: The high cost of US dairy policies," The CATO Institute, November 9, 2006.

7   McLean, Rob, "Calcium and Osteoporosis," cyberparent.com/nutrition/
     osteoporosiscausemilk.htm.
8   Yoffe, Emily, "Got osteoporosis?: Maybe all that milk you've been drink-
     ing is to blame," Aug. 3, 1999, slate.msn.com/id/32621/.
9   Harty, Sheila, *Hucksters in the Classroom: A Review of Industry
     Propaganda in Schools* (Center for Study of Responsive Law, 1979).
10   Blitz, Peggy, "Bridging the gap," *Dairy Foods* 96 (1995):1–2.
11   National Dairy Council Press Release, "Calcium summit II reunites
     national experts to strategize new solutions to reach and teach America's
     youth," Nutrition and Health News Bureau, Jan. 17, 2002.
12   Eworldwire, "UK advertising standards authority: Nestle Health and
     Nutrition claims on milk, untruthful, dishonest, and unsubstantiated,"
     Oct. 13, 2005.
13   Physicians Committee for Responsible Medicine, *Good Medicine,* Winter
     1999:23.
14   Thompson, S., "New milk effort promises fame with cap game,"
     Advertising Age Apr. 24, 2000:34.
15   Zamiska, Nicholas, "How milk got a major boost by food panel,"
     Wall Street Journal, Aug. 30, 2004, B:1.
16   digital50.com/news/itemsBW/2001/07/14/20070205006030/ca;
     "California cheese production sets new record in 2006," February 5, 2007.
17   pcrm.org; healthcentral.com/mhc/top/000276.cfm, General Health
     Encyclopedia. The American Academy of Family Physicians
     estimates that 60–80 percent of African Americans are lactose intolerant.
18   "Milk: "Got Milk?" Article, milk.com/value/innovator-spring99.html,
     originally printed in the UC Davis Innovator, spring 1999.
19   Ibid.
20   Splete, Heidi, "USDA panel skeptical about milk's health claims," *Family
     Practice News,* Dec. 5, 2001, p. 12.
21   Physicians Committee for Responsible Medicine, *Good Medicine* 2,
     Spring 2001:23.

Chapter 2

1   Advertisement, *New York Times,* Aug. 3, 1999: F6.
2   "'Calcium Crisis' Affects American Youth", National Institutes of Health,
     nih.gov/news/pr/dec2001/nichd-10.htm
3   cabotcheese.coop/pages/pressroom/?release=43

4   Ervin, R.B., et al., *Dietary intake of selected minerals for the United States population: 1999–2000. Advanced data from Vital and Health Statistics, number 341* (Hyattsville, MD: National Center for Health Statistics, 2004).

5   Feskanich D, et al., "Milk, dietary calcium, and bone fractures in women: a 12-year prospective study," *American Journal of Public Health* 87 (1997):992–97.

6   van Beresteijn, E.C., et al., "Relation of axial bone mass to habitual calcium intake and to cortical bone loss in healthy early postmenopausal women," *Bone* (1990):7–13.

7   Gethrie, Catherine, "Boning up on calcium: Are you getting enough? Too much?" *Alternative Medicine* May (2002):78–89.

8   MacLennan, W.J., "History of arthritis and bone rarefaction evidence from paleopathology onwards," *Scottish Medical Journal* 44 (1999):1–5.

9   As reported in "What about dairy: Looking behind the milk mustache," EarthSave International, earthsave.org.

10   Dunkin, A., "When brittle bones need bulking up," *BusinessWeek* Oct. 28, 1996:192.

11   Brody, J.E., "Osteoporosis threatens men as well as women," *New York Times,* Sept. 4, 1996, C:9.

12   Brody, Jane E., "Dental advice: Start early. Very early," *New York Times,* Sept. 7, 2004, D:7.

13   Lanou, Amy Joy, et al., "Dairy products and bone health in children and young adults: A reevaluation of the evidence," 115 *Pediatrics* (2005):736–43.

14   "Count on calcium," *Men's Health,* Jan–Feb. 2003, p. 93.

15   Foundations of Wellness: "Udder confusion," *Berkeley Wellness Letter,* 2002, berkeleywellness.com/html/fw/fwnut04dairy.html.

16   Nishek, Dena, "Dairy does a dieter right," *Delicious Living,* Oct. 2003, p. 15.

17   healthherbs.com/conditionitem.php?id=203

18   webcenter.health.webmd.netscape.com/medical_information/ health-e-tools/interactive/hlthyfridge_milk.

19   Weaver, C.M., et al., "Dietary calcium: adequacy of a vegetarian diet," *American Journal of Clinical Nutrition* 59 (suppl) (1994):1238–41; Heaney, R. P., et al., "Calcium absorption from kale," *American Journal of Clinical Nutrition* 51 (1990):656–57.

20   Shaw, Gina, "Superfoods everyone needs," *WebMD* Feb. 2, 2004; aolsvc.health.webmd.aol.com/content/Article/81/96952.htm.

21   Ibid.

22   Robinson, Corinne H., et al., *Normal and Therapeutic Nutrition 17*[th] ed., (New York: Macmillan, 1986) p. 448.

23   Cuatrecasas, P., et al., "Lactase deficiency in the adult: A common occurrence," *Lancet* 1 (1965):14–18; Bayless, T. M., et al., "A racial difference in incidence of lactase deficiency: A survey of milk intolerance and lactase deficiency in healthy adult males," *JAMA* 197 (1966):968–72; Huang, S. S., et al., "Milk and lactose intolerance in healthy Orientals," *Science* 160 (1968):83–84; Woteki, C. E., et al., "Lactose malabsorption in Mexican-American adults," *American Journal of Clinical Nutrition* 30 (1977):470–75; Newcomer, A. D., et al., "Family studies of lactase deficiency in the American Indian," *Gastroenterology* 73 (1977): 985–88.

24   Zamiska, Nicholas, "How milk got a major boost by food panel," *Wall Street Journal,* Aug. 30, 2004, B:1.

25   Ibid.

26   Lanou, Amy Joy, et al., "Dairy products and bone health in children and young adults: A reevaluation of the evidence," 115 *Pediatrics* (2005):736–43.; *ABC News Online,* "Conventional wisdom on milk questioned," Mar. 7, 2005.

27   Contra Costa County Child Care Council Food Program, Nutrition Edition, May 1995, 4380 Redwood Highway, B-10, San Rafael, CA 94903.

Chapter 3

1   Stein, Rob, "Bigger portions, bigger people," *San Francisco Chronicle* Jan. 23, 2003, A:4; Severson, Kim, "Obesity a threat to US security," *San Francisco Chronicle,* Jan. 7, 2003.

2   Bell, G., *Textbook of Physiology and Biochemistry,* 4th ed. (New York: Churchill Livingstone, 1954), pp. 167–70, as adapted in McDougall, John, *The McDougall Plan* (Indianappolis: New Century Publishers, 1983), p. 101.

3   Heaney, R.P., et al., "Calcium absorption from kale," *American Journal of Clinical Nutrition* 51 (1990):656–57; Weaver C.M., et al., "Dietary calcium: adequacy of a vegetarian diet," *American Journal of Clinical Nutrition* 59(suppl) (1994):1238S–41S.

4   Weaver, Connie, "Dietary calcium: Adequacy of a vegetarian diet," *American Journal of Clinical Nutrition,* 59-suppl, 1994, p1238S-41S)

5   Gilliam, Marjie, "Calcium-magnesium balance, exercise help fight osteoporosis," *Dayton Daily News,* Sept. 6, 2004, daytondailynews.com

6   Clifford, L., et al., "Chronic protracted diarrhea of infancy: A nutritional disease," Pediatrics 72 (1983):786–800.

7   Oski, F.A., "Is bovine milk a health hazard?" *Pediatrics* 75 (suppl) (1985):182–86.

8   Goldman, A.S., et al., "Milk allergy. 1. Oral challenge with milk and isolated milk proteins in allergic children," *Pediatrics* 32 (1963):425.

9   Parke, A., "Rheumatoid arthritis and food: A case study," *British Medical Journal* 282 (1981):2027.

10 Freier, S., et al., "Milk allergy in infants and young children," *Clinical Pediatrics* 9 (1970):449.

11 Soothill, J.F., et al., "Is migraine food allergy? A double-blind controlled trial of oligoantigenic diet treatment," *Lancet* (1983):865–69; Monro, J., et al., "Food allergy in migraine: Study of dietary exclusion and RAST," *Lancet,* July 5, 1980:1–5.

12 Rowe, A.H., et al., "Bronchial asthma due to allergy alone in ninety-five patients," *Journal of the American Medical Association* 169 (1959): 1158–62; Parke, A., "Rheumatoid arthritis and food: A case study," *British Medical Journal* 282 (1981):2027.

13 Lucas, A., et al., "Breast milk and subsequent intelligence quotient in children born preterm," *Lancet* 339 (1992):261–64.

14 Coombs, R.R., et al., "Allergy and cot death: With special focus on allergic sensitivity to cow's milk and anaphylaxis," *Clinical and Experimental Allergy,* July 20, 1990:359–66.

15 Adebamowo, C.A., et al., "High school dietary dairy intake and teenage acne," *Journal of the American Academy of Dermatology* 52 (2005):207–14.; Adebamowo, C.A, et al., "Milk consumption and acne in teenaged boys," *Journal of the Academy of Dermatology* 58 (2008):794–95.

16 Willett, W., et al., "Galactose consumption and metabolism in relation to the risk of ovarian cancer," *Lancet* 7 (1989):66–71; Cramer, D. W., et al., "Characteristics of women with a family history of ovarian cancer, galactose consumption and metabolism," *Cancer* 74 (1994):1309–17.

17 Waldman, T.A., et al., "Allergic gastroenterophathy. A cause of gastrointestinal protein loss," *New England Journal of Medicine* 276 (1967):761.

18 Buisseret, P.D., "Common manifestations of cow's milk allergy in children," *Lancet* 1 (1978):304.

19 Eastham, E.J., et al., "Adverse effects of milk formula ingestion on the gastrointestinal tract," *Gastroenterology* 76 (1979):365–74.

20 Feskanich, D., et al., "Milk, dietary calcium, and bone fractures in women," *American Journal of Public Health* 87 (1997):992–97; Recher, R., "The effect of milk supplements on calcium metabolism and calcium balance," *American Journal of Clinical Nutrition* 41 (1985):254.

21 Epstein, S.A., "Potential public health hazards of biosynthetic milk hormones," *International Journal of Health Services* 20 (1990):73–84.

22 Gersema, Emily, "FDA warns against use of drug in animals," *Associated Press,* Mar. 4, 2003

Chapter 4

1   Willett, Walter, *Eat, Drink, and Be Healthy* (New York: Free Press, 2001.) p.195.

2   White, G.M., "Recent findings in the epidemiologic evidence, classification, and sub-types of acne vulgaris," *Journal of the American Academy of Dermatology* 39 (1998):S34–3

3   Ayer, Jane, et al., "Acne: more than skin deep," *Postgraduate Medicine Journal* 82 (2006):500-506.

4   Velicer, Christine M., et al., "Antibiotic use in relation to the risk of breast cancer," *JAMA* 291 (2004):827–35.

5   fda.gov/Drugs/DrugSafety/PostmarketDrugSafetyInformationfor PatientsandProviders/ucm094305.htm; fda.gov/Safety/MedWatch/ Safety Information/SafetyAlertsforHumanMedicalProducts/ ucm150448.htm

6   "Dermatology: Acne, hormones & milk," April 29, 1966; time.com/time/printout/0,8816,835434,00.html

7   Adebamowo, C.A., et al., "High school dietary dairy intake and teenage acne," *Journal of the American Academy of Dermatology* 52 (2005):207–14

8   Adebamowo, C.A., et al., "Milk consumption and acne in adolescent girls," *Dermatoloy Online Journal* 12 (2006):25; ncbi.nlm.nih.govpubmed/ 17083856

9   Business Wire, "US cheese industry posts $40 billion total sales in 2003," Sept. 22, 2004.

10 Doyle, Christine, "I've ruthlessly cut back on fat," *The Telegraph*, May 13, 2003, telegraph.co.uk/health/dietandfitness/4713321/Ive-ruthlessly-cut-back-on-fat.html

11 vegsource.com/talk/awakening/messages/17526.html

12 "Addiction — drugs, alcohol, gambling," *Newsletter of the Centre of Effective Therapy*, Sept. 2002, ampersandaus.com.au/Newsletter2002_sep.html

13 Hazum, E., et al., "Morphine in cow and human milk: could dietary morphine constitute a ligand for specific morphine (mu) receptors?" *Science* 213 (1981)1010–12.

14 Ryan, Rosalind, "Do you know the whole truth about milk?" *Mail Online (Daily Mail)* February 9, 2010. dailymail.co.uk/health/article-157290/Do-know-truth-milk.html

15 Buisseret, P.D., "Common manifestations of cow's milk allergy in children," *Lancet* 1 (1978):304–5.

16 Bock, S.A., "Natural history of severe reactions to foods in young children," *Pediatrics* 107 (1985):676–80.; Schwartz, R.H., "IgE-mediated allergic reactions to cow's milk," *Immunology and Allergy Clinics of North America* 11 (1991):717–41.

17 Astor, Stephen, *Hidden Food Allergies* (New York: Avery, 1997):5.

18 Bahana, S.L., et al., "Milk hypersensitivity. I. Pathogenesis and symptomatology," *Annals of Allergy* 50 (1983):218–23; Marks, D.R., et al., "Food allergy: Manifestations, evaluation, and management," *Postgraduate Medicine* 93 (1993):191–96.; "Digesting the facts about food allergies," *Yorkshire Post*, Jan. 20, 2006., yorkshiretoday.co.uk/ViewArticle2.aspx?SectionID=105&ArticleID=1321939

19 May, C., "Food sensitivity: Facts and fancies," *Nutrition Reviews* 42 (1984):72–79.

20 Schwartz, Robert, "Allergy, intolerance, and other adverse reactions to foods," *Pediatric Annals* 21 (1992):654–74.

21 Gaby, A.R., *Preventing and Reversing Osteoporosis* (Rocklin, Calif.: Prima, 1994), p. 115.

22 Ibid.

23 Chabot, R., *Pediatric Allergy* (New York: McGraw-Hill Book Co., 1951).

24 Eastham, E.J., et al., "Adverse effects of milk formula ingestion on the gastrointestinal tract," *Gastroenterology* 76 (1979):365–74.

25 Loveless, M.H., "Milk allergy: a survey of its incidence; experiments with a masked ingestion test," *Journal of Allergy* 21 (1950):489–99.

26 Williams, Sue Rodwell, *Nutrition and Diet Therapy,* 7th Ed. (Mosby: St. Louis, 1993), p. 41.

27 Gjesing, B., et al., "Immunochemistry of food antigens," *Annals of Allergy* 53 (1984):603–8.

28 Schwarz, R., "Allergy, intolerance, and other adverse reactions to food," *Pediatric Annals* 21 (1992):654–74.

29 Hill, D.J., et al., "A study of 100 infants and young children with cow's milk allergy," 2 *Clinical Reviews in Allergy* (1984):125

30 Stefanini, G.F., et al., "Nonmigrainous headache from food allergy," *Allergy* 51 (1996):657–60.

31 Bahna, S.L., et al., "Milk hypersensitivity I. Pathogenesis and symptomatology," *Annals of Allergy* 50 (1983):218.

32 Astor, Stephen, *Hidden Food Allergies* (New York, Avery: 1997):5.

33 Levy, F.S., et al., "Adult onset of cow's milk protein allergy with small-intestinal mucosal IgE mast cells," *Allergy* 51 (1996):417–20.

34 Santiago, O., et al., "Allergy to cow's milk with onset in adult life," *Annals of Allergy* 62 (1989):185–86.

35 Wuthrich, B., et al., "Severe anaphylactic reaction to bovine serum albumin at first attempt of artificial insemination," *Allergy* 50 (1995):179–83.

36 DeBlay, F., "Urticaria and angioedema during insemination with fluid containing bovine serum albumin," *Contact Dermatitis* 28 (1993):119.

37 Schwarz, Robert H., "Allergy, intolerance, and other adverse reactions to foods," *Pediatric Annals* 21 (1992):654–74.

38 Stefanini, G.F., et al., "Nonmigrainous headache from food allergy," *Allergy* 51 (1996):657–60.

39 Ratner, D., et al., "Milk protein-free diet for non-seasonal asthma and migraine in lactase-deficient patients," *Israel Journal of Medical Sciences* 19 (1983):806–9.

40 Egger J., et al., "Is migraine a food allergy? A double-blind controlled trial of oligoantigenic diet treatment," *Lancet* 2 (1983):865–69.

41 Twogood, Daniel, *No Milk: A Revolutionary Solution to Backpain and Headaches* (Victorville, CA: Wilhelmina Books, 1992).

42 Panush, R.S., et al., "Diet therapy for rheumatoid arthritis," *Arthritis and Rheumatism* 26 (1983):462–71; Kjeldson-Kragh, J., et al., "Controlled trial of fasting and one-year vegetarian diet in rheumatoid arthritis," *Lancet* 338 (1991):889–902.

43 Ratner, D., et al., "Juvenile rheumatoid arthritis and milk allergy," *Journal of the Royal Society of Medicine* 78 (1985):410–13.

44 Parke, A.L., et al., "Rheumatoid arthritis and food: A case study," *British Medical Journal* 282 (1988):2027–30.

45 One of the more popular arthritis pain medications today, Celebrex, states in its safety information literature: "Celebrex may increase the chance of a heart attack or stroke that can lead to death ... Serious skin reactions or stomach problems such as bleeding can occur without warning and may cause death." See: celebrex.com/home/default.asp?CMP=

46 Cramer, D., et al., "Adult hypolactasia, milk consumption, and age-specific fertility," *American Journal of Epidemiology* 139 (1994):282–89.

47 *Postgraduate Medicine* 95 (1994):113–20; Carper, S., *Milk Is Not for Everybody: Living With Lactose Intolerance* (New York: Plume, 1995).

48 Flatz, G., "Genetics of lactose digestion in humans" in H. Harris and K. Hirschorn, eds., *Advances in Human Genetics* (New York: Plenum, 1980), pp 1–77.

49 *Postgraduate Medicine* 95 (1994):113–20.

50 Reuters News, as reported in "Genetically engineered dairy cows," Factoryfarming.com, Jan. 29, 1999.

51 American Academy of Opthalmology, aao.org

52 United States Environmental Protection Agency, epa.gov/sunwise/uvandhealth/html.; National Library and Information System Authority, "Effect of ozone depletion on human health," Courtesy the *Trinidad Guardian*, Oct. 4, 1999, p. 29.

53 Fackelmann, K.A., "Studies smoke out the risks of cataracts," *Science News* 142 (1992):134.; Hankinson, S.E., et al., "A prospective study of cigarette smoking and the risk of cataract surgery in women," *JAMA* 268 (1992):994–8.; "Smoking linked to cataracts: Up to 20% of cases could be caused by tobacco use," *Medical Tribune* Sept. 3, 1992, p. 3.

54 Simoons, F.J., "A geographic approach to senile cataracts: possible links with milk consumption, lactase activity, and galactose metabolism," *Digestive Disease and Science* 27 (1982):257–64.; Rinaldi, E., et al., "High frequency of lactose absorbers among adults with idiopathicsenile and presenile cataract in a population with a high prevalence of primary adult lactose malabsorption," *Lancet*, Feb. 18 (1984):355–57.; Couet, C., et al., "Lactose and cataract in humans: a review," *Journal of the American College of Nutrition* 10 (1991):79–86.

55 Winder, A.F., et al., "Partial galactose disorders in families with premature cataracts," *Archives of Disease in Childhood* 58 (1983):362–66.

56 Briggs, R.D., et al., "Myocardial infarction in patients treated with Sippy and other high-milk diets," *Circulation* 21 (1960):538–42.

57 Department of Health and Human Services, Food and Drug Administration, "Eating for a Healthy Heart," fda.gov/opacom/lowlit/hlyheart.html

58 Martin, Peter, "Milk: Nectar or Poison," article in the London Sunday Times Magazine with the cover title, "Is There a Time Bomb in Your Diet? Exploding the Myths about Milk," July 21, 2002.

59 Willett, Walter, Harvard School of Public Health, *Boston Globe,* June 8, 1999.

60 Segall, J., "Dietary lactose as a possible risk factor for ischaemic heart disease: Review of epidemiology," *International Journal of Cardiology* 46 (1994):197–207.

61 *Alternative Medicine Reviews* 3 (1998):281–94.

62 Alamgir, J., et al., "Survival trends, coronary event rates, and the MONICA Project," *Lancet* 354 (1999):862–63.

63 Ornish, D., et al., "Can lifestyle changes reverse coronary heart disease?," *Lancet* 336 (1990):129–33.

64 Report from the National Academy of Sciences Committee on Diet, Nutrition, and Cancer (Washington, D.C.: National Academy Press, 1982).

65 Health & Science, *The Week,* Dec. 27, 2003, p. 17.

66 Oster, K.A., "The treatment of bovine xanthine oxidase initiated atherosclerosis by folic acid," *Clinical Research* 24 (1976):512.

67 Ross, D.J., et al., "The presence of ectopic xanthine oxidase in athero-sclerotic plaques and myocardial tissues," *Proc Soc Exper Biol Med* 144 (1973):523–26.

68 "Study: eat leafy green veggies to help prevent cataracts," *Science Daily,* Dec. 4, 2004.

69 Martin, Charlyne Blatcher, "Bariatric surgery and pharmacology use and costs are on the rise," *Medscape Medical News,* July 14, 2005, medscape.com/viewarticle/508382

70 Tanner, Robert, "State considers using laws to fight obesity," *Associated Press,* Dec. 23, 2003.

71 Forbes.com, "Too few car seats for America's obese kids," April 3, 2006, forbes.com/lifestyle/health/feeds/hscout/2006/04/03/hscout531858.

72 Chudnoff, Scott, "Viewpoint: the connection between obesity and pelvic organ dysfunction," *Medscape Ob/Gyn & Women's Health* Febraury 21, 2006; available at: medscape.com/viewarticle/523742?src=sr; Richter, H.E, et al., "Urinary and anal incontinence in morbidly obese women considering weight loss surgery," *Obstetrics and Gynecology* 106 (2005):1272–76.

73 Fontaine, K.R., et al., "Years of life lost to obesity," *JAMA* 289 (2003): 187–93.

74 International Agency for Research on Cancer, "Weight control and physical activity," (Lyons, France: IARC, 2002).

75 CNN.com, "Too fat to fight: Army finds record number to heavy to enlist," July 4, 2005.

76 Berkey, Catherine S., et al., "Milk, dairy fat, dietary calcium, and weight gain," *Archives of Pediatrics & Adolescent Medicine* 159 (2005):543–50; *Journal of Clinical Biochemistry and Nutrition* 9 (1990):61–66.

77 Pennington, Jean A., *Bowes & Church's Food Values of Portions Commonly Used*, 17th Ed (Philadelphia: Lippincott, Williams & Wilkins, 1998).

78 Stein, Ross, "Got milk? Too much makes for a fat kid. Study blunts claim that moo juice helps people lose weight," *Washington Post*, June 7, 2005.

79 Center for Science in the Public Interest, "Dairy does diets," *Nutrition Action Health Letter*, Sept. 2004.

80 Gunther, C.W., et al. "Dairy products do not lead to alterations in body weight or fat mass in young women in a one-year intervention," *American Journal of Clinical Nutrition* 81 (2005):751–56.

81 Thompson, W.G., et al., "Effect of energy-reduced diets high in dairy products and fiber on weight loss in obese adults," *Obesity Research* 13 (2005):1344–53.

82 Barclay, Laurie, "High calcium and dairy intake may not reduce long-term weight gain," *Medscape Medical News*, March 13, 2006.

83 Warner, Melanie, "Chug milk, shed pounds? Not so fast," *New York Times*, June 21, 2005.

84 Berkey, Catherine S., et al., "Milk, dairy fat, dietary calcium, and weight gain," *Archives of Pediatrics & Adolescent Medicine* 159 (2005):543–50; Fox, Maggie, "Milk may make for heavier kids, study finds," *Reuters*, June 6, 2005.

85 Presented as part of the symposium "Dairy Product Components and Weight Regulation," given at the 2002 Experimental Biology meeting on April 21, 2002, New Orleans, LA. The symposium was sponsored by

The American Society for Nutritional Sciences and supported in part by Dairy Management Inc. and General Mills Inc., American Society for Nutritional Sciences, *Journal of Nutrition* 133 (2003): 243S–244S.

86   American Fitness Professionals and Associates, "That gut feeling," afpafitness.com/articles/Crohns Milk.htm; International Adhesions Society, adhesions.org

87   Perry, Patrick, "Unraveling the mystery of Crohn's disease," *The Saturday Evening Post,* Feb. 16, 2006.

88   APHIS Veterinary Services, Centers for Epidemiology and Animal Health, United States Department of Agriculture, Animal and Plant Health Inspection Service, "Johne's disease on US dairies, 1991–2007"; nahms.aphis.usda.gov

89   Trickett, Sarah, "Strategy to eradicate Johne's disease needed now," *Farmers Weekly Interactive,* Jan. 6, 2010.

90   Woodman, Richard, "British study links Crohn's disease to milk bug," *Reuters,* Aug. 6, 2003.

91   Gay, Lance, "Dairy industry seeks $1.3 billion to kill diseased cows," *Scripps Howard News Service,* 2001.

92   Hermon-Taylor, John, "Mycobacterium avium subspecies paratuberculosis, Crohn's disease and the Doomsday Scenario," *Gut Pathogens* 1 (2009):1–6.

93   Nauta, M. J., et al., "Human exposure to mycobacterium paratuburculosis via pasteurized milk: A modeling approach," *Veterinary Record* 143 (1998):293–96.

94   Woodman, Richard, "British study links Crohn's disease to milk bug," *Reuters,* Aug. 6, 2003.

95   Maugh, T., "Milk may be the carrier of Crohn's causes: Some argue that the bug that may cause disease is found in dairy herds," *Los Angeles Times,* Sept. 18, 2000.

96   Scientific Committee on Animal Health and Animal Welfare. "Possible links between Crohn's disease and Paratuberculosis," SANCO/B3/R16/ 2000 European Commission Directorate-General Health & Consumer Protection Directorate B — Scientific Health Opinions Unit B3, adopted Mar. 21, 2000:50–51.

97   *Cheese Reporter,* Aug. 19, 2004, cheesereporter.com

98   Perry, Patrick, "Unraveling the mystery of Crohn's disease," *The Saturday Evening Post,* Feb. 16, 2006, pp 6–9.

99 Podolsky, D.K., "Inflammatory bowel disease, Part I," *New England Journal of Medicine* 325 (1991):928.

100 Armitage, E., et al., "Increasing incidence of both juvenile-onset Crohn's disease and ulcerative colitis in Scotland," *European Journal of Gastroenterology and Hepatology* 13 (2001):1439–47.

101 "Farmers worry about disease of milk cows," *Marin Independent Journal,* May 27, 2001, A:A5.ibid.

102 Nauta, M.J., et al., "Human exposure to mycobacterium paratuburculosis via pasteurized milk: A modeling approach," *Veterinary Record* 143 (1998):293–96.

103 Hermon-Taylor, John, "Mycobacterium avium subspecies paratuberculosis, Crohn's disease and the doomsday scenario," Gut Pathogens 15 (2009):1–6.

104 24-7 PressRelease.com, "Is the dairy industry the new McDonalds?" July 3, 2005, from *Foods for Life,* 31 Eland Road, Croydon, Surrey, United Kingdom CR04LJ.

105 Chiodini, R.J., et al., "Presence of mycobacterium paratuberculosis antibodies in animal healthcare workers," Proceedings of the Fifth International Colloquium on Paratuberculosis, International Association of Paratuberculosis (1996):324-28.

106 cancer.org/docroot/STT/STT_0.asp; American Cancer Society, "Annual report to the nation on the status of cancer, 1973–98, featuring cancers with recent increasing trends," 93 (2001):824–42.

107 cancernetwork.com/display/article/10165/97413

108 National Research Council, *Diet, Nutrition, and Cancer* (Washington, DC: National Academy Press, 1982), nap.edu/books/0309032806/html/1.html

109 Madhavan, T.V., et al., "The effect of dietary protein on carcinogenesis of aflatoxin," *Archives of Pathology* 85 (1968):133–37.

110 *Journal of the National Cancer Institute* 95 (2003):1079 Cho, Eunyoung, et al., "Premenopausal fat intake and risk of breast cancer,"

111 US Department of Health and Human Services, *The Surgeon General's Report on Nutrition and Health,* Publication No. 88-50210, 1998.

112 "Big news on breast cancer," *Alternative Medicine,* Oct. 2003, p. 17.

113 Goldin, B., "Estrogen excretion patterns and plasma levels in vegetarian and omnivorous women," *New England Journal of Medicine* 307 (1982):1542–47.

114 Schindler, A., "Conversion of androstenedione to estrone by human fat tissue," *Journal of Endocrinology & Metabolism* 35 (1972):627–30.

115 MacDonald, P., "Effect of obesity on conversion of plasma androstenedione to estrone in postmenopausal women with and without endometrial cancer," *American Journal of Obstetrics and Gynecology* 130 (1978):448–55.

116 Hivley, Will, "Worrying About Milk", *Discover* 21, No. 8 (2000).

117 Grosvenor, Clark, E., et al., "Hormones and growth factors in milk," Endrocrine Reviews 14 (1993):710-28. "The Tainted Milk Mustache — How Monsanto and the FDA Spoiled a Staple Food," *Alternative Medicine,* 27 (1999):94–104.

118 Ireland, Corydon, "Hormones in milk can be dangerous," *Harvard University Gazette,* Dec. 8, 2006.

119 Plant, Jane, *Your Life in Your Own Hands* (New York: Thomas Dunne Books, 2001).; Plant, Jane, *The No-Dairy Breast Cancer Prevention Program: How One Scientist's Discovery Helped Her Defeat Her Cancer* (New York: St. Martin's Griffin, 2002).

120 Midwest Dairy Association. Jeanne Goldberg, Q&A, Mar. 2002. midwestdairy.com

121 Juskevich, J., et al., "Bovine growth hormone: Human food safety evaluation," *Science* 249 (1990):875–84; Mepham, T. B., "Bovine somatotropin and public health," *British Medical Journal* 302 (1991):4833–84.

122 "The Politics of Medicine," *Alternative Medicine* 27 (1997): 94.

123 Outwater, J.L., et al., "Dairy products and breast cancer: The IGF-1, estrogen, and BGH hypothesis," *Medical Hypothesis* 48 (1997):453–61.

124 See this story in the June/July 1998 issue of *SunCoast Eco Report.* Copies can be ordered through the editor at *SunCoast Eco Report,* PO Box 35500, Sarasota, FL 34278, or at foxBGHsuit.com

125 Xian, C., "Degradation of IGF-1 in the adult rat gastrointestinal tract is limited by a specific antiserum or the dietary protein casein," *Journal of Endocrinology* 146 (1995):215.

126 Hankinson, S. E., et al., "Circulating concentrations of insulin-like growth factor I and risk of breast cancer," *Lancet* 351 (1998):1393–96; Peyrat, J. P., et al., "Plasma insulin-like growth factor-1 (IGF-1) concentrations in breast cancer," *European Journal of Cancer* 29 (1993):492–97.

127 Ma, J., et al., "Milk intake, circulating levels of insulin-like growth factor-I, and risk of colorectal cancer in men," *Journal of the National Cancer Institute* 93 (2001):1330–36.

128 Cadogan, J., et al., "Milk intake and bone mineral acquisition in adolescent girls: Randomised, controlled intervention trial," *British Medical Journal* 315 (1997):1255–60.

129 Editorial, "A Needless New Risk of Breast Cancer," *Los Angeles Times,* Mar. 20, 1994.

130 Epstein, Samuel, "Potential public health hazards of biosynthetic milk hormones," *International Journal of Health Services* 23 (1990):73–84.

131 elanco.us/products/posilac.htm

132 Peck, Peggy, "Two or more glasses of milk may raise ovarian cancer risks, still doctors aren't advising that women stop drinking it," *WebMD Medical News,* May 5, 2000.

133 *American Journal of Epidemiology* 130 (1989):904–10.

134 "Two recent studies are souring milk's image among health authorities," *News-Medical.net,* Dec. 6, 2004. news-medical.net/?id=6697

135 Larsson, Susanna, et al., "Milk and lactose intakes and ovarian cancer risk in the Swedish Mammography Cohort," *American Journal of Clinical Nutrition* 80 (2004): 1353–57.

136 EarthSave International, PO Box 96, New York, NY, 10108; earthsave.org/health/milkletter.htm

137 Larsson, S.C., et al., "Milk, milk products, and lactose intake and ovarian cancer risk: a meta-analysis of epidemiological studies," *International Journal of Cancer* 118 (2006):431–41.

138 Liu, et al., *Reproductive Toxicology* 14 (2000):377–84.

139 Cramer, D.W., "Lactase persistence and milk consumption as determinants of ovarian cancer risk," *American Journal of Epidemiology* 130 (1989):904–10.

140 American Cancer Society, as cited in *Nutrition Action Health Letter,* Center for Science in the Public Interest 27 (May 2000):8.

141 Giovannucci, Edward, et al., "Dairy Products, calcium, and Vitamin D and risk of prostate cancer," *Epidemiologic Reviews* 23 (2001):87–92.

142 Talamini, R., et al., "Nutrition, social factors, and prostatic cancer in a northern Italian population," *British Journal of Cancer* 53 (1986):817–21; Mettlin, C., et al., "Beta-carotene and animal fats and their relationship to prostate cancer risk: a case-control study," *Cancer* 64 (1989):605–12; La Vecchia, C., et al., "Dairy products and the risk of prostatic cancer," *Oncology* 48 (1991):406–10; Talamini, R., et al.,"Diet and prostatic cancer: a case-control study in northern Italy," *Nutrition and Cancer* 18

(1992):277–86; De Stefani, E., et al., "Tobacco, alcohol, diet and risk of prostate cancer," *Tumori* 81 (1995): 315–20; Chan, J.M., et al., "Dairy products, calcium, phosphorous, vitamin D, and risk of prostate cancer," *Cancer Causes & Control* 9(1998):559–66; Jain, M.G., et al., "Plant foods, antioxidants, and prostate cancer risk: findings from case-control studies in Canada," *Nutrition and Cancer* 34 (1999):173–84; Rotkin, I.D., "Studies in the epidemiology of prostatic cancer: expanded sampling," *Cancer Treatment Reports* 61 (1977):173–80; Schuman, L.M., et al., "Some selected features of the epidemiology of prostatic cancer: Minneapolis-St. Paul, Minnesota, case-control study, 1976–79. In: Magnus, K., ed., *Trends in cancer incidence: causes and practical implications* (Washington, DC: Hemisphere Publishing, 1982),345–54; Whittemore, A.S., et al., Prostate cancer in relation to diet, physical activity, and body size in blacks, whites, and Asians in the United States and Canada," *Journal of the National Cancer Institute* 87 (1995): 652–61; Hayes, R.B., et al., "Dietary factors and risk for prostate cancer among blacks and whites in the United States," *Cancer Epidemiology, Biomarkers & Prevention* 8 (1999):25–34; Tzonou, A., et al., "Diet and cancer of the prostate: a case-control study in Greece," *International Journal of Cancer* 80 (1999):704–8; Severson, R.K., et al., "A prospective study of demographics, diet, and prostate cancer among men of Japanese ancestry in Hawaii," Cancer Research 49 (1989):1857–60; Le Marchand, L., et al., "Animal fat consumption and prostate cancer: a prospective study in Hawaii," *Epidemiology* 5 (1994):276–82; Giovannucci, E., et al., "Calcium and fructose intake in relation to risk of prostate cancer," *Cancer Research* 58 (1998):442–7; Schuurman, A.G., et al., "Animal products, calcium, and protein and prostate cancer risk in The Netherlands Cohort Study," *British Journal of Cancer* 80 (1999):1107–13; Chan, J.M., et al., "Dairy products, calcium, and prostate cancer in the Physicians' Health Study," *American Journal of Clinical Nutrition* 74 (2001):549–54; Snowdon, D.A., et al., "Diet, obesity, and risk of fatal prostate cancer," *American Journal of Epidemiology* 120 (1984):244–50; Chan, J.M. et al., "Diet and prostate cancer risk in a cohort of smokers, with a specific focus on calcium and phosphorous," (Finland) *Cancer Causes & Control* 11(2000):859–67.

143 Chan, J., et al., "Plasma insulin-like growth factor 1 and prostate cancer risk: a prospective study," *Science* 279 (1998):563–66.

144 Ibid.

145 Tzonou, A., et al., "Diet and cancer of the prostate: a case-control study in Greece," *International Journal of Cancer* 80 (1999): 704–8.

146 Mettlin, C., et al., "Beta-carotene and animal fats and their relationship to prostate cancer risk: A case-control study," *Cancer* 64 (1989):605–12.

147 Chan, J.M., et al., "Dairy products, calcium, and prostate cancer risk in the Physicians' Health Study," *American Journal of Clinical Nutrition* 74 (2001):549–54.

148 Ganmaa, D., et al., "Incidence and mortality of testicular and prostate cancers in relation to world dietary practices," *International Journal of Cancer* 98 (2002):262–67.

149 Qin, L.Q., et al., "Milk consumption is a risk factor for prostate cancer: meta-analysis of case-control studies," *Nutrition and Cancer* 481 (2004):22–27.

150 Giovannucci, Edward, et al., "Dairy Products, calcium, and Vitamin D and risk of prostate cancer," *Epidemiologic Reviews* 23 (2001):87–92.

151 Malosse, D., et al., "Correlation between milk and dairy product consumption and multiple sclerosis prevalence: a worldwide study," *Neuroepidemiology* 11 (1993):304–12.; Butcher, J., "The distribution of multiple sclerosis in relation to the dairy industry and milk consumption. *New Zealand Medical Journal* 83 (1976):427–30.

152 Malosse, D., et al., "Correlation between milk and dairy product consumption and multiple sclerosis prevalence: a worldwide study," *Neuroepidemiology* 11 (1992):304-12. Adapted from Campbell, Colin, T., The China Study. Dallas: Benbella, 2004.

153 Guggenmos, J., et al., "Antibody cross-reactivity between myelin oligo-dendrocyte glycoprotein and the milk protein butyrophilin in multiple sclerosis," *Journal of Immunology* 172 (2004): 661–68.

154 Chen, H., et al., "Diet and Parkinson's disease: a potential role of dairy products in men," *Annals of Neurology* 52 (2003):793–801.

155 Park, M., et al., "Consumption of milk and calcium in midlife and the future risk of Parkinson's disease," *Neurology* 64 (2005):1047–51.

156 MSNBC News, "Dairy intake tied to Parkinson's in Men," msnbc.msn.com/id/18203093/%23storyContinued/, April 27, 2007.

157 Menegon, A., et al., "Parkinson's disease, pesticides, and glutathione transferase polymorphisms," *Lancet* 24 (1998):1344–46.; Elbaz, A., et al., "CYP2D6 polymorphism, pesticide exposure, and Parkinson's disease," *Annals of Neurology* 55 (2004):430–34; Ossowska K., et al., "Degeneration

of dopaminergic mesocortical neurons and activation of compensatory processes induced by a long-term paraquat administration in rats: Implications for Parkinson's disease," *Neuroscience* 141 (2006): 2155–65.

158 scientificamerican.com/article.cfm?id=study-bolsters-link-betwe

159 "Costello, Sadie, et al., Parkinson's disease and residential exposure to maneb and paraquat from agricultural applications in the Central Valley of California," *American Journal of Epidemiology* 169 (2009): 919–26; Elbaz, Alexis, et al., "Professional exposure to pesticides and Parkinson disease," *Annals of Neurology* 66 (2009): 494–504.

160 Crook, W., *Ritalin: Help for the Hyperactive Child* (Jackson, TN.: Professional Books, 1991).

161 Chavarro, J.E., et al., "A prospective study of dairy foods intake and anovulatory infertility," *Human Reproduction* (2007):1–8.

162 Cramer, D., et al., "Adult hypolactasia, milk consumption, and age-specific fertility," *American Journal of Epidemiology* 139 (1994):282–89.

163 Ylikorkala, O., et al., "New concepts in dysmenorrhea," *American Journal of Obstetrics and Gynecology* 130 (1978):833–47.

164 Heber, D., et al., "Reduction of serum estradiol in postmenopausal women given free access to low-fat high-carbohydrate diet," *Nutrition* 7 (1991):137–39; Wynder, E. L., "The dietary environment and cancer," *Journal of the American Dietetic Association* 71 (1977):385–92; Ingram, D. M., et al., "Effect of a low-fat diet on female sex hormone levels," *Journal of the National Cancer Institute* (1987); Prentice, R., et al., "Dietary fat reduction and plasma estradiol concentration of healthy postmenopausal women," *Journal of the National Cancer Institute* 82 (1990):129–34; Goldin, B. R., et al., "Effect of diet on the plasma levels, metabolism and excretion of estrogens," *American Journal of Clinical Nutrition* 48 (1988):787–90.

165 Prentice, R., et al., "Dietary fat reduction and plasma estradiol concentration in healthy postmenopausal women," *Journal of the National Cancer Institute* 82 (1090):129.; Rose, D.P., et al., "Effect of a low-fat diet on hormone levels in women with cystic breast disease," *Journal of the National Cancer Institute* 78 (1987):623.

166 Northrop, Christiane, *Women's Bodies, Women's Wisdom* (New York: Bantam, 1994).

167 WHO, "*Recommendations from WHO's consultation on zoonoses,*" May 5, 2004. who.int/mediacentre/news/briefings/2004/mb3/en/

168 Dworkin, Andy, "Cattle disease fears don't cow American carnivores," *The Oregonian*, Aug. 15, 2004.; ers.usda.gov/Features/BSE/

169 "FAQ: Canadian fourth case of BSE confirmed," Jan. 23, 2006, foodconsumer.org/777/8/FAQ_Canadian_fourth_case_of_BSE_confirmed.shtml; "Mad cow case found in British Columbia," *Chicago Tribune*, Apr. 17, 2006, chicagotribune.com/news/nationworld/chi-0604170129apr17,1,6639787.story?coll= chi-newsnationworld-hed

170 Mercer, Chris, "Study highlights milk BSE risk," February 6, 2007, nutraingredients.com/news/printNewsBis.asp

171 "Report from Washington meeting on Bovine Tuberculosis," USDA Animal and Plant Health Inspection Service (APHIS), Washington, DC, Dec. 8, 2008; mirror.aphis.usda.gov/newsroom/hot_issues/bovine_tuberculosis/listening_sessions/DC_TB_LS_Summary.pdf

172 University of California Davis, Vet Views, *California Cattlemen*, "Bovine Tuberculosis: Infected Dairy Herd Identified in California," July/August 2002.

173 Mark, Jorie Green, "Bovine tuberculosis outbreaks declared national emergency," VetCentric.com, 2000.

174 "An epidemiological investigation into bovine tuberculosis," Second Report of the Independent Scientific Group on Cattle TB, Dec. 1999, Department of Environment, Food, and Rural Affairs, defra.gov.uk/animalh/tb/isg/report/contents.htm

175 "Q & A's about the bovine tuberculosis emergency declaration," aphis.usda.gov/lpa/pubs/fsheet_faq_notice.htm

176 Mark, Jorie Green, "Bovine tuberculosis outbreaks declared national emergency," VetCentric.com, 2000.

177 Meyer, Robert M., "Current status of the bovine tuberculosis eradication program in the United States, Apr. 1, 2003, USDA APHIS Veterinary Services.

178 "Bovine TB alarms health officials in Dharamshala", June 4, 2004, webindia123.com/news/showdetails.asp?id=39853&cat=India

Chapter 5

1 Chavez, Amy, "New year's resolution: self-mutilation, a trance and some milk," *Japan Times*, Feb. 18, 2006.

2 "More buyers asking: Got milk without chemicals?," *New York Times*, Aug. 1, 1999, p.6.

3   Harris, S., "Organochlorine contamination of breast milk," (Washington, D.C: Environmental Defense Fund, 1979).

4   Environmental Working Group, "Body burden: the pollution in newborns. A benchmark investigation of industrial chemicals, pollutants, and pesticides in human umbilical cord blood," July 14, 2005, executive summary available at: ewg.org/reports/bodyburden2/execsumm.php

5   Condon, Marian, "Breast is best, but it could be better: What is in breast milk that should not be?" *Pediatric Nursing* 31 (2005):333–38.

6   Chea, Terrence, "Study: Toxic chemical found in cow's milk," *Seattle Post-Intelligencer,* June 22, 2004.

7   Zhang, Husen, et al., "Perchlorate reduction by a novel chemolithoautotrophic, hydrogen-oxidizing bacterium," *Environmental Microbiology* 4 (2002):570–76.

8   Ibid.

9   "Fischer, Douglas, "Rocket fuel traces found in state milk," *Oakland Tribune,* June 22, 2004.

10 Ibid.

11 Organic Consumers Association, "Rocket fuel contaminates lettuce and milk," Nov. 29, 2004, organicconsumers.org/foodsafety/lettuce120104.cfm

12 Renner, Rebecca, "Perchlorate exposure: Tip of the iceberg?" *Foodconsumer's Agri & Environ,* Sept. 16, 2005.

13 "Rocket Science," *Environmental Working Group,* July 16, 2001. ewg.org/reports/rocketscience/; Horsham, P.A., "Oral (drinking water) two-generation (one litter per generation) reproduction study of ammonium perchlorate in rats," Argus Research Laboratories, Inc., protocol no. 1416-001 (1999). As cited in EPA 2002.

14 Ibid.

15 Haddow J.E., , et al., "Maternal thyroid deficiency during pregnancy and subsequent neuropsychological development of the child," *New England Journal of Medicine.* 341 (1999):549–55.

16 ewg.org/node/8441

17 Reich, M., "Environmental politics and science: The case of PBB contamination in Michigan," *American Journal of Public Health* 73 (1983):302–13.

18 Fischer, Douglas, "What's in you?" *Oakland Tribune,* Mar. 13, 2005, A1.

19 FDA Total Diet Study, Sept. 2004. Center for Food Safety and Applied Nutrition, Office of Plant and Dairy Foods. The Total Diet Study (TDS), sometimes called the Market Basket Study, is an ongoing FDA program

that determines levels of various contaminants and nutrients in foods. Since its inception in 1961 as a program to monitor for radioactive contamination of foods following atmospheric nuclear testing, TDS has grown to encompass additional radionuclides and residues of pesticides, industrial chemicals, toxic and nutritional elements, and folate. In all instances, analyses have been performed on foods that are prepared as they would be consumed (table-ready), so the final results can be used to provide a realistic measure of the dietary intake of these analytes.

20 pesticideinfo.org/Docs/ref_regulatoryUS.html.

21 Kiely, T., et al., *Pesticide Industry Sales and Usage: 2000 and 2001 Market Estimates,* US EPA, Office of Pesticide Programs, 2004.

22 Solomon, G., et al., *Pesticides and Human Health,* Physicians for Social Responsibility and Californians for Pesticide Reform (San Francisco, CA, 2000); psrla.org/pesthealthmain.htm.

23 Fear, N.T., et al., "Childhood cancer and paternal employment in agriculture: The role of pesticides," British Journal of Cancer 77 (1998):825–29; Sharpe, C.R., et al., "Parental exposures to pesticides and risk of Wilms' tumor in Brazil," *American Journal of Epidemiology* 141 (1995):210–17.

24 Schafer, Kristin S., et al., "Chemical trespass: Pesticides in our bodies and corporate accountability," *Pesticide Action Network,* May 2004.

25 US Center for Disease Control and Prevention, *Second National Report on Human Exposure to Environmental Chemicals,* Jan. 2003, cdc.gov

26 Environmental Working Group, *Body Burden: The Pollution in People* (Washington, D.C., 2003), ewg.org/reports/bodyburden; Bradman, A., et al., "Measurement of pesticides and other toxicants in amniotic fluid as a potential biomarker of prenatal exposure: A validation study," *Environmental Health Perspectives* 111 (2003):1179–82.

27 University of California Extension Toxicology Newsletter, "Inadvertent contamination of row crops from pesticides in fog," Vol. 9 No. 5, Dec. 1989, extoxnet.orst.edu/newsletters/n95_89.htm

28 Ames, B., "Ranking possible carcinogenic hazards," *Science* 236 (1987):272.

29 Yess, N.J., et al., "US Food and Drug Administration monitoring of pesticide residues in infant foods and adult foods eaten by infants/children," *Journal A.O.A.C. International* 76 (1993):492–507; 75 (1992):136A–158A; 74 (1991):121A–142A.

30 Dougherty, John, "Contaminated splendor" *Phoenix New Times,* Mar. 10, 2005, phoenixnewtimes.com

31 Steinman, D., *Diet for a Poisoned Planet* (New York: Ballantine, 1990).

32 "Milk: Why is its quality so low?" *Consumer Reports* 39 (1974):70.

33 Benbrook, Charles, "FAQs on pesticides in milk," The Organic Center, Dec. 2006.

34 Hedges, Stephen J., "Citing cost, USDA kills pesticide testing program," *Chicago Tribune,* September 27, 2008. archives.chicagotribune.com/ 2008/ sep/27/nation/chi-pesticidessep28

35 Corrigan, F.M., Wienburg, C.L., Shore, R.F., Daniel, S.E., and Mann, D., "Organochlorine insecticides in substantia nigra in Parkinson's disease," *Journal of Toxicology and Environmental Health* 59 (2000):229– 34; University of Rochester School of Medicine: urmc.rochester. edu/pr/News/park.html; Hileman, Bette, "The Environment and Parkinson's," *Chemical & Engineering News,* Sept. 17, 2001; Higgins, Margot, "Pesticides linked to Parkinson's disease," *Environmental News Network* (ENN), Jan. 11, 2001; *Associated Press,* "Study links pesticides, Parkinson's," Nov. 6, 2000; Chubb, Lucy, "Pesticide exposure linked to Parkinson's disease," May 6, 2000, *Environmental News Network.*

36 *Associated Press,* "Study links pesticides, Parkinson's," Nov. 6, 2000.

37 Allen, R.H., et al., "Breast cancer and pesticides in Hawaii: The need for further study," *Environmental Health Perspectives* 105, suppl. 3 (1997):679–83.

38 Sherman, J.D., "Structure-activity relationships of chemicals causing endocrine, reproductive, neurotoxic and oncogenic effects: Public health problem," *Toxicology and Industrial Health* 10 (1994):163–78.

39 Baker, D.B., "Estimation of human exposure to heptachlor epoxide and related pesticides in Hawaii," Heptachlor Research and Education Foundation (1994):1–8.

40 Brotons, J.A., et al., "Xenoestrogens released from laquer coatings in food cans," *Environmental Health Perspectives* 103 (1995):608, 612.

41 Sharpe, R.M., "Natural and anthropogenic environmental oestrogens: the scientific basis for risk assessment," *Pure and Applied Chemistry* 70 (1998):1685–1701; Colborn, T., et al., *Our Stolen Future* (Dutton, New York, 1996).

42 Reuters Health Information, Medscape, "Abbott says withdrawing attention deficit drug," Mar. 25, 2005, medscape.com/viewarticle/ 501948?src=mp; Rubin, Rita, "Warning advised on ADHD drugs; FDA

committee urges strongest notification," *USA Today,* Feb. 10–12, 2006, A1.

43 *Medscape Alert,* "FDA announces nationwide recall of all methylin chewable tablets," Feb. 14, 2005, medscape.com/viewarticle/499372

44 Physicians for Social Responsibility, psr.org; download available at: psr.igc.org/ihw-report.htm

45 Porter, Warren, et al., "Endocrine, immune and behavioral effects of aldicarb (carbamate), atrazine (triazine), and nitrate (fertilizer) mixtures at groundwater concentrations," *Toxicology and Industrial Health* 15 (1995):133–50.

46 Based upon personal discussions with the author.

47 Guillette, Elizabeth, et al., "An anthropological approach to the evaluation of preschool children exposed to pesticides in Mexico," *Environmental Health Perspectives* 106 (1998):347–53.

48 US Geological Survey, "Herbicides in ground water of the midwest: A regional study of shallow aquifers, 1991–94," July 1998.

49 Begley, Sharon, "The End of Antibiotics," *Newsweek,* Mar. 28, 1994, 47–52.

50 Heilman, Erica, "Overusing antibiotics: A serious problem," *Science Daily,* Sept. 10, 2001.

51 "Some dangers of hormones in milk," *Rachel's Hazardous Waste News* No. 382, Environmental Research Foundation, archive at: rachel.org

52 Begley, Sharon, "The End of Antibiotics," *Newsweek,* Mar. 28, 1994 p. 47–51.

53 "Rajala-Schultz, P. J., et al., "Effects of clinical mastitis on milk yield in dairy cows," *Journal of Dairy Science* 82 (1999):1213–20.

54 USDA, Animal and Plant Health Inspection Service, National Animal Health Monitoring System, Aug. 2004; Dairy 2002, Animal Disease Exclusion Practices on US Dairy Operations, 2002.

55 Ibid.

56 nahms.aphis.usda.gov/dairy/dairy07/Dairy2007_ABX.pdf

57 Perlman, D., "Doctors seek to limit antibiotics on the farm," *San Francisco Chronicle,* July 1, 2001, A16.

58 Marshall, Eliot, "Scientists endorse ban on antibiotics in feeds," *Science* 222, Nov. 11, 1983, p. 601.

59 Vickers, H.R., et al., "Dermatitis caused by penicillin in milk," *Lancet* 1 (1958):351–52; Wicher, K., et al., "Allergic reaction to penicillin present in milk," *Journal of the American Medical Association* 208 (1969):143–45.

60   Tanner, Lindsey, "Study links antibiotics and breast cancer," *Associated Press,* Feb. 16, 2004.

61   Grady, D., "A move to limit antibiotic use in animal feed," *New York Times,* Mar. 8, 1999.

62   Fox, Maggie, "US drug use in animals seen higher than thought," *Reuters News Service,* Jan. 2001.

63   *Wall Street Journal,* Dec. 29, 1989, as cited in Kradjian, Robert, "Well, at least cow's milk is pure," EarthSave International, earthsave.bc.ca/ materials/articles/health/milk_letter_p4.html; Ingersoil, Bruce, "FDA detects drugs in milk but fails to confirm results," *Wall Street Journal,* Feb. 6, 1990, A16.

64   Ingersoil, Bruce, "New York milk supply highly tainted, TV station says, based on own survey," *Wall Street Journal,* Feb. 8, 1990.

65   Kurtzweil, P., "Companies, employees answer to corrupt milk practices." Investigators' Reports, *FDA Journal,* Oct. 1991.

66   Investigator's Report, *FDA Journal* 30 (1996):34.

67   Fowler, Johnathan, "WHO: Farmers should cut antibiotic use," *Associated Press,* Sept. 16, 2003. For the full WHO report, see: who.int/salmsurv/links/gssamrgrowthreportstory/en/

68   *Food Production Daily.com* "Gene-transfer technology could increase dairy yield," Apr. 4, 2005.

69   Gersema, Emily, "FDA warns against use of drug in animals," *Associated Press,* Mar. 4, 2003.

70   Perry, Wayne, "Tainted nuke plant water reaches major NJ aquifer," *Associated Press,* May 8, 2010; google.com/hostednews/ap/article/ ALeqM5jrD4xonSoPnaXaZTftwd4RXuoA2gD9FI7LJ80

71   Lazaroff, C., "Former US nuclear weapons sites may be radioactive forever," Environment News Service, Aug. 8, 2000.

72   Caldicott, Helen, *Nuclear Madness* (New York, Norton, 1994), p. 42.

73   Ecke, Richard, "Fallout's fallout," *Great Falls Tribune–Online,* Feb. 1, 2005.

74   Caldicott, Helen, *Nuclear Madness* (New York, Norton, 1994), p. 42; also see: beyondnuclear.org for further insight into routes of human exposures.

75   Rather, J., "Babies' teeth and radiation's path," *New York Times,* June 6, 1999.

76   doh.wa.gov/hanford/publications/health/mon6.htm

77   Sternglass, E.J., et al., "Breast cancer: Evidence for a relationship to fission products in the diet," *International Journal of Health Services* 23 (1993):783–804.

78   Campbell, A., et al., Pro-inflammatory effects of aluminum in human
      glioblastoma cells," *Brain Research* 933 (2002):60–65.
79   Candy, J.M., et al., "Aluminosilicates and senile plaque formation in
      Alzheimer's disease," *Lancet* 1 (1986):354–57.
80   Soni, M.G., et al., "Safety evaluation of dietary aluminum," *Regulatory
      Toxicology and Pharmacology* 33 (2001):66–79.
81   Ibid.
82   Fernandez-Lorenzo, J.R., "Aluminum contents of human milk, cow's milk,
      and infant formulas," *Journal of Pediatric Gastroenterology and Nutrition*
      28 (1999):270–75.
83   Baumslag, Naomi, and Dia L. Michels, *Milk, Money, and Madness:
      The Culture and Politics of Breastfeeding* (London: Bergin & Garvey,
      1995).
84   "Mass treatment of humans who drank unpasteurized milk from rabid
      cows — Massachusetts, 1996–1998," *MMWR-CDC Weekly*, Mar. 26
      1999:228–29.
85   Nascenzi, Nicole, "At least 45 begin rabies treatments," Tulsa World, Dec.
      25, 2005., A1.; Nascenzi, Nicole, "42 believed at risk for rabies", *Tulsa
      World*, Dec. 24, 2005.
86   Dr. Arnold Schecter speaking at the People's Dioxin Action Summit, UC
      Berkeley, Aug. 10, 2000.
87   Pianin, Eric, "Dioxin report EPA on hold. Industries oppose finding of
      cancer link, urge delay," *Washington Post*, Apr. 12, 2001: A1.
88   Carter, Graydon, "The air at ground zero," *Vanity Fair*, Editor's Letter,
      Sept. 2004.
89   Harrison, N., "Dioxins in cow's milk," MAFF, Food Safety and Science
      Group, Oct. 1994, Food Contaminants Division, London, England,
      SW1P3JR; maff.gov.uk
90   Wired News, "Ben & Jerry's Dioxin Controversy," Aug. 18, 2000, wired.
      com/news/technology/0,1282,38302,00.html
91   National Center for Independent Information on Waste (Centre national
      d'information indépendante sur les déchets or CNIID); contact Pierre-
      Emmanuel Neurohr, at 00 33 1 43 58 68 65.
92   "FDA launches study on dioxin in fish, dairy foods," *Food Chemical News*,
      Feb. 27, 1995, as cited in *Rachel's Environment and Health Weekly*, July 17,
      1997, p. 2.
93   Rauch, Molly, "Reducing dioxin in milk," *Green Guide*, July/August 2004.

94 Center for Science in the Public Interest, "Dioxin for dinner?" *Nutrition Action Health Letter* 27, no 8 (Oct. 2000).

95 Advertisement for Promised Land Dairy products, *Vegetarian Times,* Apr. 2004, p. 22.

96 "The tainted milk mustache: How Monsanto and the FDA spoiled a staple food," *Alternative Medicine* 27 (1999):94–104.

97 Colborn, Theo, et al., *Our Stolen Future* (New York: Dutton, 1996).

98 Freeman, Aaron, "Monkeying with milk," *Multinational Monitor* 15 June, 1994; multinationalmonitor.org/hyper/issues/1994/06/freeman.html

99 Physicians Committee for Responsible Medicine, *Good Medicine,* Spring 1999.

100 "FDA approves Rumensin, WI dairy producers stand to benefit," *Wisconsin Ag Connection,* Nov. 5, 2004.

101 *Upstairs, Downstairs: Perchloroethylene in the Air in Apartments Above New York City Dry-Cleaners* (New York: Consumers Union, 1995); *Clothed in Controversy: The Risk to New Yorkers from Dry-Cleaning Emissions and What Can Be Done About It* (New York: Office of the Public Advocate for the City of New York, 1994).

102 ehp.niehs.nih.gov/; ppg.com/chm_chloralk/Bulletins/ Perchloroethylene. pdf?title=Perchloroethylene

103 nahms.aphis.usda.gov/dairy/dairy07/Dairy07_is_BLV.pdf; Hursting, S.D. Diet and human leukemia: an analysis of international data," *Preventive Medicine* 22 (1993):409–22; Buehring, G.C., et al., "Humans have anti-bodies reactive with bovine leukemia virus," *AIDS Res Hum Retroviruses* 12 (2003):1105–13; "Virus-like particles in cow's milk from herd with a high incidence of lymphosaroma," *Journal of the National Cancer Institute* 33 (1964):2055–64; Marie-Liesse, G., "Effects of brucellosis vaccination and dehorning on transmission of bovine leukemia virus in heifers on a California dairy," *Canadian Journal of Veterinary Research* 54 (1990):184; Ferrer, J., "Milk of dairy cows frequently contains leukemogenic virus," *Science* 213 (1981):1014; "Beware of the cow" (editorial), *Lancet* 2 (1974): 30; *British Medical Journal* 61 (1990):456–59; Olmstead, M., et al., "The prevalence of proviral leukemia virus in peripheral blood mono-nuclear cells at two subclinical stages of infection," *Journal of Virology* 70 (1996):2178.

104 Erskine, Ron and Lorraine Sordillo, "Bovine Leukosis Virus Update I: Prevalence, Economic Losses, and Management," *Michigan Dairy*

Review, Jan. 2009; msu.edu/~mdr/vol14no1/erskine.html

105 Ferrer, J.F., et al., "Milk of dairy cows frequently contains leukemogenic virus," *Science* 213 (1981):1014.

106 "Beware the cow" (editorial), *Lancet* 2 (1974):30; Olson, C., et al., "Transmission of lymphosarcoma from cattle to sheep," *Journal of the National Cancer Institute* 49 (1972):1463; McClure, H. M., et al., "Erythroleukemia in two infant chimpanzees fed milk from cows naturally infected with bovine C-type virus," *Cancer Research* 34 (1974):2745–57.

107 Kradjian, Robert, "The Milk Letter: A Message to My Patients," reprinted at the EarthSave website: rense.com/general29/milkt.html; Hulse, Virgil, *Mad Cows and Milkgate* (Phoenix: Marble Mountain Publishing, 1996).

108 Centers for Disease Control, "Mass treatment of humans who drank unpasteurized milk from rabid cows: Massachusetts, 1996–1998," *MMWR Weekly* 48 (1999):228–29.

109 Harris, Mark, "Got milk? Raw does a body good," *Vegetarian Times,* Sept. 2003, p.77.

110 Oski, Frank, "Is bovine milk a health hazard?" *Pediatrics* 75 (suppl) (1985):182–86.

111 Buehring, G.C., et al., "Humans have antibodies reactive with bovine leukemia virus," *AIDS Research Human Retroviruses* 12 (2003):1105–13.

112 Ibid.

113 Blair, A., "Leukemia cell types and agricultural practices in Nebraska," *Archives of Environmental Health* 40 (1985):211–14.; Donham, K.J., "Epidemiologic relationships of the bovine population and human leukemia in Iowa," *American Journal of Epidemiology* 112 (1980):80–92.

114 "Epidemiological relationships of the bovine population and human leukemia in Iowa," *American Journal of Epidemiology* 112 (1980):80.; Hursting, S.D., "Diet and human leukemia: an analysis of international data," *Preventive Medicine* 22 (1993):409–22.

115 Buehring, G.C., et al., "Bovine leukemia virus in human breast tissues," *Breast Cancer Research* 3 (2001) (Suppl 1):14.

116 Hulse, Virgil, *Mad Cows and Milkgate* (Marble Mountain Publishing, Phoenix, 1996).

117 "Tainted milk leads Japan firm to suspend dairy production," *The Honolulu Advertiser,* July 12, 2000, A10.

118 Wong, S., "Recalls of foods and cosmetics due to microbial contamination reported to the US Food and Drug Administration," *Journal of Food Protection* 63 (2000):1113–16.

119 *Reuters News*, "Study finds evidence food bug can cause arthritis," Jan. 1, 2000.

120 *American Journal of Epidemiology* 111 (1980):247–53.

121 Centers for Disease Control and Prevention, "Milk-borne salmonellosis: Illinois, update," 34 (1985):215; *FDA Consumer* 20 (1986):18.

122 *Journal of Dairy Science* 75 (1992):2330.

123 *New England Journal of Medicine* 334 (1996):1281–86.

124 Reilly, W.J., et al., "Milkborne salmonellosis in Scotland between 1980–1982," *Veterinary Record* 112 (1985):578–80.

125 Associated Press, "Missouri dairy recalls cheese," May 25, 1999.

126 Business Slant, *The Monroe Times*, Mar. 15, 2005, see themonroetimes.com/b0315bea.htm

127 Adkinson, R.W., "Implications of proposed changes in bulk tank somatic cell count regulations," *Journal of Dairy Science* 84 (2001):370–74.

128 Day, K., "Dairy, consumer groups udderly at odds on cow hormone," *The Washington Post*, May 2, 1995, D:1.

129 Brown, D., "Dairy gets an F for vitamin D content," *Washington Post*, Apr. 30, 1992.

130 Holick, M.F., et al., "The vitamin D content of fortified milk and infant formula," *New England Journal of Medicine* 326 (1992): 1178–81; Jacobus, C.H., et al., "Hypervitaminosis D associated with drinking milk," *New England Journal of Medicine* 326 (1992):1173–77.

131 *Associated Press*, "Chocolate milk recalled for vitamins," Mar. 23, 2003.

132 Ibid.

133 Taylor, W.H., "Renal calculi and self-medication with multi-vitamin preparations containing vitamin D," *Clinical Science* 42 (1972):515–22; Frost, J.W., et al., "Prolonged hypercalcemia and metastatic calcification of the sclera following the use of vitamin D in the treatment of rheumatoid arthritis," *American Journal of Medical Studies* 214 (1947):639; Forfar, J.O., et al., "Idiopathic hypercalcemia of infants: Clinical and metabolic studies with special reference to etiologic role of vitamin D," *Lancet* (1956):981–88; Facobus, C.H., et al., "Hypervitaminosis D associated with drinking milk," *New England Journal of Medicine* 326 (1992):1173–77;

"The vitamin D content of fortified milk and infant formula," *New England Journal of Medicine* 326 (1992):1178–81.

134 "Dietary calcium and idiopathic hypercalciuria," *Lancet* 1 (1981):786.

135 Byrdwell, W.C., et al., "Analyzing vitamin D in foods and supplements: methodologic challenges," *American Journal of Clinical Nutrition* 88 (2008):554S-7S.

Chapter 6

1 Tong, Vinnee, "Some schools to serve carbonated milk," *Associated Press,* Sept. 2, 2003; "Schools milk plastic bottles' popularity," *Denver Post.com,* Dec. 29, 2004.

2 Hirsch, J.M., "Schools replace milk cartons with bottles," *Associated Press.*

3 Lanou, Amy Joy, et al., "Dairy products and bone health in children and young adults: A reevaluation of the evidence," 115 *Pediatrics* (2005):736–43.

4 Winzenberg, T., et al., "Effects of calcium supplementation on bone density in healthy children: meta-analysis of randomized controlled trials," *BMJ (British Medical Journal)* 333 (2006):775–80.

5 Iacono, G., et al., "Persistent cow's milk protein intolerance in infants: The changing faces of the same disease," *Clinical and Experimental Allergy* 28 (1998):817–23; Schrander, J.J.P., et al., "Follow-up study of cow's milk protein intolerant infants," *European Journal of Pediatrics* 151 (1992):783–85; Bishop, J.M., et al., "Natural history of cow's milk allergy: clinical outcome," *Journal of Pediatrics* 116 (1990):862–67.

6 adelaide.net.au/~ndk/rhiannon.htm

7 Ryan, Rosalind, "Do you know the whole truth about milk?" *Mail Online (Daily Mail),* February 9, 2010.

8 Birch, E., et al., "Breast feeding and optimal visual development," *Journal of Pediatric Opthamology Strabismus* 30 (1993):33–38; Makrides, M., et al., Erythrocyte docosahexaenoic acid correlates with the visual response of healthy, term infants," *Pediatric Research* 34 (1993):425–27; Jorgensen, M.H., et al., "Breast-fed term infants have a better visual acuity than formula fed infants at the age of 2 and 4 months," *FASEB J* 8 (1994):2666A (abstract).

9 Lucarelli, S., et al., "Food allergy and infantile autism," *Panminera Medica* 37 (1995):137–41.

10 Schwartz, Robert, "Allergy, intolerance, and other adverse reactions to foods," *Pediatric Annals* 21 (1992):654–74.

11 Spock, B., and S. J. Parker, *Dr. Spock's Baby and Child Care* (New York: Pocket, 1998).

12 Lovegrove, J. A., et al., "Does a maternal milk-free diet prevent allergy in the "at-risk" infant?" *Proceedings of the Nutrition Society* 52 (1993):217.

13 Lehrman, Sally, "Drop milk?" *Alternative Medicine*, Apr. 2005.

14 Attwood, C., "The great American milk myth," all-creatures.org/cb/a-milk.html

15 Bertron, P., et al., "Racial bias in federal nutrition policy, part I: The public health implications of variations in lactase persistence," *Journal of the National Medical Association* 91 (1999):151–57.

16 Barnard, Neal, "Moo not necessarily good for you," *Seattle Post-Intelligencer*, Nov. 6, 2002.

17 Reilly, Jennifer, et al., "Acceptability of soymilk as a calcium-rich beverage in elementary school children," *Journal of the American Dietetic Association* 106 (2006):590–93.

18 Oski, Frank, *Don't Drink Your Milk!: New Frightening Medical Facts About the World's Most Overrated Nutrient* (New York: Teach Services, 1992).

19 Altintas, D., et al., "A prospective study of cow's milk allergy in Turkish infants," *Acta Paediatr* 84 (1995):1320–21.

20 Parish, W. E., et al., "Hypersensitivity to milk and sudden death in infancy," *Lancet* (1960):1106–10; Coombs, R.R., et al., "Allergy and cot death: With special focus on allergic sensitivity to cow's milk and anaphylaxis," *Clinical and Experimental Allergy* 20 (1990):359–66; Coombs, R.R., et al., "The enigma of cot death: Is the modified-anaphylaxis hypothesis an explanation for some cases?" *Lancet* 1(1982):1388–89; Coombs, R. R., The Jack Pepys Lecture, "The hypersensitivity reactions: Some personal reflections," *Clinical and Experimental Allergy* 22 (1992):673–80; E.A. Mitchell et al., "Cot death supplement: results from the first year of the New Zealand cot death study," *New Zealand Medical Journal* 104 (1991): 71-6.

21 Coombs, R.R., et al., "Hypersensitivity to milk and sudden death in infancy," *Lancet* 2 (1960); Coombs, R.R., et al., "Allergy and cot death: With special focus on allergic sensitivity to cow's milk and anaphylaxis," *Clinical and Experimental Allergy*, July 20, 1990:359–66.

22 Coombs, R.R., et al., "Allergy and cot death: With special focus on allergic sensitivity to cow's milk and anaphylaxis," *Clinical and Experimental Allergy*, July 20, 1990:359–66.

23 Parish, W., "Hypersensitivity to milk and sudden death in infancy," *Lancet* 2 (1960).

24 Dunea, G., "Beyond the etheric," *British Medical Journal* 285 (1982):428–29.

25 Rowe, A.H., et al., "Bronchial asthma due to food allergy alone in ninety-five patients," *Journal of the American Medical Association* 169 (1959):1158–62.

26 Kaufman, H.S., et al., "Prevention of asthma," *Clinical Allergy* 11 (1981):549–53.

27 Ibid.

28 Brasher, G.W., "Clinical aspects of infantile asthma," *Annals of Allergy* 35 (1975):216–20.

29 Ratner, D., et al., "Milk protein-free diet for nonseasonal asthma and migraine in lactase-deficient patients," *Israel Journal of Medical Sciences* 19 (1983):806–9.

30 Echechipia, B.G., et al., "Occupational asthma and rhinoconjunctivitis from inhalation of dried cow's milk caused by sensitization to lactalbumin," *Allergy* 49 (1994):189–91.

31 Fox, Stephen, "Autism on rise: no link seen with MMR vaccine," *Infections in Medicine* 18 (2001):286–87.; Loring, Dales, et al., "Time Trends in Autism and in MMR Immunization Coverage in California," *JAMA* 285 (2001):1183–85.

32 Pallarito, Karen, "US autism rates rise sharply," *HealthDay Reporter*, Mar. 7, 2005.

33 Wallis, Claudia, "New studies see a higher rate of autism: is the jump real?" *Time,* October 5, 2009; time.com/time/health/article/ 0,8599,1927824,00.html

34 Conversation with Malcolm Privette of Dr. J. Robert Cade's office at the University of Florida. Oct. 12, 2005. Malcolm shared that they receive calls from these countries and others around the world where parents are struggling with the same challenges in their children's health and the same lack of definitive answers as to the cause.

35 Communication of autism researcher J. Robert Cade, M.D., University of Florida, Departments of Physiology and Medicine, Health Science Center, Gainsville, Florida, 32610.

36 Lord, Catherine, et al., "Early diagnosis and screening of autism spectrum disorders," *Medscape Psychiatry & Mental Health* 10 (2005).

37 Deykin, E.Y., et al., "The incidence of seizures among children with autis-
    tic syndromes," *American Journal of Psychiatry* 136 (1979):1310–12.

38 Konrad, Walecia, "Dealing With the Financial Burden of Autism," *New
    York Times,* Jan. 22, 2010; nytimes.com/2010/01/23/health/ 23patient.
    html?em; Pallarito, Karen, "US autism rates rise sharply," *HealthDay
    News,* Mar. 7, 2005.

39 Wood, N.C., et al., "Abnormal intestinal permeability. An etiological
    factor in chronic psychiatric disorders?" *British Journal of Psychiatry* 150
    (1987):853–56.

40 Goodwin, M.S., et al., "Malabsorption and cerebral dysfunction: a multi-
    variate and comparative study of autistic children," *Journal of Autism and
    Childhood Schizophrenia* 1 (1971):48–62.

41 Wakefield, A.J., "Ileal-lymphoid-nodular hyperplasia, non-specific
    colitis, and pervasive developmental disorder in children," *Lancet* 351
    (1998):637–41.

42 Ibid.

43 Wakefield, A.J., et al., "Ileal-lymphoid-nodular hyperplasia, non-specific
    colitis, and pervasive developmental disorder in children," *Lancet* 35
    (1998):637–41; Wakefield, A.J., et al., "Enterocolitis in children with
    developmental disorders," *American Journal of Gastroenterology* 95
    (2000):2285–95.

44 Ibid.; Horvath, K., et al., "Gastrointestinal abnormalities in
    children with autistic disorder," *Journal of Pediatrics* 135 (1998):234–35.

45 Chang, K.J., et al., "Isolation of a specific m-opiate receptor peptide, mor-
    phiceptin, from an enzymatic digest of milk protein," *Journal of Biological
    Chemistry* 260 (1985):9706–12.

46 Panksepp, J.A., "Neurochemical theory of autism," *Trends in
    Neurosciences* 2 (1979):174–77.

47 Ross, Melanie, "Milk in diet may be linked to autism and schizophrenia,"
    University of Florida, Mar. 17, 1999; press release from the university
    found at news.ufl.edu/1999/03/15/autism

48 Ibid.

49 Cade, R., et al., "Autism and schizophrenia: Intestinal disorders,"
    Nutritional Neuroscience 3 (2000):57–72; Wakefield, A.J., "MMR
    vaccination and autism" (Letter), *Lancet* 354 (1999):949–50; Wakefield,
    A.J., "Autism, inflammatory bowel disease, and MMR vaccine," (Letter),
    Lancet 351 (1998):908.

50 Cade, J.R., et al., "A peptide found in schizophrenia and autism causes behavioral changes in rats," *Autism* 3 (1999):85–95.; Cade, J.R., et al., "Beta-casomorphin induces Fos-like immunoreactivity in discrete brain regions relevant to schizophrenia and autism," *Autism* 3 (1999): 367–83.; Dohan, F.C., et al., "Relapsed schizophrenics: Earlier discharge from the hospital after cereal-free, milk-free diet," *American Journal of Psychology* 130 (1973):685.

51 generationrescue.org.

52 Seroussi, Karyn, *The Mystery of Autism and Pervasive Developmental Disorder: A Mother's Story of Research and Recovery* (New York: Simon & Schuster, 2002).

53 The Autism Network for Dietary Intervention (ANDI), autismndi.com.

54 Personal communication with Karyn Seroussi, May 8, 2010.

55 Beckstrom, Maja, "Life, love and autism: A tale of one couple's journey," *Pioneer Press,* Jan. 11, 2004.

56 Tuohy, Wendy, "A riddle wrapped in enigma," *The Age,* Nov. 16, 2002.

57 Laidler, James R., "A stranger in a strange land: Involuntary adventures in autism," autismemtl.iquebec.com/2002/laidler_en.html

58 "Mom cures son by eliminating milk," *Derry News,* Dec. 22, 2000; conversation with Jill McIntosh, January 2001.

59 Seroussi, Karyn, *The Mystery of Autism and Pervasive Developmental Disorder: A Mother's Story of Research and Recovery* (New York: Simon & Schuster, 2002).

60 Telephone communication with Malcolm Privette of Dr. J. Robert Cade's office, Oct. 11, 2005, University of Florida, Department of Medicine and Physiology.

61 Rimland, Bernard, *Infantile Autism* (New York: Prentice Hall, 1964).

62 Summary of Defeat Autism Now (DAN!) Conference, Oct. 5–7, 2001, San Diego, California, autisminfo.com/DANOct2001.htm

63 Blaylock, Russell, "The truth behind the vaccine cover up," *Nexus New Times Magazine,* Vol. 12 Jan.–Feb. 2005.

64 Redwood, Lyn, "Poison in our vaccines: investigating mercury, thimerosal, and neurodevelopmental delay," *Mothering,* issue 115, Nov/Dec. 2002.

65 fda.gov

66 MacGregor, Hilary E., "Doctor contrarian: Parents fearful of vaccines flock to him; experts denounce his stance," *Latimes.com,* Mar. 7, 2005.

67 Olmsted, Dan, "The age of autism: Concerned in Tennessee," *Science Daily,* Nov. 8, 2005.

68 Opening statement by Congressman Daniel Burton (R-Indiana) to the House Committee on Government Reform's hearing on mercury and medicine on June 18, 2000; to view the transcripts of the hearing, visit: // vaccines.procon.org/sourcefiles/Burton_Letter.pdf; //vaccines.procon. org/sourcefiles/Burton_Report.pdf.

69 Autism and Mercury. Testimony presented by Stephanie Cave, M.D., before the Committee on Government Reform, US House of Representatives, July 18, 2000.

70 Generation Rescue, generationrescue.org/, Fact # 20.

71 Autism Society of America, "ASA & IRCA Biomedical conference addresses latest autism research," Oct. 29, 2004.

72 Dhooge, I.J., " Risk factors for the development of otitis media," *Current Allergy and Asthma Reports,* 3 (2003):321–25.

73 National Institute on Deafness and Other Communication Disorders, *Otitis media (ear infection)* (NIH Publication No. 974216). Bethesda, MD, 2002.

74 American Academy of Family Physicians, "Earaches: A painful problem for many children," familydoctor.org

75 Damoiseaux, R.A., et al., "Primary care based randomised, double blind trial of amoxicillin versus placebo for acute otitis media in children aged under 2 years," *British Medical Journal* 320 (2000):350–54.

76 Barrow, Karen, "Wait and hear: Letting ear infections clear without antibiotics," *Science Daily,* June 6, 2005; Diament, M., et al., "Abuse and timing of use of antibiotics in acute otitis media," *Archives of Otolaryngology* 100 (1974):226–32.; Yee, Daniel, "Doctors mull antibiotics for kid's ear infections: Group to recommend limited use of antibiotics for kid's ear infections," *Associated Press,* Mar. 2, 2004.

77 "Report of a survey by the Medical Research Council's Working Party for Research in General Practice: Acute otitis media in general practice," *Lancet* 2 (1957):510.

78 Pang, L Q., "The importance of allergy in otolaryngology," in *Clinical Ecology* (Springfield, Ill.: Charles Thomas, 1976).

79 Saarinen, U., "Breastfeeding prevents otitis media," *Nutrition Reviews* 41 (1983):241.

80 Rapp, Doris, *Is This Your Child?* (New York: Harper, 1992).

81 Seroussi, Karyn, *The Mystery of Autism and Pervasive Developmental Disorder: A Mother's Story of Research and Recovery* (New York: Simon & Schuster, 2002).

82 Nsouli, T.M., et al., "Role of food allergy in serious otitis media," *Annals of Allergy* 73 (1994):215–19.

83 Ibid.

84 Duncan, B., et al., "Exclusive breast-feeding for at least 4 months protects against otitis media," *Pediatrics* 91 (1993)867–72.

85 Lawrence, Ruth A., *Breastfeeding: A Guide for the Medical Profession* (St. Louis, Missouri: Mosby-Year Book, 1999).

86 Duncan, B., et al., "Exclusive breast-feeding for at least 4 months protects against otitis media," *Pediatrics* 91 (1993):867–72.

87 Dewey, Kathryn, et al., "Differences in morbidity between breastfed and formula-fed infants," *Journal of Pediatrics* 126 (1995):696–702.

88 Deid, Jessica, "Vaccine could end children's ear infections," *CNN Money. com,* Mar. 3, 2006.

89 American Academy of Otolaryngology — Head and Neck Surgery, entnet.org

90 Kleinman, L.C., et al., "The medical appropriateness of tympanos-tomy tubes proposed for children younger than 16 years in the United States," *Journal of the American Medical Association* 271 (1994).

91 Firer, M.A., et al., "Cow's milk allergy and eczema: patterns of the antibody response to cow's milk in allergic skin disease," *Clinical & Experimental Allergy* 12 (2006):385-90.

92 Oranje, A.P., et al., "Immediate contact reactions to cow's milk and egg in atopic children," *Acta Dermato-venereologica* 71 (1991):263–66.

93 Buisseret, P.D., *Lancet* (1978):304; Mueller, H.L., et al., *New England Journal of Medicine* 268 (1963):1220.

94 Jakobsson, I., et al., "Cow's milk as a cause of infantile colic in breast-fed infants," *Lancet* 2 (1978):437–39.

95 Clyne, P. S., et al., "Human breast milk contains bovine IgG: Relationship to colic?" *Pediatrics* 87 (1991):439–44.

96 Yoichi, F. et al., "Consumption of cow milk and egg by lactating women and the presence of B-lactoglobulin and ovalbumin in breast milk," *American Journal of Clinical Nutrition* 65 (1997):30–35; McClelland, D.B. L., et al., "Antibodies to cow's milk proteins in human colostrum," *Lancet*

2 (1976):1251–52; Clyne, P.S., et al., "Human breast milk contains bovine IgG: Relationship to infant colic?" *Pediatrics* 87 (1991):359–66.

97 Lamott, Anne, *Operating Instruction: A Journal of My Son's First Year* (New York: Ballantine, 1994).

98 Forget, P., et al., "Cow's milk protein allergy and gastro-oesophageal reflux," *European Journal of Pediatrics* 144 (1985):298–300.

99 Jakobsson, I., et al., "Cow's milk as a cause of infantile colic in breast-fed infants," *Lancet* 2 (1978):437–39.

100 Ibid.

101 Jakobsson, I., et al., "Cow's milk proteins cause infantile colic in breast-fed infants: a double-blind crossover study," *Pediatrics* 71 (1983):268–71.

102 Lothe, L., et al., "Cow's milk formula as a cause of infantile colic: a double-blind study," *Pediatrics* 70 (1982):7–10.

103 Wislon, J.F., et al., "Further observations on cow's milk-induced gastro-intestinal bleeding in infants with iron-deficiency anemia," *Journal of Pediatrics* 84 (1974):335–44; Woodruff, C.W., et al., "The role of fresh cow's milk in iron deficiency," *American Journal of Diseases of Children* 124 (1972):26–30; Fomon, S.J., et al., "Cow milk feeding in infancy: Gastrointestinal blood loss and iron nutritional status," *Journal of Pediatrics* 98 (1981):540–45.

104 Clein, N.W., "Cow's milk allergy in infants," *Pediatric Clinics of North America* 1 (1954):949–62.

105 Oliveira, M.A., et al., "Cow's milk consumption and iron deficiency anemia in children," *Journal of Pediatrics* 81 (2005):361–7; Anyon, C.P., et al., "Cow's milk: A cause of iron-deficiency anemia in infants," *New Zealand Medical Journal* 74 (1971):24–25.

106 Oski, Frank, *Don't Drink Your Milk* (New York: Health Services, 1983).

107 Anyon, C.P., et al., "Cow's milk: A cause of iron deficiency anemia in infants," *New Zealand Medical Journal* 74 (1971):24–25.

108 Zeigler, E., et al., "Cow milk feeding in infancy: Further observations on blood loss from the gastrointestinal tract," *Journal of Pediatrics* 116 (1990):11–18.

109 Sadowitz, P.D., et al., "Iron status and infant feeding practices in an urban ambulatory center," *Pediatrics* 72 (1983):33.

110 Oski, Frank, "Is bovine milk a health hazard?", *Pediatrics* 75 (suppl) (1985):182–86.

111 Lucas, A., et al., "Breast milk and subsequent intelligence quotient in children born preterm," *Lancet* 339 (1992):261–64.

112 Oski, Frank, *Don't Drink Your Milk* (New York: Health Services, 1983).

113 Iacono, G., et al., "Intolerance of cow's milk and chronic constipation in children," *New England Journal of Medicine* 339 (1998):110–14.

114 Giuseppe, I., et al., "Cow's milk protein allergy as a cause of anal fistula and fissures: A case report," *Journal of Allergy and Clinical Immunology* 101 (1998):125–27.

115 Iacono, G., et al., "Intolerance of cow's milk and chronic constipation in children," *New England Journal of Medicine* 339 (1998):1100–1104.

116 Eastham, E., et al., "Adverse effects of milk formula ingestion on the gastrointestinal tract," *Gastroenterology* 76 (1979):365–74; Cremin, B.J., et al., "The radiological appearance of the 'sinspissated milk syndrome': A cause of intestinal obstruction in infants," *British Journal of Radiology* 43 (1970):856–58.

117 De Peyer, E., et al., "Cow's milk intolerance presenting as necrotizing enterocolitis," *Helvetica Paediatrica Acta* 32 (1977):509–15.

118 Jenkins, H.R., et al., "Food allergy: The major cause of infantile colitis," *Archives of Disease in Childhood* 59 (1984):326–29.

119 Lovegrove, J.A., et al., "Dietary factors influencing levels of food anti-bodies and antigens in breast milk," *Acta Paediatrica* 85(1996):778–84.

120 Wilson, N.W., et al., "Severe cow's milk induced colitis in an exclusively breast-fed neonate: Case report and clinical review of cow's milk allergy," *Clinical Pediatrics* 29 (1990):77–80.

121 Juul, A., et al., "The ratio between serum levels of IGF-1 and the IGF binding proteins decreases with age in healthy patients and is increased in acromegalic patients," *Clinical Endocrinology* 41 (1994): 85–93. ; Klein I., et al., "Colonic polyps in patients with acromegaly. *Annals of Internal Medicine* 97 (1992): 27–30.

122 Akerblom, H.K., et al., "Emergence of diabetes associated autoantibod-ies in the nutritional prevention of IDDM (TRIGR) project," 59th Annual Scientific Sessions of the American Diabetic Association, June 1999, San Diego, California; Virtanen, S., et al., "Early introduction of dairy products associated with increased risk of IDDM in Finnish children," *Diabetes* 42 (1993):1786–90; Scott, F.W., et al., "Cow's milk and insulin-dependent diabetes mellitus: Is there a relationship?," *American Journal of Clinical Nutrition* 51 (1990):489–91; Savilahti, E., et al., "Children with

newly diagnosed insulin-dependent diabetes mellitus have increased levels of cow's milk antibodies," *Diabetes Research* 7 (1988):137–40; Mayer, E., et al., "Reduced risk of IDDM among breast-fed children," *Diabetes* 37 (1988):1625–32.

123 "Formula for diabetes? Cow's milk for infants may contribute to the disease," *Scientific American* (1992):24; Virtanen, S.M., et al., *Diabetologia* 37 (1994):381–87.

124 "American Academy of Pediatrics Work Group on Cow's Milk Protein and Diabetes Mellitus," *Pediatrics* 94 (1994):752–54.

125 Cavallo, M.G., et al., "Cell-mediated immune response to beta-casein in recent-onset insulin-dependent diabetes: Implications for disease pathogenesis," *Lancet* 348 (1996):926–28.

126 Dahl-Jorgenson, K., et al., "Relationship between cow's milk consumption and incidence of IDDM in childhood," *Diabetes Care* 14 (1991):1081–88.

127 Scott, F.W., "Cow milk and insulin-dependent diabetes mellitus: is there a relationship?" *American Journal of Clinical Nutrition* 51 (1990):489–91.

128 Information presented by Hans-Michael Dosch at the 59th Annual Scientific Sessions of the American Diabetic Association, June 1999, San Diego, Calif. Contact: Hans-Michael Dosch, Hospital for Sick Children, Division of Immunology and Cancer Research, Toronto, Ontario, Canada M5G 1X8.

129 Pozzilli, P., "Beta-casein in cow's milk: a major antigenic determinant for Type I diabetes?" *Journal of Endocrinological Investigation* 22 (1999):562–67.

130 Karjalainen, J., et al., "A bovine albumin peptide as a possible trigger of insulin-dependent diabetes mellitus," *New England Journal of Medicine* 327 (1992):302–7.

131 Akerblom, H.K., et al., "Emergence of diabetes associated autoantibodies in the nutritional prevention of IDDM (TRIGR) project," 59th Annual Scientific Sessions of the American Diabetes Association. June, 1999, San Diego, California.

132 Virtanen, S., et al., "Cow's milk consumption, HLA-DQB1 gentype, and Type I diabetes: a nested case-control study of siblings of children with diabetes," *Diabetes* 40 (2000):912–17.

133 O'brien, Kerry, "Juvenile diabetes linked to baby formula," Australian Broadcasting Corporation, July 29, 2004; abc.net.au/7.30/content/2004/s1165017.htm

134 "American Academy of Pediatrics Work Group on Cow's Milk Protein and Diabetes Mellitus," *Pediatrics* 94 (1994):752–54.; American Academy of Pediatrics, Committee on Nutrition, "The use of whole cow's milk in infancy," *Pediatrics* 89 (1992): 1105–09.

135 Physicians for Social Responsibility, "In Harm's Way: Toxic Threats to Child Development: Executive Summary," 2000; psr.org/chapters/boston/resources/in-harms-way.html

136 Diller, L., *Running on Ritalin: A Physician Reflects on Children, Society, and Performance in a Pill* (New York: Bantam Books, 1998).

137 *American Journal of Public Health* 89 (1999):1359–64.

138 Goode, Erica, "Reading, writing and Ritalin," *New York Times,* Apr. 9, 2000.

139 Sax, Leonard, "Ritalin: Better living through chemistry," *The world and I* (November 2000).

140 Barkley, R.A., et al., "Treating attention deficit hyperactivity disorder: medication and behavioral management training," *Pediatric Annals* 20 (1991):26–66; Centers for Disease Control and Prevention, "Mental Health in the United States: Prevalence of Diagnosis and Medication Treatment for Attention-Deficit/Hyperactivity Disorder — United States, 2003," *Morbidity and Mortality* Weekly Report 54 (2005):842–47.

141 Rubin, Rita, "Warning advised on ADHD drugs; FDA committee urges strongest notification," *USA Today,* Feb. 10–12, 2006, A1.

142 Kluger, Jeffrey, "Medicating young minds," *Newsweek,* Nov. 3, 2003, p. 48.

143 Rubin, Rita, "Warning advised on ADHD drugs; FDA committee urges strongest notification," *USA Today,* Feb. 10–12, 2006, A1.

144 "Safety and efficacy of stimulant-based therapy for ADHD: an expert interview with Robert L. Findling, MD," *Medscape Psychiatry and Mental Health,* Sept. 23, 2005; medscape.com/viewarticle/ 513204? src=sr

145 Robb, Adelaide S., "Stimulant-associated weight loss in children," *Medscape Psychiatry & Mental Health,* Feb. 8, 2006.

146 "Use of stimulants for attention deficit hyperactivity disorder," *British Medical Journal* 329 (2004):907–8.

147 Barkley, R.A., et al., "Treating attention deficit hyperactivity disorder: medication and behavioral management training," *Pediatric Annals* 20 (1991):26–66.

148 Dunnick, J.K., et al., "Experimental studies on the long-term effects of methylphenidate hydrochloride," *Toxicology* 103 (1995):77–84.

149 "Feeding minds: the impact of food on mental health," The Mental Health Foundation, 2005; Sea Containers House, 20 Upper Ground, London, England, SE19QB, www.mentalhealth.org.uk

150 Stevens, L.J., et al., "Essential fatty acid metabolism in boys with attention-deficit hyperactivity disorder," *American Journal of Clinical Nutrition* 62 (1995):761–68; Ricardson, A.J., et al. ,"The Oxford-Durham Study: a randomized, controlled trial of dietary supplementation with fatty acids in children with developmental coordination disorder," *Pediatrics* 115 (2005):1360–66; Toren, P., et al., "Zinc deficiency in attention-deficit hyperactivity disorder," *Biological Psychiatry* 40 (1996):1308–10.

151 Mira, U.K., et al., *Archives of Toxicoloy* 61 (1988):496–500; "A study of nerve conduction velocity, late responses and neuromuscular synapse functions in organophosphate workers in India," "Pesticides and Human Health: A Resource for Health Care Professionals," //psr-la.org/files/pesticides-and-human-health-solomon.pdf.

152 Christakis, D. A., et al., "Early television exposure and subsequent attentional problems in children," *Pediatrics* 113 (2004):708–13.

153 Today, Dr. Feingold's work is continued by the Feingold Association, a non-profit organization of families, educators, and health professionals. Visit the organization at feingold.org

154 Buisseret, Paul D., "Common manifestations of cow's milk allergy in children," *Lancet* 1 (1978):304–5.

155 Schauss, A.G., et al., "A critical analysis of the diets of chronic juvenile offenders," *Journal of Orthomolecular Psychiatry* 8 (1979):149.

156 Schauss, Alexander, *Diet, Crime and Delinquency* (Berkley, CA: Parker House, 1980).

157 Crook, William G., *Dr. Crook Discusses Alternatives to Ritalin in the Management of ADHD* (Washington, D.C.: Professional Books, 1997); Crook, William G., *The Yeast Connection* (Washington, D.C., Professional Books, 1985).

158 Boris, Marvin, et al., "Foods and additives are common causes of the attention deficit hyperactive disorder in children," *Annals of Allergy* 72 (1994):462–68.

159 Crook, W.G., "Can what a child eats make him dull, stupid, or hyperactive?" *Journal of Learning Disabilities* 13 (1980):53–58.

160 Rapp, Doris J., *Is This Your Child?* (New York, Harper Paperbacks, 1992); Rapp, D., "Food allergy treatment for hyperkinesis," *Journal of Learning Disabilities* 12 (1979):608–16.

161 Schauss, A.G., et al., "A critical analysis of the diets of chronic juvenile offenders," *Journal of Orthomolecular Psychiatry* 8 (1979):222.; Hoffer, A., "Behavioral nutrition," (1979):169.

162 Crook, W.G., "Can what a child eats make him dull, stupid, or hyperactive?" *Journal of Learning Disabilities* 13 (1980):53–58.

163 Organic Consumers Association, "Study indicates nutritional deficiencies lead to aggression & violence in children," Apr. 2, 2005; Sutliff, Usha, (USC Public Relations — Newsroom), "Nutrition key to aggressive behavior," Nov. 16, 2004.

164 *ABC News,* "Students behave better with healthy lunches," Jan. 22, 2002; abcnews.go.com/GMA/print?id=125404

165 "Report: Obesity rising sharply among US preschoolers," *CNN.com,* Dec. 30, 2004. heart.org/HEARTORG/GettingHealthy/Overweight- in-Children_UCM_304054_Article.jsp

166 Eaton, D.K., et al. "Associations of body mass index and perceived weight with suicide ideation and suicide attempts among US high school students," *Archives of Pediatrics & Adolescent Medicine* 1599(2005): 513–19.

167 Fox, Maggie, "Milk may make for heavier kids, study finds," *Reuters,* June 6, 2005.

Chapter 7

1 Kelly, Alice Lesch, "The dairy debate: Does milk build strong bones?" *Los Angeles Times,* Mar. 7, 2005.

2 Recer, P., "Every body *still* needs milk," *Oakland Tribune,* Aug. 14, 1997, A1.

3 Ibid.

4 Owen, R.A., et al., "Incidence of Colles' fractures in a North American community," *American Journal of Public Health* 72 (1982): 604–7.

5 Melton, L.J., et al., " Bone density and fracture risk in men," *Journal of Bone and Mineral Research* 13 (1998):1915; Melton, L.J., et al., "Perspective. How many women have osteoporosis?" *Journal of Bone and Mineral Research* 7 (1992):1005.

6 Wardlaw, G.M., "Putting osteoporosis in perspective," *Journal of the American Dietetic Association* 93 (1993):1000–6.

7   Greendale, G.A., et al., "Physical and functional effects of osteoporotic fractures in women: the Rancho Bernardo Study," *Journal of the American Geriatric* Society 43 (1995): 955–61.

8   Cummings, Steven, et al., "Epidemiology of osteoporosis and osteoporotic fractures," *Epidemiologic Reviews* 7 (1985):179–208.

9   WHO Study Group on Assessment of Fracture Risk and Its Application to Screening for Post Menopausal Osteoporosis, "Assessment of fracture risk and its application to screening for post menopausal osteoporosis: report of a WHO study group," WHO Technical Series, No. 843 (Geneva, WHO, 1994).

10 Moynihan, Ray, et al., "Selling sickness: the pharmaceutical industry and disease mongering," Commentary: Medicalisation of risk factors, *British Medical Journal* 324 (2002): 886–91.

11 Haentjens, P., et al., "The economic cost of hip fractures among elderly women," *American Journal of Bone and Joint Surgery* 83 (2001): 493–500; Braithwaite, R.S., et al., "Estimating hip fracture morbidity, mortality and costs," *Journal of the American Geriatric Society* 51 (2003):364–70.

12 *PR Newswire,* "The market for osteoporosis therapies will exceed $9 billion by 2007, according to Decision Resources, Inc." June 29, 1999; prnewswire.com

13 Melton, L., et al., "Secular trends in the incidence of hip fractures," *Calcified Tissue International* 41 (1987):57–64; Wallace, W. A., "The increasing incidence of fractures of the proximal femur: An orthopedic epidemic," *Lancet* 1 (1983):1413–14; Johansson, C., et al., "Prevalence of fractures among 10,000 women from the 1900 to 1940 birth cohorts resident in Gothenburg," *Maturitas* 14 (1991):65–74; Lees, B., et al., "Differences in proximal femur density over two centuries." *Lancet* 341 (1993):673–75; Boyce, W.J., et al., "Rising incidence of fracture of the proximal femur," *Lancet* 19 (1985):150–51.

14 Gullberg, B., et al., "World-wide projections for hip fracture," *Osteoporosis International* 7 (1997):407.

15 Kong, Dolores, "Seeing milk in a different light," *Boston Globe,* Dec. 13, 1999.

16 Willett, Walter, *Eat, Drink, and Be Healthy* (New York: Free Press, 2001), p 159.

17 whitakerwellness.com/html/osteoporosis.html

18 Cummings, R. G., et al., "Case-control study of risk factors for hip fractures in the elderly," *American Journal of Epidemiology* 139 (1994):493–503.

19 Kanis, John A., et al., "A meta-analysis of milk intake and fracture risk: low utility for case finding," *Osteoporosis International* 16 (2004):799–804.

20 Feskanich, D., et al., "Milk dietary calcium and bone fractures in women: A 12-year prospective study," *American Journal of Public Health* 87 (1997):992–97.

21 Cumming, R.G., et al., "Case-control study of risk factors for hip fractures in the elderly," *American Journal of Epidemiology* 139 (1994):493–503.

22 Kelly, Alice Lesch, "The dairy debate: Does milk build stronger bones?" *LA Times.com,* Mar. 7, 2005.

23 Campbell, T. Colin, *The China Study : The Most Comprehensive Study of Nutrition Ever Conducted and the Startling Implications for Diet, Weight Loss and Long-Term Health* (Dallas: Benbella Books, 2005).

24 *New York Times,* May 8, 1990, interview with Jane Brody.

25 Springen, Karen, "Calcium overload," *Newsweek,* Aug. 14, 2000, p. 64.

26 Cumming, R.G., et al., "Calcium intake and fracture risk: results from the Study of Osteoporotic Fractures," *American Journal of Epidemiology* 145 (1997):926–34.

27 *Calcified Tissue International* 41 (1985):14–18.

28 LeRoy, Bob, "Milk and strong bones: The weak link," *Vegetarian Voice* 21 (1996):8.

29 Mazess, R., "Bone-mineral content of North American Eskimoes," *American Journal of Clinical Nutrition* 27 (1980):916–25.

30 Riggs, B., "Dietary calcium intakes and rates of bone loss in women," *Journal of Clinical Investigation* 80 (1987):979–82.

31 Lloyd, T., "Adult female hip bone density reflects teenage sports-exercise patterns, but not teenage calcium intake," *Pediatrics* 106 (2000):40–4; Welten, D.C., et al., "Weight-bearing activity during youth is a more important factor for peak bone mass than calcium intake," *Journal of Bone Mineral Research* 9 (1994):1089–96.

32 Springen, Karen, "Calcium overload," *Newsweek,* Aug. 14, 2000:64.

33 Ettinger, B., "Postmenopausal bone loss is prevented by treatment with low-dosage estrogen with calcium," *Annals of Internal Medicine* 106 (1987):40–45; Nilas, L., "Calcium supplementation and postmenopausal bone loss," *British Medical Journal* 289 (1984):1103–6.

34 Porthouse, J., et al., "Randomised controlled trial of calcium and supplementation with cholecalciferol (vitamin D3) for prevention of fractures in primary care," *British Medical Journal* 330(2005.):1003.

35 Riis, B., et al., "Does calcium supplementation prevent postmenopausal bone loss? A double-blind, controlled clinical study," *New England Journal of Medicine* 316 (1987):173–77.

36 Hegsted, D.M., "Calcium and osteoporosis," *Journal of Nutrition* 116 (1986):2316-19; Yoffe, Emily, "Got osteoporosis? Maybe all that milk you've been drinking is to blame," *Slate,* Aug. 3, 1999.

37 Cook, J., "Calcium supplementation: Effect on iron absorption," *American Journal of Clinical Nutrition* 53 (1991):106–11; Hallberg, L., "Calcium: Effect of different amounts of non-heme and heme iron absorption in humans," *American Journal of Clinical Nutrition* 53 (1991):112–19.

38 Burros, M., "Testing Calcium Supplements for Lead," *New York Times,* June 4, 1997, C:5; Bourgoin, Bernard P., et al., "Lead content in 70 brands of dietary calcium supplements," *American Journal of Public Health* 83 (1993):1155–60.

39 Wilkin, Terence, "Changing perceptions in osteoporosis," *British Medical Journal* 318 (1999):862–65.

40 Kubena, Karen S., et al., "Nutrition and the immune system: A review of the nutrient-nutrient interactions," *Journal of the American Dietetic Association* 96 (1996):1156–64.

41 Zemel, M., "Calcium utilization: Effect of varying level and source of dietary protein," *American Journal of Clinical Nutrition* 48 (1988):880–83; Schuette, S., "Studies on the mechanism of protein-induced hypercalciuria in older men and women," *Journal of Nutrition* 110 (1980):305–15; Hegsted, M., "Long-term effects of level of protein intake on calcium metabolism in young adult women," *Journal of Nutrition* 111 (1981):244–51.

42 Associated Press, "Students sour on longer-lasting milk," Sept. 19, 2004; www.heraldonline.com

43 Sellmeyer, D.E., et al., "A high ratio of dietary animal to vegetable protein increases the rate of bone loss and the risk of fracture in postmenopausal women," *American Journal of Clinical Nutrition* 73 (2001):118–22; Barzel, U.S., Osteoporosis (New York, Grune & Stratton: 1970); Barzel, U.S., "The effect of excessive acid feeding on bone," *Calcified Tissue Research* 4 (1969):94-100.

44 Lemann, J., et al., "Studies of the mechanism by which chronic metabolic acidosis augments urinary calcium excretion in man," *Journal of Clinical Investigation* 46 (1967):1318-28; Barzel, U.S., "Acid-induced osteoporosis: an experimental model of human osteoporosis," *Calcified Tissue Research* 21 (suppl) (1976):417–22.

45 Ibid.

46 Frassetto, L.A., et al., "Effect of age on blood acid-base composition in adult humans: role of age-related renal functional decline," *American Journal of Physiology* 271 (1996):1114-22.

47 Frassetto, L.A., et al., "Worldwide incidence of hip fracture in elderly women: Relation to consumption of animal and vegetable foods," *The Journals of Gerontology* 55 (1999):585-92; Heaney, R.P., "Protein intake and the calcium economy," *Journal of the American Dietetic Association* 93 (1993):1259–60; Chu, J.Y., et al., "Studies in calcium metabolism. II. Effects of low calcium and variable protein intake on human calcium metabolism," *American Journal of Clinical Nutrition* 28 (1975):1028; Margen, S., et al., "Studies in calcium metabolism. I. The calciuretic effect of dietary protein," *American Journal of Clinical Nutrition* 27 (1974):584; Johnson, N., et al., "Effect of level of protein intake on urinary and fecal calcium and calcium retention of young adult males," *Journal of Nutrition* 100 (1970):1425.

48 Breslau, A.A., et al., "Relationship of animal protein-rich diet to kidney stone formation and calcium metabolism," *Journal of Clinical Nutrition & Endocrinology* 66 (1988):140–46.

49 Lindsay, A.H., et al., "Protein-induced hypercalciuria: A longer-term study," *American Journal of Clinical Nutrition* 32 (1979):741–49.

50 Ornish, Dean, *Dr. Dean Ornish's Program for Reversing Heart Disease: The Only System Scientifically Proven to Reverse Heart Disease Without Drugs or Surgery* (New York, Ivy Book: 1995).

51 Itoh, Roichi, et al., " Dietary protein intake and urinary excretion of calcium: a cross-sectional study in a healthy Japanese population," *American Journal of Clinical Nutrition* 67 (1998):438–44.

52 Recker, R.R., et al., "The effect of milk supplements on calcium metabolism, bone metabolism, and calcium balance," *American Journal of Clinical Nutrition* 41 (1985):254–63; Abelow, B.J., et al., "Cross-cultural associations between dietary animal protein and hip fracture: A hypothesis," *Calcified Tissue International* 50 (1992):14–18; Riggs, B.L., et al., "Dietary

calcium intake and rates of bone loss in women," *Journal of Clinical Investigation* 80 (1987):979–82; *Journal of Nutrition* 116 (1986):2316.

53 Heaney, R.P., "Protein intake and the calcium economy," *Journal of the American Dietetic Association* 93 (1993):1259–60.

54 US Department of Agriculture, 1984 Nationwide food consumption survey. Nutrient intakes: individuals in 48 states, year 1977–1978. Hyattsville, MD: USDA, Consumer Nutrition Division, Human Nutrition Information Service, Report No. 1–2.

55 Atkins, C., *Dr. Atkins' New Diet Revolution* (New York, NY: Dell Publishing Co, 1967); Sears, Barry, *The Zone* (New York: Harper Collins, 1995); Eades, M.R., *Protein Power* (New York: Bantam Books, 1996).

56 Hegsted, M. et al., "Long-term effects of level of protein intake on calcium metabolism in young adult women," *Journal of Nutrition* 111 (1981):244–51.

57 Avery Ince, B., et al., "Lowering dietary protein to US recommended dietary allowance levels reduces urinary calcium excretion and bone resaborption in young women," *The Journal of Clinical Endocrinology & Metabolism* 89 (2004): 3801–7.

58 Marsh, A.G., et al., "Cortical bone density of adult lacto-ovo-vegetarian women and omnivorous women," *Journal of the American Dietetic Association* 76 (1980):148–51.

59 Robertson, W.G., et al., "Should recurrent calcium oxalate stone formers become vegetarians?" *British Journal of Urology* 51 (1979):427–31.

60 Feskanich, D., et al., "Milk, dietary calcium, and bone fractures in women: a 12-year prospective study," *American Journal of Public Health* 87 (1997):992–97.

61 Abelow, B.J., et al., "Cross-cultural association between dietary animal protein and hip fracture: A hypothesis," *Calcified Tissue International* 50 (1992):14–18.

62 World Health Organization, "Population nutrient intake goals for preventing diet-related chronic diseases: Recommendations for preventing osteoporosis," who.int/nutrition/topics/5_population_nutrient/en/index25.html

63 Frassetto, Lynda A., et al., "Worldwide incidence of hip fracture in elderly women," *The Journal of Gerontology* 55 (2000): 585–92.

64 LeRoy, Bob, "Milk does not build strong bones," *Vegetarian Voice 21* (1996):17.

65 Freidrich, Bruce, "Osteoporosis," Guest Editorial:
    notmilk.com/calbones.html

66 Sellmeyer, Deborah E., et al., "A high ratio of dietary animal to veg-
    etable protein increases the rate of bone loss and the risk of fracture
    in postmenopausal women," *American Journal of Clinical Nutrition* 73
    (2001):118–22.

67 Frassetto L.A., et al., " Worldwide incidence of hip fracture in
    elderly women: relation to consumption of animal and vegetable foods,"
    Journal of Gerontology 55 (2000):M585–92; Abelow, B.J., et al., "Cross-
    cultural association between dietary animal protein and hip fracture: a
    hypothesis," *Calcified Tissue International* 50 (1992):14–18.

68 Sellmeyer, D.E., et al., "A high ratio of dietary animal to vegetable protein
    increases the rate of bone loss and the risk of fracture in postmenopausal
    women," *American Journal of Clinical Nutrition* 73 (2001):118–22.

69 Hegsted, D., "Calcium and osteoporosis," *Journal of Nutrition* 116
    (1986):2316–19.

70 Zemel, M., "Calcium utilization: effect of varying level and source of
    dietary protein," *American Journal of Clinical Nutrition* 48 (1988):880–83;
    Breslau, N., "Relationship of animal-protein-rich diet to kidney stone for-
    mation and calcium metabolism," *Journal of Clinical Endocrinology and
    Metabolism* 66 (1988):140–46.

71 Xu, L., et al. ,"Very low rates of hip fracture in Beijing, People's Republic
    of China: the Beijing Osteoporosis Project," *American Journal of
    Epidemiology* 144 (1996):901–7.

72 Schwartz, A.V., et al., "International variation in the incidence of hip
    fractures: Cross-National Project on Osteoporosis for the World Health
    Organization Program for Research on Aging," *Osteoporosis International*
    9 (1999):242–53.

73 Walker, A., "The influence of numerous pregnancies and lactations
    on bone dimensions in South African Bantu and Caucasian mothers,"
    Clinical Science 42 (1972):189–96.

74 Campbell, T. Colin, et al., "Diet and chronic degenerative diseases: per-
    spectives from China," *American Journal of Clinical Nutrition* 59 (suppl)
    (1994):1153S–61S.

75 Remer, T., et al., "Estimation of the renal net acid excretion by adults con-
    suming diets containing variable amounts of protein," *American Journal
    of Clinical Nutrition* 59 (1994):1356–61.

76 Krieger, N.S., et al., "Acidosis inhibits osteoblastic and stimulates osteo-clastic activity in vitro," *American Journal of Physiology-Renal Physiology* 262 (1992): F442–48.

77 Hara, Y., et al., "Acidosis, not azotemia, stimulates branched-chain, amino acid catabolism in uremic rats," *Kidney International* 32 (1987):808–14; May, R.C., et al., "Mechanisms for defects in muscle protein metabolism in rats with chronic uremia: Influence of metabolic acidosis," *Journal of Clinical Investigation* 79 (1987):1099–103.

78 Nordin, B., et al., "The nature and significance of the relationship between urinary sodium and urinary calcium in women," *Journal of Nutrition* 123 (1993):1615–22.

79 Kok, D.J., et al., "The effects of dietary excesses in animal protein and in sodium on the composition and the crystalization kinetics of cal-cium oxalate monohydrate in urines of healthy men," *Journal of Clinical Endocrinology and Metabolism* 71 (1990):861–67.

80 Nordin, B.E., et al., "The nature and significance of the relationship between urinary sodium and urinary calcium in women," *Journal of Nutrition* 123 (1993):1615–22; Goulding, A., et al., "Effects of varying dietary intake on the fasting excretion of sodium, calcium and hydroxyproline in young women," *New Zealand Medical Journal* 96 (1983):853-4.

81 Devine, A., et al., *American Journal of Clinical Nutrition* 62 (1995): 740–45; Shortt, C., et al., *European Journal of Clinical Nutrition* 42 (1988):595–603.

82 Shank, F.R., et al., "Perspectives of the Food and Drug Administration on dietary sodium," *Journal of the American Dietetic Association* 80 (1982):29–35.

83 Bibbins-Domingo, Kirsten, et al., "Projected effect of dietary salt reduc-tions on future cardiovascular disease," *New England Journal of Medicine,* Jan. 20, 2010; content.nejm.org/cgi/content/full/NEJMoa0907355

84 Hernandez-Avila, Mauricio, et al., "Caffeine, moderate alcohol intake, and risk of fractures of the hip and forearm in middle-aged women," *American Journal of Clinical Nutrition* 54 (1991):157–63.

85 Baran, D., et al., "Effect of alcohol ingestion on bone and mineral metab-olism in rates," *American Journal of Physiology* 238 (1980):507–10.

86 Hopper, J.L., et al., "The bone density of female twins discordant for tobacco use," *New England Journal of Medicine* 330 (1994):387–92.

87 Law, M.R., et al., "A meta-analysis of cigarette smoking, bone mineral density and risk of hip fracture: recognition of a major effect," *British Medical Journal* 315 (1997):841–46.

88 Ibid.

89 Brody, J.E., "Osteoporosis can threaten men as well as women," *New York Times*, Sept. 4, 1996, C9.

90 Holl, M., et al., "Sucrose ingestion, insulin response, and mineral absorption in humans," *Journal of Nutrition* 117 (1987):1229–33.

91 Heaney, R.P., et al. "Carbonated beverages and urinary calcium excretion," *American Journal of Clinical Nutrition* 74 (2001):343–7.

92 Massey, L.K., et al., "Caffeine, urinary calcium, calcium metabolism and bone," *Journal of Nutrition* 123 (1993):1611–4.; Harris, S., "Caffeine and bone loss in healthy postmenopausal women," *American Journal of Clinical Nutrition* 60 (1994):573–78.

93 "Rapuri, Prema B., "Caffeine intake increases the rate of bone loss in elderly women and interacts with vitamin D receptor genotypes," *American Journal of Clinical Nutrition* 74(2001):694–700; Bauer, D.C., et al., "Factors associated with appendicular bone mass in older women: The study of Osteoporotic Fractures Research Group," *Annals of Internal Medicine* 118 (1993):657–65.

94 Kiel, D.P., et al., "Caffeine and the risk of hip fracture: the Framingham Study," *American Journal of Epidemiology* 132 (1990):675–84.

95 cbsnews.com/stories/2002/11/14/Sunday/main529388.html

96 Hernandez-Avila, Mauricio, et al., "Caffeine, moderate alcohol intake, and risk of fractures of the hip and forearm in middle-aged women," *American Journal of Clinical Nutrition* 54 (1991):157–63.

97 Abrams, S.A., et al., "Mineral balance and bone turnover in adolescents with anorexia nervosa," *Journal of Pediatrics* 123 (1993):326–31.

98 Garcia, C., et al., "Preservation of the ovary: A reevaluation," *Fertility & Sterility* 42 (1984):510–14.

99 Ikeda, K., "Inhibition of in vitro mineralization by aluminum in a clonal osteoblast like line," *Calcified Tissue International* 39 (1986).

100 Spencer, H., et al., "Effect of small doses of aluminum-containing antacids on calcium and phosphorus metabolism," *American Journal of Clinical Nutrition* 36 (1982):32–40.

101 Eastwood, J.B., et al., "Aluminum deposition in bone after contamination of drinking water supply," *Lancet* 336 (1990).

102 Hahn, T.J., et al., "Effect of chronic corticosteroid administration on diaphyseal and metaphyseal bone mass," *Journal of Clinical Endocrinology and Metabolism* 39 (1974):274–81; Hahn, T.J., "Corticosteroid-induced osteopenia," *Archives of Internal Medicine* 138 (1978):882–85.

103 Ettinger, B., et al., "Thyroid supplements: effect on bone mass," *Western Journal of Medicine* 136 (1982):472–76.

104 Spencer, H., et al., "Effect of small doses of aluminum-containing antac-ids on calcium and phosphorus metabolism," *American Journal of Clinical Nutrition* 36 (1982):32–40.

105 Gage, Brian F., et al., "Risk of osteoporotic fracture in elderly patients tak-ing Warfarin," *Archives of Internal Medicine* 166 (2006):241–46.

106 Becker, R., et al., *The Body Electric: Electromagnetism and the Foundation of Life* (New York: William Morrow, 1988).

107 Lane, N., "Long-distance running, bone density, and osteoarthritis," *Journal of the American Medical Association* 225 (1986):1147–51.

108 Lloyd, T., et al., "Adult female hip bone density reflects teenage sports-exercise patterns but not teenage calcium intake," *Pediatrics* 106 (2000):40–44.

109 Nieves, J.W., et al., "A case-control study of hip fracture: evaluation of selected dietary variables and teenage physical activity," *Osteoporosis International* 2 (1992):122–27.

110 Dalsky, G., "Weight-bearing exercise training and lumbar bone mineral content in post-menopausal women," *Annals of Internal Medicine* 108 (1988):824–38.

111 Notelovitz, M., and D. Tonnessen, *Menopause and Midlife Health* (New York: St. Martin's, 1993).

112 Chow, Raphael, et al., "Effect of two randomized exercise programs on bone mass of healthy postmenopausal women," *British Medical Journal* 295 (1987):231–34.

113 Demarco, C., "Take charge of our body," in *Women's Health Advisor* (Winlaw, B.C., Canada: Well Women Press, 1994).

114 Jacobsen, B.K., et al. "Exercise and other factors in the prevention of hip fracture: The Leisure World Study," *Epidemiology* 12 (1991):16.

115 Randall, Teri, "Longitudinal study pursues questions of calcium, hor-mones, and metabolism in life of skeleton," *JAMA* 268 (1992): 2353–57.

116 Lloyd, T., et al., "Adult female hip bone density reflects teenage sports-exer-cise patterns but not teenage calcium intake," *Pediatrics* 1 (2000):40–44.

117 Lanou, Amy Joy, et al., "Calcium, dairy products, and bone health in children and young adults: a reevaluation of the evidence," *Pediatrics* 115 (2005):736–43.

118 Heidrich, R., *A Race for Life* (New York: Lantern Books, 2000).

119 Locker, D., "Benefits and Risks of Water Fluoridation. An Update of the 1996 Federal-Provincial Sub-committee Report," Prepared for Ontario Ministry of Health and Long Term Care, 1999; Levy, S.M., et al., "Total fluoride intake and implications for dietary fluoride supplementation," *Journal of Public Health Dentistry* 59 (1999):211–23; McDonagh, M., et al., "A Systematic Review of Public Water Fluoridation," NHS Center for Reviews and Dissemination, University of York, 2000.

120 Sogaard, C.H., et al., "Marked decrease in trabecular bone quality after five years of sodium fluoride therapy — assessed by biomechanical testing of iliac crest bone biopsies in osteoporotic patients," *Bone* 15 (1994): 393–99; Lee, John R., "Fluoridation and osteoporosis," *Fluoride* 25 (1992):162–64.

121 Jacobsen, S., et al., "Regional variation in the incidence of hip fracture: US white women aged 65 years and older," 264 *JAMA* (1990):500–502; Cooper, C., et al., "Water fluoride concentration and fracture of the proximal femur," 44 *Journal of Epidemiological Community Health* (1990):17–19; Cooper, C., et al., "Water fluoridation and hip fracture," 266 *JAMA* (1991):513–14; Colquhoun, J., et al., "Water fluoridation and fractures," *New Zealand Medical Journal* 104 (1991):343; Danielson, C., et al., "Hip fractures and fluoridation in Utah's elderly population," *JAMA* 268 (1992):746–48; Lee, John R., "Fluoridation and hip fractures," *Earth Island Journal,* Earth Island Institute 13, Spring 1998.

122 Sowers, M.R., et al., "The relationship of bone mass and fracture history to fluoride and calcium intake: a study of three communities," *American Journal of Clinical Nutrition* 44 (1986):889–98.

123 Sowers, M.R., et al., "A prospective study of bone mineral content and fracture in communities with differential fluoride exposure," *American Journal of Epidemiology* 133 (1991):649–60.

124 Jacobsen S.J., J. Goldberg, T.P. Miles, *et al.* Regional variation in the incidence of hip fracture. *Journal of American Medical Association* 264 (1990):500–502; Jacobsen, S.J., et al., "The association between water fluoridation and hip fracture among white women and men aged 65 years

and older. A national ecologic study," *Annals of Epidemiology* 2 (1992): 617–26.

125 Cooper, C., et al., "Water fluoridation and hip fracture" (Letter), *Journal of the American Medical Association* 266 (1991): 513–14.

126 Keller, C., "Fluorides in drinking water," Paper presented at the Workshop on Drinking Water Fluoride Influence on Hip Fractures and Bone Health, Bethesda, MD, Apr. 10, 1991.

127 May, D.S, and M.G. Wilson, "Hip fractures in relation to water fluoridation: an ecologic analysis," presented at the Workshop of Drinking Water Fluoride Influence on Hip Fractures and Bone Health, Apr. 10, 1991, Bethesda, MD.

128 Danielson, C., et al., "Hip fractures and fluoridation in Utah's elderly population," *Journal of the American Medical Association* 286 (19912):746–48.

129 Jacmin-Gedda, H., et al., "Fluoride concentration in drinking water and fractures in the elderly" (Letter), *Journal of the American Medical Association* 273 (1995):775–76.

130 Breslau, A.A., et al., "Relationship of animal protein-rich diet to kidney stone formation and calcium metabolism," *Journal of Clinical Nutrition & Endocrinology* 66 (1988):140–46.

131 Originally reported in Jacqmin-Gadda, H., et al., "Fluoride concentration in drinking water and fractures in the elderly," *Fluoride* 28 (1995), and abstracted in a letter in *Journal of the American Medical Association* 273 (1995):775–76.

132 News release from the National Federation of Federal Employees (NFFE) local 2050, July 2, 1997. This organization consists of toxicologists, chemists, and biologists at the United States Environmental Protection Agency in Washington, D.C. Contact J. William Hirzy, Ph.D., senior vice president, (202) 260-4683; Li, X.S., et al., "Effects of fluoride exposure on intelligence in children," *Fluoride* 28 (1995):189–92.

Chapter 8

1 Spock, Benjamin, *Dr. Spock's Baby and Childcare: Seventh Edition* (New York: Pocket, 1998).

2 RockyMountainNews.com, Apr. 10, 2004.

3 Martin, Peter, "Milk: Nectar or Poison," London *Sunday Times* Magazine, and also, "Is there a timebomb in your diet? Exploding the myths about milk," July 21, 2002.

4   Robbins, John, *Diet for a New America* (Walpole, NH: Stillpoint, 1987).

5   Waters, Jen, "Udderly-computerized," *Washington Times*, Apr. 14, 2005.

6   Associated Press "Chatfield cow produces more than 70,000 pounds of milk," *Star Tribune*, Aug. 31, 2004.

7   "FDA approves Rumensin, WI dairy producers stand to benefit," *Wisconsin Ag Connection*, Nov. 5, 2004.

8   Anderson, J. and D. Van Atta, "Stray voltage killing US dairy cows," *The Washington Post*, Aug. 9, 1989.

9   Martin, Peter, "Milk: Nectar or poison?", *The Sunday Times Magazine*, July 21, 2002.

10 USDA, Animal and Plant Health Inspection Service, National Animal Health Monitoring System, Aug. 2004; Dairy 2002, Animal Disease Exclusion Practices on US Dairy Operations, 2002, www.aphis.usda.gov/vs/ceah/cahm/Dairy_Cattle.

11 *ABC News*, "Darker side of dairy farming," Jan 26, 2010; blogs.abcnews.com/nightlinedailyline/2010/01/darker-side-of-dairy-farming.html "Cow torture video: Willet dairy caught burning off cow's horns, chopping calf's · tail in Mercy for Animals expose," www.huffingtonpost.com/2010/01/27/cow-torture-video-willet-_n_ 438403.html; www.mercyforanimals.org/ohdairy/

12 www.cnn.com/video/#/video/us/2010/01/29/hln.jvm.dairy.cow.abuse.cnn?iref=allsearch

13 www.mercyforanimals.org/ohdairy/

14 Petrie, N.J., et al., "Cortisol responses of calves to two methods of tail docking used with or without local anesthetic," *New Zealand Veterinarian Journal* 44 (1996):4–8.

15 Tucker, C.B., et al., "Tail docking dairy cattle: Effects on cow cleanliness and udder health," *Journal of Dairy Science* 84 (2001):84–87.

16 Barnett, J.L., et al., "Tail docking and beliefs about the practice in the Victorian dairy industry," *Australian Veterinarian Journal* 77 (1999):742–47.

17 Department of Animal Science, University of Minnesota, *Practical Techniques for Dairy Farmers*, 3rd Edition.

18 Petrie, N.J., et al., "Cortisol responses of calves to two methods of dis-budding used with or without local anesthetic," *New Zealand Veterinary Journal* 44 (1995):9–14.

19 Faulkner, P.M., et al., "Reducing pain after dehorning in dairy calves," *Journal of Dairy Science* 83 (2000):2037–41.

20 Carlson, K.R., et al., "Caring for dairy animals — On-the-Dairy Self-Evaluation Guide," Agri-Education, Inc., Stratford, IA, 2004, p 48.

21 "OSU scientists develop test to detect 'dead-gut' in dairy cows," *Science Daily,* Jan. 19, 2005.

22 Montague, Peter, "Making milk; basic choices," *Rachel's Environmental and Health Weekly,* No. 384, Apr. 7, 1994.

23 Ibid.

24 Ibid.

25 *Consumer Reports,* May (1992): 330–32.

26 "Got money? The dairy industry milks Congress for yet another bailout," *Washington Post,* Friday, Oct. 9, 2009; washingtonpost.com/wp-dyn/content/article/2009/10/08/AR2009100803578.html

27 Chite, Ralph, "Dairy policy issues," *Congressional Research Service,* June 16, 2006, p.7.

28 Cone, Marla, "State dairy farms try to clean up their act," *Los Angeles Times,* Apr. 28, 1998, A1.

29 Copeland, Claudia and Jefferey Zinn, Senate Committee on Agriculture, Nutrition, and Forestry, "Animal waste pollution in America: an emerging problem," 104th Congress, Dec. 1997, updated May 12, 1998, available at: ncseonline.org/nle/crsreports/agriculture/ag-48.cfm

30 US Environmental Protection Agency, Office of Water Standards and Applied Sciences Division, "Environmental impacts of animal feeding operations," Dec. 31, 1998.

31 Cone, Marla, "State dairy farms try to clean up their act," *Los Angeles Times,* Apr. 28, 1998, A1.

32 "Massive cow manure mound burns for third month," CNN.com, Jan. 28, 2005. Smoaky.com/forum/lofiversion/index.php/t31193.html

33 Romney, Lee, "Deaths of 3 immigrant workers dog state's dairy industry," *San Francisco Chronicle,* Jan. 3, 2003, A3.

34 "Animal waste pollution in America: An emerging national problem," report compiled by the minority staff of the United States Senate Committee on Agriculture, Nutrition and Forestry for Senator Tom Harkin, Dec. 1997.

35 Illinois Environmental Protection Agency, "Understanding the pollution potential of livestock waste," 1991.

36 Husar, John, "Manure spill claims 100,000 fish," *Chicago Tribune,* Mar. 16, 1998.

37 Bischoff, Laura A., "Illinois megafarm neighbors sound alarm on waste," *Dayton Daily News,* Dec. 2, 2002.

38 Associated Press, "Dairy accused of dumping cow waste," Sept. 25, 1998.

39 Letson, David, et al., "Confined animal production and the manure problem," *Choices* (1995), p.18.

40 Testimony of Thomas P. Bonacquisti, "An Examination of the Potential Human Health, Water Quality, and Other Impacts of the Confined Animal Feeding Operation Industry," US Senate Committee on Environment and Public Works, Sept. 6 2007; epw.senate.gov/public/index.cfm?FuseAction=Files.View&FileStore_id=60afb942-8320-4d34-98ac-b23e4de96cc5

41 Diringer, Elliot, "Regulators go after polluting dairies," *San Francisco Chronicle,* July 19, 1997, A1.

42 Jacobson, L.D., et al., "Generic environmental impact statement on animal agriculture: Summary of the literature related to air quality and odor," Prepared for the Minnesota Environmental Quality Board, 1999. Minneapolis, MN: University of Minnesota, College of Agriculture, Food, and Environmental Sciences. Available: mnplan.state.mn.us/pdf/1999/eqb/scoping/aircha.pdf

43 Raloff, J., "Environmental concerns reemerge over steroids given to livestock," *Science News,* Jan. 5, 2002.

44 Clover, Charles, "Flower may hold key to methane," *The Times* London, Sept. 7, 2007.

45 "Dairy cow is nature's milk factory," *Bristol Herald Courier,* July 21, 1983.

46 California Farm Bureau Federation, "How much water does it take to make a glass of milk?" cfbf.com/info/milk.cfm, accessed May 4, 2010.

47 Grady, D., "A move to limit antibiotic use in animal feed," *New York Times,* May 20, 1999, A20, and Nov. 4, 1999, A15; *New England Journal of Medicine* 19 (1999):1420–25; *New England Journal of Medicine* 20 (1999):1525–32.

48 Glynn, K., et al., "Emergence of multi-drug-resistant salmonella enterica serotype typhimurium DT104 infections in the United States," *New England Journal of Medicine* 19 (1998):1333–38.

49 USFDA, Center for Veterinary Medicine, "Human-use antibiotics in livestock production," fda.gov/cvm/HRESP106_157.htm; State

Environmental Resource Center, "Antibiotics in agriculture,"
serconline.org/antibiotics/background/html

50 O'neil, Kathleen, "Animals on drugs," *The Environmental Magazine*
Nov. 2000., emagazine.com/view/?877&printview&imagesoff; Umrigar,
Thrifty, "Antibiotics in food now major health threat," *Beacon Journal,*
Apr. 1, 2002; Falcon, Mike, "Brad Whitford fights antibiotic resistance,"
USA Today, May 13, 2002.

51 Segelken, Roger, "CU veterinarians: revised farm practices could slow
salmonella strain," *Cornell Chronicle,* Feb. 5, 1998, news.cornell.edu/
Chronicle/98/2.5.98/salmonella.html

52 "The hunt for the odourless pig," *The Economist,* Nov. 24, 2007, p 60.

Chapter 9

1 ams.usda.gov/AMSv1.0/ams.fetchTemplateData.do?template=
TemplateC&navID=PesticideDataProgram&rightNav1=
PesticideDataProgram&topNav=&leftNav=ScienceandLaboratories&pag
e=PesticideDataProgram&resultType

2 Eaton, S. B., et al., "Paleolithic nutrition: a consideration of its nature
and current implications," *New England Journal of Medicine* 312
(1985):283–89.

3 Harvard School of Public Health, Nutrition Source, "Calcium and Milk,"
hsph.harvard.edu/nutritionsource/calcium.html; DRI: Dietary Reference
Intakes For Calcium, Phosphorus, Magnesium, Vitamin D, and Fluoride,
Standing Committee on the Scientific Evaluation of Dietary Reference
Intakes, Food and Nutrition Board, Institute of Medicine, National
Academy Press, Washington, D.C. 1999, books.nap.edu/html/dri_calcium/

4 www.nhs.uk/Conditions/Osteoporosis/Pages/Prevention.aspx;
www.nos.org.uk/NetCommunity/Document.doc?id=395

5 who.int/dietphysicalactivity/publications/trs916/en/gsfao_osteo.pdf

6 Prentice, A., "What are the dietary requirements for calcium and vitamin
D?" *Calcified Tissue International* 70 (2002): 83–8.

7 Harvard School of Public Health, Nutrition Source, "Calcium and Milk,"
hsph.harvard.edu/nutritionsource/calcium.html

8 Morr, Simon, et al., "How Much Calcium Is in Your Drinking Water? A
Survey of Calcium Concentrations in Bottled and Tap Water and Their
Significance for Medical Treatment and Drug Administration," *HSS
Journal 2* (2006):130–35.

9   Matsuoka, L.Y., et al., "Chronic sunscreen use decreases circulating concentrations of 25-hydroxyvitamin D. A preliminary study," *Archives of Dermatology* 124 (1988):1802–04.

10 Wortsman, J., et al., "Decreased bioavailability of vitamin D in obesity," *American Journal of Clinical Nutrition* 72 (2000):690–93.

11 Bushinsky, D.A., et al., "The effects of acid on bone," *Current Opinion in Nephrology and Hypertension* 9 (2000):369-79.

12 Remer, Thomas, et al., "Dietary potential renal acid load and renal net acid excretion in healthy, free-living children and adolescents," *American Journal of Clinical Nutrition* 77 (2003):1255-60.

13 Welten, D.C., et al., "Weight-bearing activity during youth is a more important factor for peak bone mass than calcium intake," *Journal of Bone Mineral Research* 9 (1994):1089–96.

14 Tinetti, M., "Preventing falls in elderly persons," *New England Journal of Medicine* 348 (2003): 42–49; Resnick, B., "Falls in a community of older adults: Putting research into practice," *Clinical Nursing Research* 8 (1999):251–66.

15 Voukelatos, Alexander, et al., " A randomized, controlled trial of tai chi for the prevention of ills: The Central Sydney tai chi Trial," *Journal of the American Geriatrics Society* 55 (2007):1185–91; Li, F., et al., "Tai chi and fall reductions in older adults: A randomized controlled trial," *Journal of Gerontology: Biological Sciences* 60 (2005):187–194.

Index

Page numbers in **bold** indicate information in tables.

About the Author

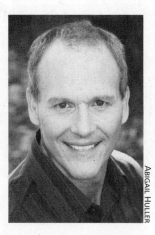

ABIGAIL HULLER

A wellness consultant for more than 25 years, Joseph Keon holds a doctorate degree in nutrition, fitness expert certifications by both the Cooper Institute for Aerobics Research in Dallas, Texas, and the American Council on Exercise, and is a member of the American College of Lifestyle Medicine. He is past chairman of the board of directors for Dr. Helen Caldicott's Nuclear Policy Research Institute, and past member of the Marin Health Council, an advisory to the Marin County Board of Supervisors. Dr. Keon has spearheaded important consumer environmental awareness campaigns, including the effort to eliminate the use of the ozone-depleting soil fumigant methyl-bromide in strawberry farming.

Dr. Keon has been featured in numerous magazines and newspapers internationally and has also appeared on local and national news broadcast, including CBS Evening News with Dan Rather and ABC News. He works closely with several environmental and public health organizations and is the author of three other books: *Whole Health: The Guide to Wellness of Body and Mind; The Truth About Breast Cancer: A Seven-Step Prevention Plan;* and the forthcoming *Questions That Matter.*

If you have enjoyed *Whitewash,* you might also enjoy other

BOOKS TO BUILD A NEW SOCIETY

Our books provide positive solutions for people who want to make a difference. We specialize in:

Sustainable Living • Green Building • Peak Oil
Renewable Energy • Environment & Economy
Natural Building & Appropriate Technology
Progressive Leadership • Resistance and Community
Educational & Parenting Resources

New Society Publishers

ENVIRONMENTAL BENEFITS STATEMENT

New Society Publishers has chosen to produce this book on recycled paper made with **100% post consumer waste,** processed chlorine free, and old growth free.

For every 5,000 books printed, New Society saves the following resources:[1]

33	Trees
3,020	Pounds of Solid Waste
3,322	Gallons of Water
4,334	Kilowatt Hours of Electricity
5,489	Pounds of Greenhouse Gases
24	Pounds of HAPs, VOCs, and AOX Combined
8	Cubic Yards of Landfill Space

[1]Environmental benefits are calculated based on research done by the Environmental Defense Fund and other members of the Paper Task Force who study the environmental impacts of the paper industry.

For a full list of NSP's titles, please call 1-800-567-6772 *or check out our website* at:

www.newsociety.com

NEW SOCIETY PUBLISHERS
Deep Green for over 30 years